Passing the Final FFICM

This innovative resource serves as a fusion of an MCQ guide and a textbook, providing essential content for postgraduate trainees gearing up for the FFICM Final exam, a vital part of the CCT in Intensive Care Medicine.

Crafted to meet the unique requirements of the MCQ while also addressing the necessity for concise, well-structured responses in the OSCE, this book prioritises quick topic transitions, delivering focused, streamlined learning across a range of ICM topics. Its uniqueness lies in its unorthodox structure; rather than having a conventional table of contents, it gives you the freedom to start your learning adventure from any page.

Each of the 1,400 facts is structured as a question, reflecting the format of both exams. Answers are conveniently positioned just below, eliminating the need for constant page-flipping. The material is carefully curated to cover the breadth of the ICM curriculum, weaving in valuable insights from the author's and colleagues' exam experiences. Random questions replicate the unpredictability of both exams and enhance the reader's capacity to swiftly switch between topics during self-assessment. This balances knowledge application and active recall while using memory-enhancing methods like self-quizzing, chunking, and spaced repetition.

Muzzammil Ali, a graduate of the University of Birmingham, UK, currently holds the position of Senior Registrar in Intensive Care and Acute Internal Medicine in the West Midlands. His dedication extends to leadership roles at Queen Elizabeth Hospital Birmingham, an honorary Clinical Lecturer position at the University of Birmingham, and representing the West Midlands as the trainee representative for Intensive Care Medicine.

MasterPass Series

For more information about this series, please visit: https://www.routledge.com/MasterPass/book-series/CRCMASPASS

Passing the Final FFICM

High-Yield Facts for the MCQ
& OSCE Exams

Muzzammil Ali

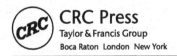

CRC Press
Taylor & Francis Group
Boca Raton London New York

CRC Press is an imprint of the
Taylor & Francis Group, an **informa** business

First edition published 2024
by CRC Press
2385 NW Executive Center Drive, Suite 320, Boca Raton FL 33431

and by CRC Press
4 Park Square, Milton Park, Abingdon, Oxon, OX14 4RN

CRC Press is an imprint of Taylor & Francis Group, LLC

ISBN: 9781032590622 (hbk)
ISBN: 9781032590608 (pbk)
ISBN: 9781003452751 (ebk)

DOI: 10.1201/9781003452751

Typeset in Century Gothic Pro
by KnowledgeWorks Global Ltd.

Dedication

To my beloved family,
Amina, Nizam, and Nura,
for your unwavering belief in me.

And to my dearest, Joanna,
for your enduring support, endless inspiration,
and reliable companionship throughout this journey.

Also, to my esteemed colleagues,
for your invaluable mentorship, constant encouragement,
and for fostering an environment that has nurtured my growth.

Contents

This book does not contain separate chapters but comprises a compilation of bite-sized question-and-answer segments, designed to emulate the unpredictable and erratic nature of both exam components.

With a collection of 1,400 essential facts, each fact functions as a multi-purpose instrument for self-review and study, applicable to a diverse range of postgraduate Intensive Care exams.

How to Use This Book

The key is simple: Cover up!

To get the most out of this book, active mental engagement is essential. Simply skimming through the answers without first attempting the questions hinders the learning process.

I advise using a bookmark, a piece of paper, or even your hand to cover the answers while you tackle each question. Don't be afraid of making mistakes; view them as invaluable opportunities for learning. Keep in mind that making errors while studying is completely acceptable.

I also recommend keeping a notebook close by to jot down any challenging facts or topics that you encounter. This practice will assist you in recognising and subsequently addressing specific knowledge gaps.

You'll notice that some text is intentionally bolded to create acronyms, which are designed to aid in memory retention. I've included this feature because I found it to be particularly helpful during my own review process.

When to Use This Book?

Crafted for quick, digestible learning, this book offers you the flexibility to dive into any section that piques your interest. I highly recommend taking advantage of 'hidden moments' throughout your day – be it while waiting for a train, picking up your kids from school, or queuing for your morning brew. Whether you're studying alone or with peers, these brief moments can be converted into productive revision opportunities. A mere five-minute commitment can deliver tangible progress. This adaptable format is especially useful for making your study routine less daunting, particularly after exhausting on-call shifts.

To drive the point home, consider this succinct example:

Question:

*Which substances primarily cause crystal nephropathy in **tumour lysis syndrome (TLS)**?*

Answer:

Uric acid and calcium phosphate

It's a quick read, but it offers crucial knowledge: in TLS, acute kidney injury can arise from crystal nephropathy, primarily driven by uric acid and calcium phosphate. Consequently, should you face an OSCE question like, 'Why may acute kidney injury occur in TLS?', you are well-prepared to offer an insightful answer.

But this book is more than an exam-prep tool; it acts as a catalyst for lifelong learning. Consistent interaction with the content, even after your exams, ensures that the knowledge remains fresh in your memory. Avoid the trap of letting your acquired knowledge diminish by incorporating this resource into the 'hidden moments' of your daily life.

Disclaimer

- This book serves as a fusion of an MCQ guide and a textbook, primarily intended as a supplementary study resource rather than a comprehensive reference. I highly suggest pairing this book with specialised MCQ and OSCE question banks for a well-rounded study approach. If you discover particular areas where your knowledge is lacking while using this book, I recommend seeking out additional resources that concentrate on those topics to enhance your understanding.
- It's important to underscore that this book includes a limited number of images, which may not fully cover certain image-intensive aspects of the OSCE exam, where you may encounter numerous ECGs and radiological images.
- The frequent use of the phrase 'most likely' aligns with the style of exam questions, indicating that while other diagnoses are possible, the provided answer is the most probable one.
- The information presented is up-to-date as of the book's publication, including details such as the new global definition of ARDS, the revised definition of pulmonary artery hypertension, and the Sepsis-3 definition of sepsis. However, it's important to be aware that information may change or become outdated over time.
- For the sake of brevity, standard medical acronyms like MRI, JVP, CXR, and ECG are used without further elaboration.

Preface

Tackling the FFICM exam was a rigorous endeavour that pushed the boundaries of my medical expertise and adaptability. As I prepared, I noticed an intriguing parallel between the MCQ and OSCE. Despite their differences, both components shared elements of unpredictability, and the occasional inclusion of niche subjects. Achieving success required more than just a fundamental understanding of common topics; it necessitated a distinctive perspective and approach.

This book was specifically crafted to meet the unique requirements of the MCQ, while also addressing the necessity for concise, well-structured responses in the OSCE. It prioritises quick topic transitions, delivering focused, streamlined learning across a range of ICM topics. Its uniqueness lies in its unorthodox structure; rather than having a conventional table of contents, it gives you the freedom to start your learning adventure from any page.

Each of the 1,400 facts is structured as a question, reflecting the format of both exams. Answers are conveniently positioned just below, eliminating the need for constant page-flipping. The material is carefully curated to cover the breadth of the ICM curriculum, incorporating valuable insights from my own exam experiences and those of my colleagues. It truly offers a little bit of everything. Random questions replicate the unpredictability of both exams and enhance your capacity to swiftly switch between topics during self-assessment. My objective is to balance the application of knowledge with active recall, while incorporating memory-boosting techniques such as self-quizzing, chunking and spaced repetition.

When composing this book, I drew upon a wide range of resources to ensure its relevance in the constantly evolving field of medicine. Depending on your clinical experience, you may find some facts either elementary or complex. Yet, virtually any topic, including esoteric ones like 'fire safety', can appear in the exam. Getting acquainted with these topics, even without memorising them, will enhance your likelihood of success. This book also covers specialised topics such as mechanical cardiovascular support and rare conditions like HLH. While these topics may not regularly appear in your day-to-day clinical practice, they are crucial for exam preparation. That said, the emphasis on basic sciences has been scaled back, in alignment with the FICM's assumption of your proficiency through your primary base-specialty exams.

As you work through this resource, you'll find that some of the longer facts can serve as valuable material for the Short Oral Examination (SOE). Consequently, comprehensive preparation for the MCQ and OSCE will undeniably elevate your performance in the SOE. It's worth noting, however, that this book lacks visual aids like ECGs or radiological scans, crucial for OSCE readiness. For this purpose, I recommend using a separate image repository.

My dedication to you goes beyond merely helping you pass the FFICM exam; consider this book a resource for continuous learning. Whether you need a knowledge refresher or a confidence boost, a quick glance at any section of the book should suffice. It also serves as a handy guide for ward rounds, enabling you to deepen your understanding and engage in informed discussions with colleagues.

I extend my warmest wishes to you on your journey.

Muzz

About the Author

Muzzammil Ali, a University of Birmingham UK graduate, currently holds the position of Senior Registrar in Intensive Care and Acute Internal Medicine within the West Midlands. He is a fervent advocate for medical education, committed to supporting trainees in achieving point-of-care ultrasound accreditation and excelling in their medical exams.

Renowned as the author of the medical textbook *MRCP Facts* and the creator of @ mrcpfacts, the largest verified Instagram page dedicated to MRCP-related content, Muzzammil's dedication to education extends to leadership roles at the Queen Elizabeth Hospital Birmingham. He also holds an honorary position as a Clinical Lecturer at the University of Birmingham and represents the West Midlands as the trainee representative for Intensive Care Medicine.

Drawing upon his expertise in postgraduate exams, including FFICM, MRCP, and the Acute Medicine SCE, Dr Ali has written this book with the sincere aspiration of guiding others toward success.

Resources

Websites

- BMJ OnExamination: https://www.onexamination.com/
- Brain Trauma Foundation (BTF): https://braintrauma.org/
- British National Formulary (BNF): https://bnf.nice.org.uk/
- British Society of Echocardiography: https://www.bsecho.org/
- British Thoracic Society: https://www.brit-thoracic.org.uk
- Clinical Key: https://www.clinicalkey.com/
- Cochrane: https://www.cochrane.org/
- Deranged Physiology: https://derangedphysiology.com/
- EMCrit Project: https://emcrit.org/
- European Society of Cardiology (ESC): https://www.escardio.org/
- Faculty of Intensive Care Medicine (FICM): https://www.ficm.ac.uk/
- Fire Service: https://www.fireservice.co.uk/
- Focused Ultrasound in Intensive Care (FUSIC): https://ics.ac.uk/learning/fusic.html
- GP Notebook: https://gpnotebook.com/
- Intensive Care National Audit and Research Centre (ICNARC): https://www.icnarc.org/
- Intensive Care Society (ICS): https://ics.ac.uk/guidance
- Life in the Fast Lane: https://litfl.com
- NICE Guidelines: https://www.nice.org.uk/guidance
- Passmedicine: https://passmedicine.com/
- Patient.info: https://patient.info/patientplus
- Pubmed Central: https://pubmed.ncbi.nlm.nih.gov
- Resuscitation Council UK: https://lms.resus.org.uk/
- ScienceDirect: https://www.sciencedirect.com/
- StatPearls: https://www.statpearls.com/
- The Bottom Line: https://www.thebottomline.org.uk/
- UpToDate: https://www.uptodate.com

Textbooks

- Abbas, S., Herod, R., & Horner, D. (2015). Intensive Care Medicine MCQs. tfm Publishing Limited.
- Ali, M. (2021). MRCP Facts.
- Benington, S., Nightingale, P., & Shelly, M. P. (2009). Multiple Choice Questions in Intensive Care Medicine. Tfm.
- Bersten, A. D., & Handy, J. M. (2019). Oh's Intensive Care Manual (8th ed.). Elsevier.
- Davies, E. (2022). The Final FFICM Structured Oral Examination Study Guide (1st ed.). CRC Press.
- Davies, K., Gough, C., King, E., Plumb, B., & Walton, B. (2017). Single Best Answer Questions for the Final FFICM. Cambridge University Press.
- Eyre, L., Bodenham, A., & Anaesthesia, in Critical. (2021). MCQs and SBAs in Intensive Care Medicine. Oxford University Press.
- Feather, A., Randall, D., & Waterhouse, M. (2020). Kumar And Clark's Clinical Medicine (10th ed.). Elsevier Health Sciences.
- Flavin, K., Morkane, C., & Marsh, S. (2018). Questions for the Final FFICM Structured Oral Examination. Cambridge University Press.
- Gillon, S., Wright, C., Knott, C., Mcphail, M., & Camporota, L. (2016). Revision Notes in Intensive Care Medicine. Oxford University Press.

- Hersey, P., O'connor, L., Sams, T. E., & Sturman, J. (2020). OSCEs for Intensive Care Medicine. Oxford University Press.
- Jeyanathan, J., Johnson, C., & Haslam, J. (2018). Viva and Structured Oral Examinations in Intensive Care Medicine. Tfm Publishing Ltd.
- Jeyasankar Jeyanathan, & Owens, D. (2016). Objective Structured Clinical Examination in Intensive Care Medicine. tfm Publishing Limited.
- Kalra, P. A. (2014). Essential revision notes for MRCP. Pastest.
- Lane, N., Powter, L., & Samir Patel. (2016). Best of Five MCQs for the Acute Medicine SCE. Oxford University Press.
- Lobaz, S., Hamilton, M., Glossop, A. J., & Raithatha, A. H. (2015). Critical Care MCQs. tfm Publishing Limited.
- McCombe, K., & Wijayasiri, L. (2017). The Primary FRCA Structured Oral Exam Guide 1. CRC Press.
- McCombe, K., & Wijayasiri, L. (2017). The Primary FRCA Structured Oral Exam Guide 2. CRC Press.
- Nichani, R., & McGrath, B. (2016). OSCEs for the Final FFICM. Cambridge University Press.
- Sprigings, D., & Chambers, J. (2017). Acute Medicine: A Practical Guide to the Management of Medical Emergencies. Wiley Blackwell/John Wiley & Sons, Inc.
- Wilkinson, I. B., Raine, T., Wiles, K., Goodhart, A., Hall, C., & O'Neill, H. (2017). Oxford Handbook of Clinical Medicine (10th ed.). Oxford University Press.

Fact 1:

What causes a high and low **mixed venous oxygen saturation (S_vO_2)**?

S_vO_2 is obtained from a pulmonary artery catheter. It measures the end result of O_2 consumption and delivery, and contains blood from both the SVC and IVC. The normal range is approximately 65–70%.

↑ S_vO_2	↓ S_vO_2
• ↑ O_2 delivery, e.g. ↑ FiO_2, hyperbaric O_2 • ↓ O_2 extraction, e.g. hypothermia, general anaesthetic, neuromuscular blockade • ↑ Flow states, e.g. sepsis, thyrotoxicosis, severe liver disease	• ↓ O_2 delivery, e.g. shock states, hypoxemia, anaemia • ↑ O_2 extraction, e.g. hyperthermia, shivering, pain, seizures

$S_{cv}O_2$, on the other hand, measures oxygen saturation in the SVC, taken from an internal jugular, subclavian or axillary vein catheter and is sometimes used as a surrogate for S_vO_2.

Typically, in healthy individuals, $S_vO_2 > S_{cv}O_2$ because the brain (SVC-drained) has a higher oxygen demand compared to organs like the kidneys (IVC-drained) with lower oxygen demands.

$S_{cv}O_2$ can surpass S_vO_2 in cases where the brain's metabolic requirement decreases, such as during anaesthesia, in TBI, or in shock, when body oxygen extraction increases, which leads to reduced oxygen saturation in the IVC.

Fact 2:

What factors affect **functional residual capacity (FRC)**?

- FRC = expiratory reserve volume + residual volume.
- It is the volume of air in the lungs after normal expiration, measured by either gas dilution or body plethysmography.

↑ FRC	↓ FRC
• Standing position • Asthma/COPD • PEEP/CPAP	• Supine position • Obesity • Pregnancy • Restrictive lung disorders • General anaesthesia

Fact 3:

Which should be the normal **cuff pressure** of a tracheostomy?

20–30 cm H_2O – should be checked every 8–12 hours, or more frequently depending on the clinical picture

Higher cuff pressures may compress tracheal capillaries, limit blood flow, and predispose to tracheal necrosis (ischaemic damage).

Fact 4:

What is the difference between **cardiac output** and **cardiac index**?

- Cardiac Output = Heart Rate x Stroke Volume
  Normal range ~ 4–8 L/min
- Cardiac Index = Cardiac Output/Body Surface Area
  Normal range ~ 2.5–4 L/min

Fact 5:

What is the physiological role of **C-reactive protein**?

- A pentraxin protein synthesised in the liver
- ↑ In response to inflammation
- Binds to phosphocholine on the surface of dead/dying cells, which activates the complement system

Fact 6:

Which cardiac structural abnormality may the presence of a **right bundle branch block** in a young adult indicate?

Atrial septal defect

DOI: 10.1201/9781003452751-1

Fact 7:

What are some of the causes of a **raised MCV**?

D	**D**rugs, e.g. anticonvulsants, antimicrobials, chemotherapy
R	**R**eticulocytosis
A	**A**lcohol abuse
M	**M**egaloblastic anaemia, e.g. pernicious anaemia, B_{12}/folate deficiency
A	**A**rtefact, e.g. aplasia, myelofibrosis, hyperglycaemia, cold agglutinins
T	**T**hyroid (hypothyroidism)
I	**I**mmature bone marrow cells, e.g. myelodysplastic syndrome
C	**C**hronic liver disease

Fact 8:

What is the dose of IV salbutamol in treating **life-threatening asthma**, and what are some side effects?

- Dose: 3–20 mcg/min
- Side effects: tachycardia, arrhythmias, tremors, hyperglycaemia, hypokalaemia, and type B lactic acidosis

Fact 9:

What are the mechanisms of **drug-induced hyperkalaemia**?

K⁺ supplements	• Sando-K • IV fluids with K⁺
Drugs that impair K⁺ distribution	• **B**eta blockers • **A**rginine • **D**igoxin • **S**uxamethonium
Drugs that ↓ renal K⁺ excretion	• Calcineurin inhibitors, e.g. tacrolimus and ciclosporin • Potassium-sparing diuretics, e.g. spironolactone, eplerenone • Some antibiotics, e.g. trimethoprim
Drugs that impact on the RAAS	• NSAIDs • ACE inhibitors, ARBs • Heparin

Fact 10:

When do you control hypertension in the first 24 hours after an **acute ischaemic stroke** according to NICE?

NICE advises against actively managing hypertension during this period, except in the following situations:

- To facilitate thrombolysis–target BP < 185/110.
- In cases of pre-eclampsia, aortic dissection, or hypertensive encephalopathy/nephropathy/cardiac failure.

Fact 11:

What percentage TBSA **burn** would meet the criteria for referral to a burns centre on area alone?

>40% Total Body Surface Area (TBSA)

Fact 12:

Where is **propofol** predominantly metabolised?

Hepatic metabolism, primarily via glucuronidation and sulfation pathways.

Fact 13:

What is the dose of IV magnesium in the management of **acute asthma**, and how does it work as a bronchodilator?

Dose: 1.2–2 g IV over 20 minutes

Mechanism as a bronchodilator:

1. Calcium blocker in bronchial smooth muscle
2. ↓ Ach release at the NMJ
3. ↑ Sensitivity of β-receptors to catecholamines

Fact 14:

What is the **Parkland formula** for IV fluid replacement after a burn, and does it take into account pre-hospital fluid administration?

Volume of IV fluids =
4 mL/kg / %TBSA over 24 hours

Half of total is given in the first 8 hours after the injury.

This formula takes into account pre-hospital fluid administration. Therefore, any prehospital fluid is subtracted from total.

When calculating TBSA, erythematous regions are omitted unless there is additional blistering or underlying evidence of a partial-thickness burn.

Fact 15:

What did the **PROPPR trial (2015)** demonstrate for blood product administration in a 1:1:1 ratio compared to a 1:1:2 plasma:platelet:red cell ratio in patients with severe trauma and major bleeding?

- No difference in all-cause 24-hour or 90-day mortality
- Post-hoc analysis found a significant reduction in death by exsanguination within the first 24 hours and a higher rate of achieving haemostasis in the 1:1:1 group compared to the 1:1:2 group.

Fact 16:

What are the 12 physiological variables of the **APACHE II score**?

CNS	CVS	RESP	RENAL	MICRO/HAEM
GCS	MAP HR	RR PaO_2	Arterial pH Na$^+$ K$^+$ Creatinine	Temperature WCC Hct
The worst of these variables within the first 24 hours of critical care admission is used				

Effects of age and chronic health are incorporated to give a single score with a maximum of 71. A score of >25 represents a predicted mortality of >50%.

Fact 17:

What dose of adrenaline do you give in adult **anaphylaxis**?

0.5–1 mL of 1:1,000 IM (0.5–1 mg)

OR

0.5–1 mL of 1:10,000 IV (50–100 mcg)

Fact 18:

What is the difference between **intra-abdominal hypertension (IAH)** and **abdominal compartment syndrome (ACS)**, and how do you measure intra-abdominal pressure (IAP)?

- IAH: sustained or repeated pathological elevation of IAP ≥ 12 mmHg
- ACS: sustained IAP > 20 mmHg + new organ dysfunction/failure +/– abdominal perfusion pressure (APP) < 60 mmHg

IAP is measured:

- Direct: puncture of the abdominal cavity
- Indirect: via a urinary catheter in the bladder or a balloon-tipped catheter inserted into the stomach. Correlates well with direct measurements but can be inaccurate when there are adhesions, pelvic fractures, and abdominal packs.

Fact 19:

Where in adults does the **trachea** start and divide anatomically?

- Starts at C6
- Extends to T4 where it bifurcates
- It is approximately 10–12 cm long
- The right main bronchus separates at a 25° angle and the left main bronchus separates at a 45° angle.

Fact 20:

What are the differences between a **Minnesota tube (MT)** and **Sengstaken–Blakemore tube (SBT)**?

Both are used for bleeding UGI varices resistant to medical and/or endoscopic treatment.

- SBT has three ports – oesophageal balloon, gastric balloon, and gastric aspiration port. MT has an additional port for oesophageal suction to ↓ the risk of aspiration.
- The MT has a higher-volume gastric balloon (450–500 mL vs. 250–300 mL).

Fact 21:

What is the evidence for a **decompressive hemicraniectomy (DH)** in malignant middle cerebral artery syndrome according to the DECIMAL (2007), HAMLET (2009) and DESTINY II (2011) trials?

- **Mortality**: Decompressive hemicraniectomy significantly reduces mortality compared to conservative treatment in all three studies. This benefit appears to be particularly strong when surgery is performed early (within 48 hours) after stroke onset. This was observed in younger patients (18–55 years in DECIMAL) and older patients (≥61 years in DESTINY II), as well as in the varied population of HAMLET.
- **Neurological Disability**: The findings on functional outcome are more complex and are potentially dependent on factors like age, stroke severity, and time to surgery:
  - Decompressive hemicraniectomy did not significantly improve the proportion of patients achieving a 'good' functional outcome (mRS ≤ 3) at 6 or 12 months in DECIMAL and HAMLET.
  - However, it significantly increased the proportion of patients achieving a 'moderate' functional outcome (mRS ≤ 4) at six months in DECIMAL and DESTINY II.

- Notably, no surviving patients in DESTINY II achieved the best possible functional outcome (mRS 0–2).
- **Overall**: Decompressive hemicraniectomy offers a clear and substantial mortality benefit. While it may not guarantee good recovery and return to pre-stroke levels of function, it can increase the chances of achieving moderate disability as opposed to severe disability or death. This decision requires individualised assessment and MDT involvement.

Fact 22:

How do you distinguish between moderate, severe and life-threatening **acute asthma**?

Moderate	Severe
PEFR > 50%	PEFR 33–50%
	RR ≥ 25
	HR ≥ 110
	Inability to complete sentences in one breath
	Life-threatening
No features of severe asthma	Features of severe asthma + at least one of: • PEFR < 33% • SpO_2 < 92% • Normal or ↓ PCO_2: implies poor ventilation • **C**yanosis, **c**onfusion or **c**oma • **H**ypotension or ↓ HR • **E**xhaustion or poor respiratory effort • **S**ilent chest • **T**achy(arrhythmia)

Fact 23:

When is it safe to use **suxamethonium** after a significant burn injury?

- Within the first 24 hours after the burn
- One year after the burn

Fact 24:

How do you calculate the internal diameter of an **endotracheal tube** in the paediatric population?

Cuffed : [age / 4] + 3.5
Uncuffed : [age / 4] + 3.5 + 0.5

Fact 25:

What is the recommended therapeutic management for a **variceal haemorrhage** that continues to bleed despite pharmacological intervention, endoscopic banding and balloon tamponade?

Transjugular Intrahepatic Portosystemic Shunt (TIPS)

Fact 26:

When is **damage control surgery** more preferable than definite surgery in trauma?

When there is severe haemorrhagic shock and/or ongoing bleeding. This is particularly necessary if the **lethal diamond** is present (hypothermia, acidosis, coagulopathy and hypocalcaemia) and in patients who have inaccessible major venous injuries or those who require time-consuming procedures.

Fact 27:

What risk is associated with the administration of **suxamethonium** after a spinal cord injury, and how soon after the injury does this risk occur?

- Life-threatening hyperkalaemia
- 72 hours after spinal cord injury

Fact 28:

How is the **rapid shallow breathing index (RSBI)** useful as a weaning predictor?

RSBI = RR / Tv

- RSBI < 105: 80% chance of successful extubation
- RSBI >105: strongly suggests weaning failure

Fact 29:

What are the approximate proportions of Na$^+$ and K$^+$ in some commonly used **crystalloid solutions**?

Fluid	Na$^+$ (mmol/L)	K$^+$ (mmol/L)
0.9% N. saline	154	0
Hartmann's	131	5
5% Dextrose	0	0
0.18% N. saline + 4% dextrose	30	0
0.45% N. saline + 5% dextrose	77	0

Fact 30:

What happens to pulmonary artery pressure after a **cardiac arrest**?

↑ Multifactorial reasons why this may occur include:

- Post-ROSC
  - ↑ PVR secondary to hypoxia/acidosis
  - ↑ PAP secondary to cardiac dysfunction as part of post-cardiac arrest syndrome
- Precipitant of cardiac arrest
  - ↑ PAP secondary to cardiac dysfunction (e.g. STEMI) or pulmonary embolism

Fact 31:

What **adrenaline** dose would you give to a three-year-old in cardiac arrest?

10 mcg / kg = 0.1 mL / kg of 1 in 10,000 solution

Formula for weight	Calculation	Estimated weight (kg)
3 (age) + 7	3(3) + 7	16
2 (age + 4)	2(3 + 4)	14

Using the average weight of 15 kg, this is 150 mcg, which is **1.5 mL of 1:10,000 of adrenaline solution.**

Fact 32:

What is meant by **intention to treat** analysis in a randomised controlled trial?

- All participants are analysed based on their originally assigned treatment groups, regardless of whether they completed or received the intended treatment.
- This approach helps maintain the randomisation and avoids biases caused by crossover or dropout.

Fact 33:

What are the differences in **relative humidity** in a ventilator circuit when using an ultrasonic nebuliser as opposed to a heat and moisture exchanger (HME)?

- Ultrasonic nebuliser: exceeds 100% relative humidity
- HME: achieves approximately 70% relative humidity

Fact 34:

Which clinical features in someone with a **burn** may indicate the need for early intubation?

- GCS < 8
- Respiratory distress or failure
- Noticeable swelling or blistering in the lips, tongue or oropharynx
- Voice changes, e.g. hoarseness or stridor
- Singed nasal hair
- Carbonaceous sputum
- Extensive burns of the face or neck, including circumferential burns

Fact 35:

How does **digoxin** work in treating atrial fibrillation with a fast ventricular rate?

Direct	Indirect
Inhibits cardiac Na^+/K^+-ATPase ▼ ↑ Intracellular Na^+ ▼ Exchange of Na^+ for Ca^{2+} via the Na^+/Ca^{2+} pump ▼ ↑ Intracellular Ca^{2+} ↓ Intracellular Na^+	↑ Acetylcholine at cardiac muscarinic receptors
↑ **Intracellular Ca^{2+} causes** ↑ **cardiac contraction** ↓ **Intracellular Na^+ prolongs refractory time of the bundle of His**	**Results in prolongation of the refractory period at the AV node and bundle of His**

Fact 36:

Which alternative drug can be used in the management of AVNRT if **adenosine** is contraindicated?

Verapamil 2.5–5 mg IV

Fact 37:

Why may someone with **primary hyperaldosteronism (Conn's syndrome)** develop muscle weakness and tetany?

Due to hypokalaemic metabolic alkalosis

Conn's syndrome causes a low renin hypertension.

It is diagnosed by a ↑ aldosterone:renin ratio.

Fact 38:

What modifications have been implemented in advanced life support algorithms for resuscitating individuals with **hypothermia**?

- Refrain from administering adrenaline or any other drugs until the temperature is >30°C.
- When the temperature ranges from 30°C to 35°C, double the dose intervals for ALS drugs.
- In cases of VF, consider delivering up to three shocks if needed, but hold off on further shocks until the temperature is >30°C.

Fact 39:

What is the most likely diagnosis if someone develops **hypocalcaemia and seizures** two days after starting chemotherapy?

Tumour lysis syndrome (TLS) – electrolyte abnormalities can precipitate neurological dysfunction.

Common abnormalities include:

- ↓ Calcium
- ↑ Phosphate, potassium, urate, LDH, lactate

TLS is due to the sudden and large-scale death of cells following the initiation of chemotherapy. It is often associated with acute leukaemias and high-grade lymphomas, e.g. Burkitt's.

Fact 40:

What are the most likely causes for developing drowsiness one week after undergoing endovascular coiling for a **subarachnoid haemorrhage**, when a CT scan indicates no rebleeding, infarction or hydrocephalus?

- Delayed cerebral ischaemia (DCI)
  - o Cerebral vasospasm
  - o Local hypoperfusion or disordered autoregulation
- Non-convulsive seizures

Fact 41:

What's the rationale for including **clindamycin or linezolid** alongside broad-spectrum antibiotics in the treatment of necrotising fasciitis?

For the termination of toxin production

Fact 42:

Besides **hypothermia**, what are some alternative reasons for the presence of J-waves on an ECG?

Normal variant (early repolarisation)

Hypercalcaemia
Angina – vasospastic
Brain injury including a subarachnoid haemorrhage
Idiopathic ventricular fibrillation
Type 1 Brugada syndrome

Fact 43:

When would you consider placing an inferior vena cava (IVC) filter after a **pulmonary embolism (PE)**?

- If anticoagulation is contraindicated, e.g. the bleeding risk is very high
- If thrombosis has recurred despite adequate anticoagulation
- If temporary cessation of anticoagulation within one month is anticipated, e.g. pregnant patients within one month of the expected date of delivery

IVC filters have no long-term mortality benefit. As foreign material, they are thrombogenic (↑ incidence of DVT).

Fact 44:

What is the utility of the **LRINEC (Laboratory Risk Indicator for Necrotising Fasciitis)** score?

- The LRINEC score distinguishes necrotising fasciitis from other soft tissue infections, e.g. cellulitis.
- The score incorporates CRP, WCC, Hb, sodium, creatinine and glucose.
- A LRINEC score of ≥6 could be used as a potential tool to rule in necrotising fasciitis, but a score <6 should not be used to rule out the diagnosis.
- A score ≥8 has a positive predictive value >90%.

Fact 45:

Is it necessary to check digoxin levels during and after administering **digoxin-specific antibody fragments** for digoxin toxicity?

No – the assay measures both digoxin bound to antibody fragments and free digoxin. This overestimates free levels.

Fact 46:

What fibrinogen level may warrant administering **cryoprecipitate** in a trauma patient?

Fibrinogen < 1.5–2 g/L

Fact 47:

What is the normal axis for left ventricular depolarisation in an adult, and what are the Sokolow-Lyon criteria for **left ventricular hypertrophy (LVH)**?

- Normal axis: −30 to +90 degrees
- LVH: If the height of the R wave in $V_{5/6}$ + the depth of the S wave in $V_{1/2}$ is ≥35 mm
- The most common cause of LVH is hypertension

Fact 48:

What are the two pathways of **coagulation**?

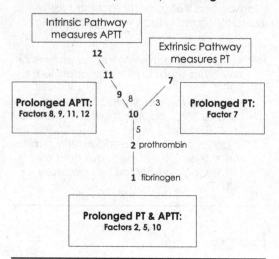

Fact 49:

Which substances are primarily responsible for crystal nephropathy in **tumour lysis syndrome**?

Uric acid and calcium phosphate

↑ Cell turnover → ↑ purine metabolism → ↑ serum urate

↑ Cell lysis → ↑ serum phosphate which binds to calcium

Uric acid precipitates readily in the presence of calcium phosphate, and calcium phosphate precipitates readily in the presence of uric acid.

Fact 50:

According to the BTS guidelines, when do you insert a chest drain for a **spontaneous pneumothorax (PTX)**?

1. Primary PTX when aspiration fails. Aspiration is indicated for a primary PTX when breathless and/or size is >2 cm.
2. Secondary PTX when aspiration fails. Aspiration is indicated for a secondary PTX when the size is 1–2 cm.
3. Secondary PTX when the patient is breathless and/or the size of the pneumothorax is >2 cm.

Fact 51:

What clinical feature would indicate a **haemodynamically unstable pulmonary embolism** (previously called a massive or high-risk PE)?

Significant hypotension:

Blood pressure of <90 mmHg <u>OR</u> a drop of >40 mmHg from baseline, which is not explained by something else, e.g. arrhythmia, hypovolaemia or sepsis.

Fact 52:

What makes **ketamine** effective in enhancing lung function and alleviating bronchospasm in asthma?

It is a bronchodilator.

It is a phencyclidine derivative. It has little effect on the laryngeal reflexes, and a patent airway can often be maintained. However, it can induce ↑ secretion production, potentially leading to laryngospasm due to these retained reflexes.

Fact 53:

What CT features are associated with an increased severity of **acute pancreatitis**?

- Extensive fat stranding
- Peri-pancreatitis fluid collections
- Pancreatic necrosis

Fact 54:

On which side of the body do traumatic **diaphragmatic injuries** tend to occur?

Left side

Fact 55:

What are the principles of ventilating someone with **life-threatening asthma** and which strategies can achieve this?

Principles	Strategies
Lung protective ventilation: • Limit peak and mean airway pressures • Allow for a prolonged expiratory time • Maintain adequate oxygenation	• ↓ Tidal volume • ↓ RR • ↓ Or removal of extrinsic PEEP • ↓ Inspiratory time or ↑ expiratory time • Permissive hypercapnia • Intermittent disconnection from ventilator and manual chest decompression

Fact 56:

Why should care be taken when giving **flumazenil**?

It reverses the effects of benzodiazepines.

It has a relatively short half-life when compared to benzodiazepines and has a risk of provoking seizures when administered.

Fact 57:

What do the **Berlin criteria** for ARDS entail, and what are the four key recommendations of the **New Global Definition of ARDS** that expand upon these criteria?

Berlin criteria:

Timing	Within one week of a known clinical insult or new/worsening respiratory symptoms
Oxygenation (P/F ratios)	$PaO_2/FiO_2 < 40$ kPa ($\leq$300 mmHg) with a minimum PEEP of 5 cm H_2O: • Mild ≤ 39.9 kPa • Moderate ≤ 26.6 kPa • Severe ≤ 13.3 kPa
CXR or CT	Bilateral opacities not explained by effusions/collapse/nodules
Origin of oedema	Respiratory failure NOT fully explained by cardiac failure or fluid overload

Four key recommendations:

- Intubation is not required for making a diagnosis. This includes patients on high-flow nasal oxygen (HFNO) ≥ 30 L/min or NIV/CPAP with end-expiratory pressure ≥ 5 cmH$_2$O.
- Uses SpO_2/FiO_2 as an alternative to P/F to assess oxygenation. A SpO_2/FiO_2 ≤ 315 + SpO_2 ≤ 97% is indicative of compromised oxygenation.
- The requirement of bilateral lung opacities as an imaging criterion remains, but now includes using ultrasound, provided it is performed by a well-trained operator.
- In settings with limited resources, the following are not essential for diagnosis: PEEP, specific oxygen flow rates, or particular types of respiratory support devices.

Fact 58:

Which ion has the most significant impact on the **resting potential** of neural tissue?

Potassium – This has a large concentration gradient across the cell membrane *and* the greatest permeability at rest.

Every cell membrane has a transmembrane potential difference of –70 mV. This difference is dependent on two factors: The transmembrane concentration gradient *and* the permeability of the membrane to the ions.

Fact 59:

What are some general respiratory changes that occur by the third trimester of **pregnancy**?

Tidal volume		Chest wall compliance	
Respiratory rate		Airway resistance	
pH	↑	FRC	↓
PaO_2		HCO_3^-	
Maternal 2,3-DPG		$paCO_2$	

Lung compliance remains largely the same.

Fact 60:

What is the pathogenesis of **hepatic encephalopathy (HE)** in chronic liver disease and what are some treatment options?

- **Pathogenesis**: HE occurs when the liver cannot remove ammonia from enteric sources. This ammonia enters the systemic circulation. It goes to the brain to cause neurotoxicity and cerebral oedema.
- **Management**:
  - Treat any precipitating factor, e.g. SBP, UGIB, electrolyte disturbances. May also need organ support on ICU, e.g. for ↓ GCS in Grade 4 HE
  - Lactulose & Rifaximin: ↓ Ammonia levels in the gut by ↑ transit time and ↓ bacterial numbers
  - LOLA: Removes ammonia from the blood through extrahepatic metabolism of ammonia to glutamine. This treatment is not widely available and has little evidence of benefit.

Fact 61:

Which parameters on a **blood gas** are directly and indirectly measured?

- Direct: pH, PaO_2, $PaCO_2$
- Indirect: Standard bicarbonate, base excess, SaO_2

Fact 62:

How do you treat **prilocaine** toxicity?

Methylthioninium chloride (methylene blue) 1 mg/kg IV

- Prilocaine is metabolised in the liver to O-toluidine.
- O-toluidine oxidises haemoglobin into methaemoglobin.
- Methaemoglobin has ↓ oxygen-carrying capacity resulting in cyanosis.
- Methylene blue accelerates the reduction of methaemoglobin.

Fact 63:

How do you distinguish between **hyperacute, acute and subacute liver failure** using the O'Grady classification?

Acute liver failure is triad of jaundice, coagulopathy and encephalopathy. It is classified according to the time from the onset of jaundice to the development of encephalopathy:

- Hyperacute disease: <7 days
- Acute disease: 1–4 weeks
- Subacute disease: 4–12 weeks

Fact 64:

What is meant by **pulsus paradoxus** and in which clinical contexts may it be present?

An amplification of the typical drop in systolic BP during inhalation by >10 mmHg. When severe, the radial pulse vanishes during inspiration. The 'paradox' is that the pulse disappears despite cardiac contraction. It is often due to pericardial disease, particularly cardiac tamponade, but can occur in many contexts including ('PRACTICE'):

- **P**ulmonary embolism
- **R**V infarction and **R**estrictive cardiomyopathy
- **A**sthma and COPD (severe)
- **C**ardiac tamponade and **C**onstrictive pericarditis
- **T**ension pneumothorax
- **I**atrogenic during surgery
- **C**ompression (obesity, pectus excavatum)
- **E**ffusions (large bilateral pleural effusions)

Fact 65:

What ECG pattern has developed if a person who took a large quantity of **cocaine** now has ST elevation in V_{1-3} and T-wave inversion in V_{1-2}?

Drug-induced Brugada

Fact 66:

What type of lung injury does a titrated PEEP strategy aim to decrease when treating **ARDS**?

↓ Atelectotrauma

Fact 67:

What are the King's criteria for **non-paracetamol-induced acute liver failure**?

		Any three of the following:
INR > 6.5 (PT > 100 seconds)	OR	• Aetiology: Non-A, non-B hepatitis or idiosyncratic drug reaction • Bilirubin > 300 µmol/L • Age < 11 or > 40 years • INR > 3.5 (PT > 50 seconds) • Time from onset of jaundice to encephalopathy > 7 days

---

Fact 68:

Which three clinical signs make up Beck's triad in acute **pericardial tamponade**?

* ↓ BP
* ↓ Heart sounds (quiet/muffled)
* ↑ CVP – distended neck veins

Fact 69:

How does **mannitol** reduce intracranial pressure (ICP)?

Mannitol is a diuretic and 'free radical scavenger'. It is freely filtered through the glomerulus and is not re-absorbed. It decreases ICP in two main ways:

Immediate effect (Plasma expansion)	Slightly delayed effect (Osmotic gradient)
Plasma expansion results in: • ↓ Blood viscosity • ↑ Intravascular volume • ↑ Cardiac output Overall, these effects result in ↑ regional cerebral blood flow and compensatory cerebral vasoconstriction in brain regions where autoregulation is intact → ↓ ICP	↑ Plasma osmolality → shifts water from cerebral extracellular space into plasma → ↓ cerebral oedema (if the BBB is intact)

Fact 70:

Which arrhythmias can cause **cannon-A** waves in the JVP waveform?

* Complete heart block
* Ventricular tachycardia
* Junctional rhythms including AVNRT

Fact 71:

Which complication of **heparin** therapy carries the highest mortality?

Type 2 HIT (heparin-induced thrombocytopaenia) due to arterial/venous thrombotic complications

	Type 1 HIT	Type 2 HIT
Onset (days)	1–4	5–14
Nadir platelet count	>100,000	50–100,000
Immune complexes	No	Yes (IgG-Heparin-platelet factor 4)
Thrombosis	No	Arterial and venous
Treatment	Observation	Stop heparin Change to an alternative anticoagulant to prevent thromboses, e.g. direct thrombin inhibitors (lepirudin, argatroban, bivalirudin) or anti-thrombin-dependent factor Xa inhibitors (fondaparinux, danaparoid)

Fact 72:

How may **somatosensory evoked potentials (SSEPs)** suggest poor neurological outcome post-cardiac arrest?

They test the somatosensory pathway integrity.

Stimulating a peripheral nerve, e.g. median nerve can be detected at the cortical level. The bilateral absence of the N20 spike on SSEP testing can be used as part of neuro-prognostication in predicting poor neurological outcome in comatosed patients following cardiac arrest.

Fact 73:

What is the classical CSF finding in **Guillain–Barré syndrome (GBS)**?

Albuminocytological dissociation

(↑ CSF protein, normal glucose and no pleocytosis)

GBS is a post-infectious immune-mediated acute inflammatory demyelinating polyneuropathy (AIDP). The majority of cases occur within one month of a respiratory or GI infection, e.g. *Campylobacter jejuni, Mycoplasma pneumoniae*, CMV or EBV. The pathogenesis is a cross reaction of antibodies with gangliosides in the peripheral nervous system. Anti-ganglioside antibodies (e.g. anti-GM1) are present in 25% of patients. The majority of cases exhibit Landry's ascending paralysis, areflexia and autonomic dysfunction. Sensory symptoms tend to be mild/absent.

Fact 74:

Which reversal agent can you use to manage major bleeding in someone who takes **dabigatran**?

Idarucizumab–5 mg IV bolus

This is humanised monoclonal antibody fragment that binds to dabigatran and its metabolites.

HD or HF can also remove dabigatran.

Fact 75:

What are the **RIFLE criteria** for acute kidney injury?

	Creatinine	GFR	Urine output
Risk	↑ Cr × 1.5	>25% ↓	<0.5 mL/kg/hr for 6 hrs
Injury	↑ Cr × 2	>50% ↓	<0.5 mL/kg/hr for 12 hrs
Failure	↑ Cr × 3		<0.3 mL/kg/hr for 24 hrs <u>OR</u> Anuria for 12 hrs
Loss	Loss of renal function > Four weeks		
End stage	Loss of renal function > Three months		

Fact 76:

What is the **GCS** if someone with a head injury is opening his eyes to painful stimuli, is saying occasional inappropriate words and is extending his limbs to pain?

GCS = 7

Score	Eye opening	Verbal response	Motor response
6	-	-	Obeys commands
5	-	Alert and orientated	Localises to pain
4	Spontaneous	Confused	Withdrawal from pain
3	On speech	**Inappropriate words**	Flexion to pain
2	**On pain**	Incomprehensible sounds	**Extension to pain**
1	None	None	None

Fact 77:

Why is **atropine** ineffective for treating bradycardia in a heart transplant?

The heart is completely denervated. Therefore, the lack of a vagal input would prevent any anticholinergic effects of atropine. Sympathomimetic agents are used instead for chronotropy or inotropy.

Fact 78:

Which organism is most likely to cause right-sided **infective endocarditis** in an intravenous drug user?

Staphylococcus aureus

Fact 79:

How may hyperoxia cause harm in an **acute myocardial infarction**?

- Through free radical production
- Through coronary vasoconstriction

Fact 80:

What are the four mechanisms of AKI in **rhabdomyolysis**?

1. Myoglobin combines with Tamm–Horsfall protein to form insoluble casts and tubular obstruction.
2. Hyperuricaemia worsens this tubular obstruction.
3. The haem moiety is directly nephrotoxic.
4. There is inappropriate renal vasoconstriction because of hypovolaemia and third-spacing.

Fact 81:

What is the $PaCO_2$ level in **life-threatening asthma**?

Normal or ↓ $PaCO_2$

Fact 82:

Why may peripheral oedema develop in **cor pulmonale** if there is preserved ventricular function?

Chronic hypoxia causes sympathetic stimulation. This activates the renin–angiotensin–aldosterone system (RAAS) which results in fluid retention.

Fact 83:

What is meant by **FVC, FEV₁/FVC ratio, TLC and DLCO**?

- FVC: Volume from maximal inspiration to maximal expiration
- FEV$_1$/FVC ratio: The portion of FVC exhaled in the first second
- TLC: The total volume of gas in the lungs at maximal inspiration
- DLCO: Lung diffusion capacity for carbon monoxide, approximating oxygen transfer from alveoli to red blood cells

---

Fact 84:

Which **laxative** class is least likely to cause diarrhoea?

Bulk-forming laxatives, e.g. psyllium, methylcellulose

These laxatives work by absorbing water in the intestine, which increases stool bulk and stimulates peristalsis.

Fact 85:

What is meant by **pre-excitation** in electrophysiology?

There is an accessory pathway between the atria and ventricles. This prematurely activates the ventricles.

Fact 86:

What is the **static compliance** if the expired tidal volume is 800 mL, plateau pressure is 50 cmH$_2$O and PEEP is 10 cm H$_2$O?

$$C_{stat} = V_t / (P_{plateau} - PEEP)$$

$$C_{stat} = 800 / 50 - 10 = 20 \text{ mL} / cmH_2O$$

Static compliance represents pulmonary compliance during periods without gas flow, e.g. inspiratory hold

---

Fact 87:

What are the two types of **amiodarone-induced thyrotoxicosis (AIT)**?

	Type 1 AIT	Type 2 AIT
Pre-existing thyroid disease	Often	No
Pathology	Excessive hormone synthesis due to excess iodine found in amiodarone	Excessive release of preformed hormones due to thyroiditis
Goitre	Mostly multinodular	Absent or small
Radi-oiodine isotope uptake	Normal	↓/ absent
Thyroid ABS	Present	Absent
IL-6	Normal/mildly raised	Very high
Treatment options	• Stop amiodarone • Antithyroid drugs • K⁺ perchlorate • Thyroidectomy	• Stop amiodarone • Anti-inflammatory drugs, e.g. prednisolone

Fact 88:

When should you send blood for mast cell tryptase in **anaphylaxis**?

- Initial sample as soon as possible
- Second sample at 1–2 hours
- Third sample at 24 hours or in convalescence

Mast cells are found within many tissues including lung, intestine and skin. Tryptase is a protease enzyme which acts via PARs (protease-activated receptors). Mast cell tryptase is a reliable marker of mast cell degranulation.

Fact 89:

Why may **Torsades de Pointes (TdP)** develop after giving amiodarone to treat atrial fibrillation?

Amiodarone prolongs the QT interval.

QT prolongation increases the risk of TdP.

- If there are adverse features: Synchronised DCCV
- If no adverse features:
  - o   Stop all drugs that prolong the QT.
  - o   Correct any electrolyte abnormalities.
  - o   Give IV magnesium (2 g over 10 minutes).

Fact 90:

What are the five different types of **myocardial infarction (MI)**?

Type 1 MI	Acute coronary syndrome	Caused by coronary artery disease with atherothrombotic plaque rupture or erosion leading to either an occlusive or partially occlusive thrombus
Type 2 MI	Supply–demand imbalance	• Myocardial cell death secondary to an oxygen supply–demand imbalance to the myocardium, e.g. septic shock, hypoxia or hypovolaemia • Management focuses on optimisation of oxygen delivery
Type 3 MI	MI causing death	• Symptoms indicative of MI with presumed new ECG changes or ventricular fibrillation, but biomarker samples not obtained before death • MI detected at autopsy examination
Type 4 MI	PCI-related	• Type 4a: Procedure-related MI occurring 48 hours after PCI • Type 4b: MI due to stent or scaffold thrombosis following PCI • Type 4c: Restenosis associated with PCI
Type 5 MI	CABG-related	Procedural myocardial injury during or ≤ 48 hours after CABG/cardiac surgery

Fact 91:

What is normal **pleural fluid** pH and what pH would you expect in a parapneumonic effusion?

Normal pleural pH	Uncomplicated parapneu-monic effusion	Complicated parapneumonic effusion
7.60–7.66	pH ≥ 7.2	pH < 7.2
Normal	Sterile pleural fluid	Bacterial invasion without pus

An empyema is pus in the pleural space.

Fact 92:

How would you manage someone with **longstanding atrial fibrillation** with adverse signs if their INR was 1.3?

Sedation + synchronised DC cardioversion

The risk of embolisation (~6.8%) is outweighed by the need for urgent HR control. There is no difference in the incidence of embolic phenomena between chemical or electrical; electrical cardioversion occurs faster.

Fact 93:

What are the grades of **hepatic encephalopathy (HE)**?

HE is reversible impairment of brain function. Severity is graded according to the West Haven criteria:

Grade	Level of consciousness	Cognition/ Behaviour	Neurological examination
1	Mild confusion	↓ Attention	Mild asterixis/ tremor
2	Lethargy	Disorientation, inappropriate behaviour	Asterixis, slurred speech
3	Somnolent but rousable	Bizarre behaviour	Rigidity, clonus, hyperreflexia
4	Coma		Abnormal posturing

Fact 94:

What are some causes of an **overdamped** A-line trace?

- *Tubing*: Overly compliant, narrow or kinked
- *Obstruction*: Air bubbles, blood clots
- *Pressure bag*: Underinflated or low flush bag pressure
- *Connections*: Loose connections in the fluid-filled part of the electronic monitoring system
- *Artery*: Arterial spasm

Fact 95:

What kind of inspiratory pattern does **volume-controlled ventilation** produce?

Square inspiratory flow pattern

Fact 96:

What is the first line treatment if someone presents with central crushing chest pain, a blood pressure of 75/45 mmHg and **sinus bradycardia** at 38 bpm?

Atropine 500 mcg IV – repeat every 3–5 minutes up to a maximum of 3 mg in an attempt to ↑ HR and ↑ cardiac output.

If bradycardia persists despite atropine, consider cardiac pacing. If pacing cannot be achieved promptly, consider the use of second-line drugs (adrenaline, dobutamine or isoprenaline).

In some settings, second line drugs may be appropriate before cardiac pacing, e.g. using glucagon for an overdose of a beta-blocker or calcium channel blocker.

Fact 97:

What makes noradrenaline a suitable option to manage hypotension following elective surgery in someone with known **severe aortic stenosis (AS)** with a peak transvalvular gradient of 80 mmHg?

Noradrenaline → ↑ SVR → ↑ DBP → ↑ coronary perfusion

In severe AS, maintaining good coronary perfusion is essential as the LV is hypertrophied and prone to ischaemia if the DBP falls.

Drugs that ↓ afterload or ↑ heart rate (↓ diastolic time) should be avoided.

Fact 98:

What is the difference between Charcot's triad and Reynold's pentad in **acute cholangitis**?

Charcot's triad	Reynold's pentad
Fever + Jaundice + Right upper quadrant pain	Charcot's triad + Altered mental status + Shock

Fact 99:

How do you diagnose **peritoneal dialysis (PD) peritonitis** and which organisms are implicated?

Two of the following:

- The presence of signs/symptoms such as fever, abdominal pain, nausea, vomiting or cloudy effluent
- A white cell count >100 per mL of effluent with >50% neutrophils after a 2-hour dwell
- A positive culture from the effluent

The most common organisms are coagulase-negative Staphylococcus, non-Pseudomonas Gram-negative organisms and *Staphylococcus aureus*. Treatment should include intra-peritoneal antibiotics.

Fact 100:

What are the absolute contraindications to **full face mask NIV** in an acute exacerbation of COPD?

- Patient refusal
- Severe facial deformity
- Facial burns
- Fixed upper airway obstruction
- Pneumothorax (unless a chest drain is inserted)
- Recent upper GI surgery

Fact 101:

Which **Mapleson circuits** are best suited for neonates?

Mapleson E and F

Fact 102:

Which pathophysiological mechanism would increase **peak airway pressure** but not plateau pressure?

↑ Airway resistance

Fact 103:

What is the **mixed venous oxygen content** if a pulmonary artery catheter generates these results:

Haemoglobin	10 g/dL
Mixed venous oxygen saturation	70%
Mixed venous oxygen tension (PvO_2)	6.67 kPa

$CvO_2 = (1.34 \times Hb \times SvO_2) + (0.003 \times PvO_2)$

$CvO_2 = (1.34 \times 10 \times 70) + (0.003 \times 6.67)$

$CvO_2 = (938) + (0.02)$

$CvO_2 = \textbf{938.02 mL / dL}$

Fact 104:

Which drugs are recommended to treat **cocaine-associated hypertension,** and why are beta-blockers not recommended first-line?

- Benzodiazepines (e.g. diazepam)
- Nitrates (e.g. glyceryl trinitrate)
- Alpha-blockers (e.g. phentolamine)

Cocaine is an indirectly acting sympathomimetic. It causes hypertension due to ↓ reuptake of noradrenaline at sympathetic nerve terminals.

Beta blockade results in unopposed alpha stimulation. This can worsen coronary artery vasoconstriction and systemic hypertension.

Fact 105:

Which triggers are used to support a **patient-initiated breath** on a ventilator?

- *Flow*: A pre-set flow rate generated by the patient triggers a supported breath.
- *Pressure*: A ↓ in pressure below a pre-set value within the ventilator circuit triggers a supported breath.

Fact 106:

Which **anion and cation** are the most prevalent intracellularly?

- *Anion*: Phosphate
- *Cation*: Potassium

Fact 107:

Which chromosome contains the predisposing gene for **malignant hyperthermia (MH)**?

Chromosome 19 – close to the gene for the ryanodine/dihydropyridine receptor complex

- During anaesthesia, abnormal skeletal muscle contraction and metabolism lead to ↑ temperature and ↑ muscle rigidity.
- Triggers are volatile agents and suxamethonium.
- A rapid ↑ in $ETCO_2$ is one of the earliest signs. Other features may include CVS instability and cyanosis. The reaction can be delayed for several hours.
- Muscle biopsies may appear histologically normal, and the caffeine halothane contracture test is the gold standard for diagnosis.
- Treatment is with IV dantrolene.

Fact 108:

How do you define a **sub-massive pulmonary embolism (PE)** (intermediate-risk PE)?

PE + RV dysfunction/myocardial necrosis without systemic hypotension/ haemodynamic instability

- RV dysfunction: dilated RV on CT/TTE, new RBBB, $S_1Q_3T_3$, ↑ BNP
- Myocardial necrosis: ↑ Cardiac enzymes, e.g. Troponin

Fact 109:

What is **central cord syndrome** and what are its main clinical features?

Bleeding, infarction or oedema involving the central grey matter of the spinal cord.

Features:

Upper limbs	Lower limbs
Motor loss in upper limbs > motor loss in lower limbs	
Mixed UMN and LMN signs	UMN signs
Loss of pain and temperature	Variable sensory changes

Fact 110:

In an adult, where should the balloon tip of an **intra-aortic balloon pump (IABP)** be situated when it's properly positioned?

In the descending thoracic aorta approximately 2 cm distal to the origin of the left subclavian artery

Fact 111:

What **bispectral index (BIS)** should be targeted for a change of dressing in someone with an extensive burn?

40 – 60 (for GA and amnesia)

BIS values range from 0 to 100.

0 is no brain activity and 100 is wide awake.

Fact 112:

What accounts for **alfentanil's** faster onset of action in comparison to fentanyl, even though alfentanil has a lower lipid solubility than fentanyl?

Alfentanil's faster onset of action is attributed to its lower pKa value (6.5) compared to fentanyl's pKa of 8.4. At physiological pH, this lower pKa means that more alfentanil exists in a non-ionised form. Non-ionised drugs are more lipophilic and can cross the blood-brain barrier more easily, leading to a faster onset of action.

Fact 113:

What is the most likely diagnosis if a lady presents with **breathlessness**, a raised JVP, a cough with clear sputum and bilateral infiltrates on her chest X-ray 10 days after a C-section?

Postpartum cardiomyopathy

Presentation and treatment are similar to congestive cardiac failure. An echo will often show diastolic dysfunction. It can present up to five months post-delivery.

Fact 114:

What is the effect of constipation on the efficiency of **peritoneal dialysis (PD)**?

Constipation will ↓ the efficiency of PD.

- A Tenckhoff catheter delivers dialysate into the peritoneum, where it stays to remove waste and fluid before being drained.
- The characteristics of the dialysate and the duration it stays in the peritoneum can be modified to affect clearance and salt/water balance.
- Constipation affects the efficiency of PD as it ↓ dialysate flow.

Fact 115:

Where does the fresh gas flow (FGF) enter a **Mapleson C** or Water's circuit?

Between the reservoir bag (RB) and the adjustable pressure limiting (APL) valve:

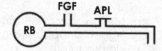

It needs 15 L/min O_2 to prevent rebreathing. The APL valve controls pressures and PEEP (up to ~ 60 cmH_2O).

Fact 116:

Which muscle can be coinfected in **pyelonephritis**?

- Psoas muscle – an abscess can form – because the kidneys are retroperitoneal.
- A psoas abscess is best imaged with an MRI.

Fact 117:

What is the best way to confirm placement of **endotracheal tube** immediately after intubation?

Continuous waveform end-tidal capnography

Fact 118:

What is the best treatment to manage someone who developed a **LV aneurysm** and LVEF 22% following a STEMI and has just received amiodarone for an episode of VT?

ICD implantation

A ↓ ejection fraction and LV aneurysm ↑ the risk of recurrent VT and sudden cardiac death.

Aneurysm excision is reserved as a last line for those with recurrent VT despite other interventions.

Fact 119:

What are the initial BiPAP settings for an **acute exacerbation of COPD**?

- Indication: Respiratory acidosis (pH < 7.35, $PaCO_2$ > 6 kPa) after 1 hour of medical treatment
- IPAP: 10
- EPAP: 4–5
- Target SpO_2: 88–92%

The IPAP is gradually increased until therapeutic response and/or patient tolerability.

Fact 120:

Is there evidence for implanting **left ventricular assist devices (LVADs)** in patients with end-stage heart failure?

Yes

REMATCH trial (2001) compared permanent LVAD insertion with best medical management in those not eligible for transplant. It demonstrated a ↓ one-year and two-year all-cause mortality with permanent LVAD insertion.

Fact 121:

What are the primary functions of an **intra-aortic balloon pump (IABP)** and what does the balloon contain?

Primary functions:
↑ Myocardial oxygen supply
↑ LV ejection fraction and cardiac output
↓ Myocardial oxygen demand
↓ LV afterload
↓ LV wall stress

Balloon:
- Filled with helium which has ↓ viscosity. This allows it to travel quickly through the connecting tubes.
- Compared to air, there is a ↓ risk of air embolism if ruptured.
- When inflated, the balloon should partially occlude the descending aorta (not >80–90% of its diameter).

Fact 122:

Which **Lindegaard ratio** is suggestive of vasospasm on transcranial Doppler studies in someone with a subarachnoid haemorrhage (SAH)?

A ratio > 3 is suggestive of vasospasm.

The Lindegaard ratio is the ratio of flow velocity in the ipsilateral middle cerebral and internal carotid artery:

$$\frac{\text{Mean flow velocity in MCA}}{\text{Mean flow velocity in ICA}}$$

It helps to distinguish hyperaemia from vasospasm. It is based on the principle that as an artery narrows, the blood flow velocity within it increases:

- <3 suggests alternative aetiology, e.g. hyperaemia
- >3 suggests mild to moderate vasospasm
- >6 suggests severe vasospasm

Vasospasm is a narrowing of the intracranial arteries and can occur following a SAH. Incidence peaks at 3–10 days post-SAH, persists for several days and is associated with a worse outcome.

Fact 123:

In a post-operative patient with ongoing bleeding and a **prolonged R-time**, which blood product would you give?

FFP

The R (reaction)-time reflects the concentration of soluble clotting factors in the plasma. An ↑ R-time suggests a deficiency in clotting factors.

Fact 124:

Why does excessive tube length lead to an **underdamped** trace on invasive BP monitoring?

It lowers the natural frequency in the system.

Fact 125:

Which transplacental autoantibodies are associated with **congenital complete heart block** in a mother who has systemic lupus erythematosus during pregnancy?

Anti-Ro (SSA) antibodies

Fact 126:

What are the possible routes by which **temporary pacing** can be delivered?

Transcutaneous, transvenous, epicardial, oesophageal

Fact 127:

What pathophysiological mechanism causes an increase in the **plateau pressure**?

↓ Lung compliance

Fact 128:

What are the types of **patient evacuation** in the event of a fire?

Horizontal evacuation	To an adjacent area
Vertical evacuation	To a lower floor
External evacuation	Outside of the building

Fact 129:

What are the key features of a **scleroderma renal crisis (SRC)** and how do you treat it?

Renal failure
Accelerated hypertension
Microangiopathic haemolytic anaemia

SRC complicates systemic sclerosis in 10% of patients. It is a life-threatening complication characterised by endothelial dysfunction and RAAS activation. As RAAS activation plays a central role in this condition, treatment is with ACE inhibitors.

Fact 130:

What is the mechanism of action of the primary class of **antibiotics** frequently employed as first-line treatment in an 18-year-old patient with a headache, photophobia, fever and confusion?

Inhibition of cell wall synthesis

First-line antibiotics for possible bacterial meningitis are cephalosporins.

Penicillins, cephalosporins, carbapenems and monobactams all act via inhibition of cell wall synthesis.

Fact 131:

What happens to the HR and SVR in someone with a cervical injury and **neurogenic shock**?

- ↓ HR: Sympathetic input to the heart originates from T1 to T4, so injuries above this level lead to unopposed parasympathetic activity and a ↓ heart rate.
- ↓ SVR: Peripheral vasodilation occurs due to impaired sympathetic innervation, resulting in warm extremities and disrupted temperature regulation with heat loss.

In cervical injuries, the loss of spinal and autonomic reflexes below the injury level is linked to flaccid paralysis, absence of reflexes and sensory disruptions below the lesion.

Fact 132:

What is the **ejection fraction** if the end-diastolic volume (EDV) is 60 mL and end-systolic volume (ESV) is 40 mL?

33%

EF = Stroke volume / EDV

Stroke volume (SV) = EDV − ESV = 60 − 40 = 20

Therefore EF = 20 / 60 = 1/ 3 = **33%**

Fact 133:

What are the **endocrine effects** of losing brainstem function?

- ↓ ADH: Pituitary ischaemia leads to cranial diabetes insipidus.
- ↓ T3: Hypothalamic dysfunction leads to hypothermia and functional hypothyroidism.

Fact 134:

When is haemodialysis recommended on presentation in someone with an **aspirin** overdose?

- Plasma salicylate > 700 mg/L (5.1 mmol/L)
- Severe metabolic acidosis

Fact 135:

How far would you typically advance an **oesophageal Doppler probe** via the nose and mouth?

- Nose: 40–45 cm
- Mouth: 35–40 cm

Fact 136:

Which drug augments the release of Factor 8 and vWF in **Von Willebrand's disease**?

Desmopressin (DDAVP) – a synthetic drug that increases Factor 8 and vWF and improves platelet function

Fact 137:

In which aortic disease is an **intra-aortic balloon pump (IABP)** contraindicated?

Aortic regurgitation

For blood to be ejected antegradely to perfuse the tissues and retrogradely to perfuse the coronaries, the aortic valve must be closed and competent.

Fact 138:

What is the effect of low erythropoietin (Epo) in **chronic kidney disease (CKD)**?

↓ Red cell survival and ↓ red cell production

Fact 139:

How do you treat a **variceal bleed**?

Pharmacological
- Fluid resuscitation
- Transfusion
  - Non-exsanguinating haemorrhage: Target Hb > 70 g/L
  - Blood products in coagulopathy or in massive transfusion
- Drugs to ↓ portal pressure:
  - Terlipressin (splanchnic vasoconstrictor): ↓ variceal bleeding, rebleeding rates and mortality rates.
  - Somatostatin or its analogue, octreotide, have also been used.

Endoscopic
- Endoscopic treatments favour band ligation over sclerotherapy, especially in controlling bleeding and improving mortality, although it may be more challenging during active bleeding.

Rescue therapy
- A Sengstaken–Blakemore tube for ongoing massive haemorrhage when the above treatments fail. The oesophageal balloon is used if the gastric balloon fails to adequately control bleeding. This is a temporary measure (to allow repeat endoscopy, TIPS or transplant), and it has a high rebleed rate after removal (50% risk of re-bleeding following balloon deflation).
- Stent procedures, typically a percutaneous TIPS, offer definitive treatment to ↓ portal pressure but come with an ↑ risk of encephalopathy.

Fact 140:

What problem does a **continuous-flow LVAD** pose when inserting a peripheral arterial cannula in a radial artery?

- Patients will not have normal pulsatile flow.
- This makes A-line insertion more difficult.

Fact 141:

What attributes of drugs render them appropriate for elimination through **renal replacement therapy**?

- ↑ Water solubility
- ↓ Molecular weight (HD: ≤500 Da, HF: ≤40 kDa)
- ↓ Volume of distribution (<1 L/kg)
- ↓ Degree of protein-binding (free fraction is removed)
- ↓ Endogenous clearance (<4 mL/min/kg)
- Extraction ratio > endogenous elimination

Fact 142:

Why is **etomidate** not used as maintenance sedation in critically ill patients on ICU?

It causes adrenal suppression (inhibits 11β-hydroxylase).

Fact 143:

What were the findings of the **HALT-IT trial (2020)** concerning the use of tranexamic acid (TXA) in upper GI bleeding?

- No benefit of using TXA in GI bleeding
- Associated with a significantly higher risk of venous thromboembolism

Fact 144:

When should you consider intraosseous access in a **cardiac arrest**?

- If IV access cannot be gained within 2 minutes.
- The tibial or humeral sites should be tried first.

Fact 145:

What are the features of **hypertensive retinopathy**?

Grade 1	Arterial narrowing
Grade 2	AV nicking
Grade 3	Haemorrhages, exudates and cotton wool spots
Grade 4	All of the above + papilloedema

Fact 146:

How is it possible to get both a pansystolic and ejection systolic murmur in **Tetralogy of Fallot (TOF)**?

- The ventricular septal defect (VSD) causes a pansystolic murmur.
- Pulmonary stenosis causes an ejection systolic murmur.

The four features of TOF are:
Septal defect (VSD)
Aortic displacement (overriding aorta)
Stenosis of pulmonary valve
Hypertrophy of right ventricle

Fact 147:

How would you manage a symptomatic **secondary pneumothorax** of 3 cm in a chronic smoker?

Insert a small-bore chest drain (8–14 Fr) and attach to an underwater seal drain

Needle aspiration would have been appropriate if the pneumothorax was 1–2 cm in this risk group.

Fact 148:

Which metabolic abnormalities are commonly seen in **gastric outlet obstruction (GOO)**?

- Metabolic alkalosis: Vomiting results in the loss of H^+.
- Hypochloraemia: Vomiting results in the loss of Cl^-.
- Hypokalaemia: Renal loss of K^+ as H^+ are exchanged for K^+ in the distal tubule and through activation of the RAAS as a consequence of dehydration

The two most common causes of GOO in adults are peptic ulcer disease and gastric carcinoma.

Fact 149:

What is meant by **positive predictive value (PPV)** and **negative predictive value (NPV)**?

- *PPV*: How likely is it that the patient has the disease, given that the test is positive?
- *NPV*: How likely is it that the patient has the disease, given that the test is negative?

For example, D-dimer has a good NPV but a poor PPV:
- If D-dimer is negative, PE is unlikely (low false-negative rate)
- If D-dimer is positive, who knows? (high false-positive rate)

Fact 150:

What ECG changes may you see in **cardiac tamponade**?

- ↓ Amplitude electrical signals
- Electrical alternans – cyclical variations in QRS amplitude (more specific for tamponade)

Echocardiography is the single most important investigation for pericardial tamponade.

The pericardial sac normally contains 30–50 mL of serous fluid. This fluid is produced by the visceral mesothelial cells and is drained by the lymphatic system.

Fact 151:

How may **isoprenaline** be used to manage someone with bradycardia-dependent Torsades de Pointes secondary to acquired QT prolongation?

To ↑ the HR

Isoprenaline is a non-selective β_1/β_2 agonist. When used, it causes an ↑ in the HR. This shortens the QT interval. It is useful as a bridge to temporary pacing in patients unresponsive to magnesium sulphate.

Fact 152:

What are the main cardiovascular abnormalities that are associated with **Turner's syndrome**?

- Bicuspid aortic valve
- Coarctation of the aorta

Fact 153:

Where would you zero the transducer of an **arterial line**?

The phlebostatic axis – this corresponds roughly with the position of the right atrium and the aortic root.

Fact 154:

What is the basic management of **diabetic ketoacidosis (DKA)**?

- Intravenous fluids with potassium replacement
- Fluid boluses if shocked (SBP < 90 mmHg)
- Fixed rate insulin infusion (FRII) 0.1 units/kg/hr. If glucose/ketone/bicarbonate targets are not being met, then the rate can be increased.
- Long-acting insulin should be continued.
- If glucose <14 mmol/L, 10% glucose should be added.
- Precipitating cause should be identified and treated.

Fact 155:

How can the **NEXUS criteria** assist in determining which trauma patients do not need cervical spine imaging?

No cervical imaging is needed if all of these are present ('NSAID'):

- No focal **N**eurologic deficit
- No midline **S**pinal tenderness
- No **A**ltered level of consciousness
- Not **I**ntoxicated
- No **D**istracting injury

The NEXUS criteria have a sensitivity of 99.6% for ruling out cervical spine injury in the original study validating the criteria. It may not be reliable in patients > 65 years of age. The Canadian C-spine rules is an alternative tool.

Fact 156:

Why is it necessary to exercise caution when employing **pulmonary vasodilators** in patients with COPD-related cor pulmonale?

- Pulmonary vasodilators reverse the chronic effects of hypoxic pulmonary vasoconstriction.
- Using them can paradoxically worsen hypoxaemia.

Fact 157:

What are the estimated **daily nutritional requirements** in critical illness?

Energy	25–35 kcal/kg
Carbohydrate	2 g/kg
Protein	0.8–1.5 g/kg
Lipid	1.0–1.5 g/kg
Water	30 mL/kg
Na^+, Cl^-, K^+	1 mmol/kg
PO_4^{3-}	0.4 mmol/kg
Mg^{2+}, Ca^{2+}	0.1 mmol/kg
Selenium	100 µg
Zinc	10 mg
Vitamin B1 (thiamine)	100 mg

Fact 158:

What is the **mean**, **median** and **mode** for data that are normally distributed, and what is a **parametric test**?

Mean (μ) = Median = Mode

The curve is bell-shaped and equal on both sides.

A parametric test is a statistical test which assumes that data is normally distributed.

Fact 159:

What are the six components of the **Sequential Organ Failure Assessment (SOFA) Score**?

1	2	3	4	5	6
CNS	CVS	Resp	Clotting	Liver	Renal
GCS	MAP or use of vasopressors	PaO_2/FiO_2	Platelet count	Bilirubin	Creatinine

- The SOFA score is a mortality prediction score that is based on the degree of dysfunction of six organ systems. It scores the degree of dysfunction of each between 0 and 4 with a total possible score of 0–24.
- The score is calculated on admission and every 24 hours until discharge using the worst parameters measured during the prior 24 hours.
- A score of >15 correlates with a mortality rate of 90%.

Fact 160:

What is the difference between the Well's score and **PE Severity Index (PESI)** for a pulmonary embolism?

- Well's score: The clinical likelihood of having a PE
- PESI: Once the diagnosis of a PE is made, this is risk stratification tool to determine 30-day mortality (class 3–5 are high risk)

Fact 161:

What is the classical triad seen in acute **Graft versus Host Disease (GvHD)** following an allogeneic haematopoietic cell transplant?

Hepatitis
Enteritis
Dermatitis

Occurs when antigen presenting cells of the recipient interact with donor T-cells.

Chronic graft versus host disease on the other hand is a diverse syndrome with varying clinical features resembling autoimmune disorders. It can present with multiple organ involvement.

Fact 162:

How would you treat **Panton–Valentine Leukocidin (PVL) staphylococcus**?

- Toxin clearance: Clindamycin and/or linezolid
- Intracellular clearance: Rifampicin
- IVIg: Adjunct to neutralise exotoxins/ superantigens

PVL is one of many toxins produced by *Staphylococcus aureus* (can be MSSA or MRSA). It is usually associated with skin and soft tissue infections but can also result in necrotising haemorrhagic pneumonia.

Fact 163:

Why should **0.9% NaCl** be used as the infusion fluid in arterial lines instead of glucose-containing fluids?

Pseudohyperglycaemia may occur, potentially leading to hypoglycaemia if insulin treatment is initiated.

Fact 164:

What is the most sensitive indication of respiratory muscle dysfunction in **Guillain–Barré syndrome**?

Forced vital capacity

Fact 165:

Why is thiopentone contraindicated as an induction agent in patients with **acute intermittent porphyria (AIP)**?

Thiopentone, like other barbiturates, significantly induces the enzyme ALA synthetase.

This leads to ↑ production of delta-ALA from succinate and glycine within the mitochondria, exacerbating the symptoms of AIP.

Fact 166:

What are some causes of **pulmonary fibrosis**?

	Upper lobe		Lower lobe
C	Coal-workers pneumoconiosis	C	Cryptogenic fibrosing alveolitis (now IPF)
H	Histiocytosis	A	Asbestosis
A	ABPA	R	Rheumatoid arthritis
A	Ankylosing spondylitis	D	Drugs (bleomycin, methotrexate, amiodarone)
R	Radiation pneumonitis	S	Scleroderma
T	Tuberculosis		
S	Silicosis		
S	Sarcoidosis		

Fact 167:

Why should individuals who have a **CYP2D6 gene duplication** not be given codeine?

They are ultrarapid metabolisers.

Individuals who have more than two normally functioning copies of the CYP2D6 gene are able to metabolise codeine to morphine more rapidly and more completely. As a result, even with therapeutic doses of codeine, these individuals experience the symptoms of morphine overdose.

Fact 168:

How would you represent a **1% solution** in mg per 100 mL?

1% solution = 10 mg / mL

Therefore 100 mL = 10 × 100
= 1,000 **mg per 100 mL**

Fact 169:

How does the effect of **carvedilol** on reducing the hepatic venous pressure gradient (HVPG) compare to that of propranolol?

In the secondary prophylaxis of variceal bleeding, carvedilol produces more pronounced reductions in HVPG compared to propranolol.

Fact 170:

Why may you consider adding vancomycin to cefuroxime for an 85-year-old nursing home resident who presents **septic arthritis**?

Nursing home residents are at risk of MRSA.

Fact 171:

Which organism often causes **Lemierre's disease**?

Fusobacterium necrophorum (Gram –ve anaerobe)

Characterised by thrombophlebitis of the internal jugular vein (IJV) and bacteremia following an oropharyngeal infection. This can cause the development of a thrombus in the IJV which can migrate inferiorly to the subclavian vein or superiorly to the venous sinuses. Treatment is with 2–6 weeks of antibiotics +/– anticoagulation.

Fact 172:

What impact does **hypophosphataemia** have the oxygen dissociation curve?

- Hypophosphataemia can deplete 2,3-DPG.
- This shifts the oxygen dissociation curve to the left with ↓ oxygen delivery to peripheral tissues.

Fact 173:

Which **thyroid hormone** is the most physiologically active?

T3 – from peripheral 5'-deiodination of T4 by deiodinases

Fact 174:

Which gases are absorbed by **infrared analysers**?

Gases with molecules that contain at least two dissimilar atoms absorb radiation in the infrared region of the electromagnetic spectrum, e.g. carbon dioxide, nitrous oxide and all halogenated volatile anaesthetic agents.

Oxygen, nitrogen, helium and the inert (or noble) gases do not absorb infrared light and cannot be measured using this technology.

Fact 175:

Which agent that is used to treat **typhoid fever** can also cause aplastic anaemia?

Chloramphenicol

Fact 176:

How do you define **death**?

Irreversible loss of the capacity for consciousness + irreversible loss of the capacity to breathe

Fact 177:

Why may patients with high spinal injury develop **gastroparesis**?

Unopposed vagal activity to stomach

Enteral feeding may therefore lead to abdominal distension and aspiration.

Fact 178:

What are some of the systemic complications of a **subarachnoid haemorrhage**?

- *Cardiac:* Myocardial injury, dysrhythmias, global and regional wall motion abnormalities including Takotsubo cardiomyopathy
- *Respiratory:* Neurogenic pulmonary oedema, aspiration pneumonitis
- *Endocrine:* Hyperglycaemia, pyrexia, hyponatraemia (due to cerebral salt-wasting syndrome or SIADH)
- *Gastrointestinal:* Stress ulceration
- *Haematological:* Venous thromboembolism

Fact 179:

Apart from an elevated lithium dosage, what are some other factors that can lead to **chronic lithium toxicity**?

- Dehydration
- Renal impairment
- ↓ Renal clearance of lithium, e.g. ACE inhibitors, angiotensin II receptor antagonists and thiazide diuretics
- Diabetes insipidus and hypothyroidism (both of these can also be caused by chronic lithium therapy)

Fact 180:

Is there a role for early commencement of RRT in stage 3 **acute kidney injury**?

- No mortality benefit has been shown by commencing RRT early.
- Not all patients in stage 3 AKI will require RRT.
- RRT also has associated morbidity, e.g. risks of line insertion, haemodynamic instability and anticoagulation.
- Initiation may result in dependence and possible RRT-related kidney injury.

Fact 181:

How is using ultrasound to determine **optic nerve sheath diameter** (ONSD) useful in predicting ICP?

ONSD > 5 mm predicts ICP > 20 mmHg with a sensitivity and specificity of 90%

Fact 182:

Is there a place for gut decontamination and the use of lactulose in the treatment of encephalopathy associated with **acute liver failure**?

Nope

Fact 183:

How is **atracurium** metabolised?

Via two main pathways independent of renal and hepatic function:

- Hoffman degradation (30–70%): Non-enzymatic spontaneous process. There is ↓ Hoffman degradation at ↓ temperature and ↓ pH
- Ester hydrolysis: Catalysis by non-specific plasma esterases

Fact 184:

What are some condition-specific reasons why someone with **Marfan's syndrome** may develop breathlessness?

S	**S**pontaenous pneumothoraces
T	**T**MJ dislocation because of a high arched palpate (and potential for difficult airway)
A	**A**ortic regurgitation (due to cystic medial necrosis)
M	**M**itral valve disease (valve prolapse or regurgitation) which can lead to pulmonary hypertension and heart failure
P	**P**ectus deformities and kyphoscoliosis (which can cause respiratory failure)

Marfan's syndrome is caused by an autosomal dominant mutation on chromosome 15 involving the glycoprotein fibrillin-1 gene

Fact 185:

How long should **clopidogrel, prasugrel,** or **ticagrelor** be stopped for before doing a lumbar puncture?

Seven days before performing the lumbar puncture

Fact 186:

Which investigation would you perform in someone who had **coronary stents** 5 hours ago, and these are his most recent observations:

- HR 120 with electrical alternans & low-voltage QRS
- BP 75/40
- CVP 25

TTE – the most likely diagnosis is cardiac tamponade

The pericardial fluid initially compresses the lowest pressure chamber – the RA – and this impairs atrial filling, causing hypotension but with an ↑ CVP (distended neck veins). Electrical alternans occurs due to movement of the heart within the fluid-filled pericardial sac.

Fact 187:

Which cranial nerve is usually first to be affected by a **raised intracranial pressure**?

Abducens Nerve (CN6) because of its long course

This supplies the lateral rectus muscle, which is responsible for ipsilateral aBduction of the eye.

In a CN6 palsy, the tonic unopposed action of the medial rectus muscle causes the eye to be aDducted at rest. The affected person is unable to aBduct the eye fully when asked.

Fact 188:

How does **aprotinin** work?

- Inhibits fibrinolysis via inactivation of free plasmin
- Inhibits trypsin and kallikrein

Given prior to cardiac bypass to ↓ blood loss as it prevents clot activation, factor consumption and platelet dysfunction. There is evidence for and against its use, e.g. ↑ risk of MI, stroke, renal failure and heart failure.

Fact 189:

What happens to the pulmonary vascular resistance, intrapleural pressure, intracranial pressure and cardiac output in **abdominal compartment syndrome (ACS)**?

- ↓ Lung compliance → ↑ intrathoracic pressures → hypoxic vasoconstriction → ↑ **PVR**
- ↑ **intrapleural pressure** → ↑ CVP and ↑ PAOP
- ↓ Cranial venous outflow → ↑ **ICP**
- ↓ Venous return → ↓ **CO** → ↓ organ perfusion, e.g. renal → ↑ organ venous congestion

---

Fact 190:

What are the components of the **Model for End-Stage Liver Disease (MELD) score**?

- **B**ilirubin
- **I**NR
- **C**reatinine
- **S**odium

MELD predicts three-month mortality in patients with cirrhosis. The original version was created to estimate survival in patients undergoing elective TIPS. The components are entered into a formula to give a score from 6 to 40. The higher the score, the greater the mortality, e.g. a score ≤ 9 is has a predicted three-month mortality of 1.9%. It has since been validated to predict short-term mortality in patients with cirrhosis with variceal bleeding, acute alcoholic hepatitis or undergoing non-transplant surgeries.

Fact 191:

What methods exist for **sterilising** medical equipment, and what are some examples of these?

Heat	Dry heat	e.g. incineration, hot air oven, baking
	Moist heat	e.g. autoclave
Chemical		e.g. ethylene oxide
Irradiation		e.g. gamma, ultraviolet

Fact 192:

How does **sodium zirconium cyclosilicate** work in the management of hyperkalaemia?

It is a non-absorbed cation-exchange compound that acts as a selective potassium binder in the gastro-intestinal tract.

Fact 193:

What does the **Delphi method** evaluate?

Expert consensus – it is a recognised approach to reach a consensus on real-world expertise gathered from experts in specific subject areas.

Fact 194:

What may the presence of **ruminococcus** in the blood suggest?

Possible gut pathology, e.g. GI perforation. These bacteria belong to the Clostridia class, are anaerobic and are Gram-positive gut microbes.

Fact 195:

What are the treatment priorities in **massive pulmonary haemorrhage (MPH)**?

A	Airway protection
B	Ensuring adequate gas exchange, including considering lung isolation in unilateral disease to avoid contamination of the 'good' lung
C	Blood product resuscitation and correction of coagulopathy
	Identifying the source of bleeding and stopping it

Fact 196:

How useful is a **synacthen test** performed in critical illness to diagnose adrenal insufficiency?

Not very useful as it may be confounded by critical illness

Fact 197:

Why may the urinary ketones be negative in **diabetic ketoacidosis**?

Impaired urinary clearance in DKA

Fact 198:

Why are obstetric patients at an increased risk of **regurgitation**?

↓ Tone of the lower oesophageal sphincter
↓ Gastric emptying
↑ Intra-abdominal pressure due to gravid uterus

Fact 199:

What specific treatment options are there for *Clostridium difficile*?

Antibiotics	**First line**	Vancomycin 125 mg QDS (enteral)
	Second line/ relapse	Fidaxomicin 200 mg BD (enteral)
	Third line/ life-threatening	Vancomycin 500 mg QDS (enteral) +/− IV metronidazole 500 mg TDS
Surgery	May be required for life-threatening disease	
Faecal microbiota transplant	Considered in recurrent disease > 2 episodes	

Fact 200:

What is **hepatopulmonary syndrome**?

Hypoxemia due to dilated intrapulmonary vasculature in the presence of liver disease (more common in chronic liver disease). Occurs due to ineffective clearance of mediators that cause intrapulmonary vasodilatation.

Patients present with dyspnoea, platypnea and orthodeoxia. Contrast-enhanced echocardiography with agitated saline is the gold standard for diagnosing pulmonary vascular dilatation. It will demonstrate a right to left intrapulmonary shunt after 3–4 cardiac cycles in patients with hepatopulmonary syndrome.

Fact 201:

What is the current recommendation for using **high-frequency oscillatory ventilation (HFOV)** in ARDS?

FICM and ICS strongly recommended against it after the **OSCILLATE** and **OSCAR** trials. Potential harms include barotrauma, hypotension and oxygenation failure.

- OSCAR 2013: No mortality benefit to HFOV
- OSCILLATE 2013: Significantly higher in-hospital mortality (trial was stopped early)

HFOV is still used in paediatrics when conventional ventilation fails.

Fact 202:

What are the four categories of the **Maastricht classification** of Donation after Circulatory Death (DCD)?

DCD applies after death is confirmed using cardio-respiratory criteria. There are two types of DCD:

- *Controlled*: Planned withdrawal of life-sustaining treatments
- *Uncontrolled*: Organ retrieval after a cardiac arrest that is unexpected.

The clinical circumstances in which DCD can occur are described by the Maastricht classification:

Category	Type	Circumstances	Typical location
1	Uncontrolled	Dead on arrival	Emergency department
2	Uncontrolled	Unsuccessful resuscitation	Emergency department
3	Controlled	Cardiac arrest follows planned withdrawal of life sustaining treatments	Intensive care unit
4	Either	Cardiac arrest in a patient who is brain dead	Intensive care unit

Fact 203:

Why is **amiodarone** not suitable for removal through renal replacement therapy?

- Large volume of distribution
- Eliminated in bile
- Highly protein-bound

Fact 204:

What is **acalculous cholecystitis?**

Gallbladder inflammation without gallstones. It is caused by dysfunction or hypokinesis of gallbladder emptying. It is life-threatening and has a higher risk of perforation and necrosis compared to calculous disease.

Stasis of the gallbladder results in the build-up of intraluminal pressure. This eventually results in ischaemia of the gallbladder wall, inflammation and colonisation with bacteria. If the pressure is not relieved, the gallbladder wall will become progressively ischaemic eventually resulting in gangrene and perforation. Diagnosis is made with US, CT or a HIDA scan. In unstable patients, percutaneous drainage may be used initially, followed by cholecystectomy when feasible.

Fact 205:

How do you diagnose **acute pancreatitis** and how do you classify its severity according to the revised Atlanta classification?

Diagnosis	Severity
Diagnosis requires two or more of the following: • Pain consistent with acute pancreatitis • A rise in biochemical markers – amylase or lipase (more specific) > 3 times upper limit of normal • Imaging confirming acute pancreatitis	The revised Atlanta classification quantifies severity as: • **Mild:** Absence of organ failure or complications • **Moderate:** Transient organ failure or local/systemic complications without persistent organ failure • **Severe:** Persistent > 48 hours organ failure

Fact 206:

What are the possible effects of **amiodarone** on the thyroid and liver?

- *Thyroid*: Both hypothyroidism and hyperthyroidism
- *Liver:* Hepatotoxicity

Fact 207:

In addition to **spontaneous bacterial peritonitis (SBP)**, what other diagnosis should you consider if someone grows multiple organisms from their ascitic fluid and has an ascitic neutrophil count > 1,000 cells/mm³?

Secondary Bacterial Peritonitis – due to bowel perforation or inflammation of intra-abdominal organs

Performing a CT to detect perforation is recommended in cases of suspected secondary bacterial peritonitis.

Fact 208:

Which conditions require notification due to **Group A β-streptococcus (GAS)** infection?

Scarlet fever, invasive GAS (iGAS), toxic shock syndrome

Fact 209:

How can catheter ablation for drug-refractory atrial fibrillation result in an **atrial oesophageal fistula**?

Heat from ablation → ulceration/necrosis of thin-walled left atrium → fistula formation to oesophagus which lies just posterior to the LA

Fact 210:

What is level of the **thyroid cartilage** and **cricoid cartilage**?

- Thyroid cartilage: C4–C5
- Cricoid cartilage: C6

The cricothyroid membrane connects the cricoid and thyroid cartilages and serves as the location for cricothyrotomy.

Fact 211:

What is the recommended time frame to initiate **aspirin** therapy after administering thrombolysis for an acute ischaemic stroke?

Aspirin should be withheld for 24 hours after thrombolysis.

Fact 212:

What type of **ECMO** would a lung transplant patient with early graft failure and refractory hypoxaemia require?

Veno-venous ECMO (VV-ECMO)

Fact 213:

What drug can you give for **intraabdominal hypertension** in someone with high volumes of nasogastric aspirates?

Prokinetics, e.g. metoclopramide, erythromycin

Fact 214:

What modifiable factors can lead to **secondary brain injury** in cases of traumatic brain injury?

- ↑ ICP, ↑ temperature, ↑ pCO_2
- ↓ BP (CVS instability), ↓ pO_2

Fact 215:

Why may a ventilator try to support a respiratory rate of 80 breaths per minute in someone who is on **pressure support ventilation** when the actual respiratory rate is 20 breaths per minute and the flow trigger is 200 mL/min?

The ventilator may be sensing the heartbeat as the beginning of a spontaneous breath.

This is because the trigger may be too low. Therefore, to remedy this, the flow trigger can be ↑.

Fact 216:

How would you manage someone who has developed an **intracerebral bleed** on warfarin with an INR of 6.4?

Prothrombin complex concentrate (PCC) 25–50 units/kg, e.g. Beriplex or Octaplex + IV Vitamin K

- PCC contains clotting factors 2, 7, 9, 10, protein C, and S. It rapidly reverses INR but has a short half-life, so IV vitamin K should be given to aid clotting factor synthesis, which takes about 6 hours.
- If PCC is not available, FFP can be an alternative, but it provides suboptimal INR reversal due to diluted clotting factors, requires a 20–30-minute thawing period and carries transfusion-related risks.

Fact 217:

How does **rivaroxaban** work?

Rivaro**Xa**ban is a highly selective direct factor **Xa** inhibitor, capable of inhibiting both unbound factor Xa and factor Xa within the prothrombinase complex.

It belongs to the oxazolidinone derivative class and exhibits excellent gut absorption.

Fact 218:

How would you pre-operatively manage someone for an elective **total hip replacement (THR)** if they had a STEMI six months ago, had a drug eluting stent inserted at the time and is now on dual antiplatelet therapy (DAPT)?

Postpone the THR for one year from stent insertion

DAPT should be continued for one year following the insertion of a drug eluting stent unless the surgery is urgent. The risk of stent thrombosis is ↑ if DAPT is discontinued. Stent thrombosis is associated with a significantly ↑ morbidity and mortality.

Fact 219:

What is the typical triad of clinical features seen in **serotonin syndrome**?

Altered mental status	Neuromuscular dysfunction	Autonomic dysfunction
Anxiety Agitation Delirium Seizures Coma	Hyperreflexia Tremor Myoclonus ↑ Tone	Hyper/ hypotension Tachycardia Mydriasis Diarrhoea Sweating

Fact 220:

What are the main indications for a **ventricular assist device (VAD)**?

- An LVAD takes blood from the LV and ejects it into the ascending or descending aorta.
- An RVAD takes blood from the RV and ejects into the pulmonary artery.
- A BVAD supports both sides.

Indications:

- Bridge to recovery, e.g. cardiogenic shock following myocarditis, graft-failure post-transplant, post-MI
- Bridge to candidacy
- Bridge to transplant, e.g. heart failure despite maximal medical management
- Destination (permanent) therapy, e.g. patients in whom transplantation is required but contraindicated

Fact 221:

What has happened to the serum ADH if someone has **hypernatremia and polyuria** following a head injury?

↓ ADH – this is cranial diabetes insipidus.

Diabetes insipidus is characterised by ↑ plasma osmolality and ↓ urine osmolality

Fact 222:

How does **levosimendan** work as an inodilator?

Inotropy
↑ Sensitivity of troponin C to intracellular Ca^{2+} without increasing intracellular calcium concentration. This ↑ inotropy without a significant ↑ in oxygen consumption. Does not impair diastolic relaxation.
Vasodilatation

Opens ATP-sensitive K^+ channels → vascular smooth muscle relaxation:
• ↓ Preload
• ↓ Afterload
  o Systemic circulation (↓ SVR)
    ■ ↓ LV work → ↓ LV O_2 consumption
    ■ ↓ Coronary vascular resistance → ↑ coronary flow and O_2 supply
    ■ ↑ Renal blood flow
  o Pulmonary circulation (↓ PVR)
    ■ ↓ PAP and ↓ PCWP→ ↓ RV work → ↓ RV O_2 consumption

Other effects
Anti-inflammatory effects, anti-apoptotic effects, cAMP-PDE inhibitory effects

Overall:

- ↑ Cardiac output, stroke volume, heart rate, coronary blood flow, renal blood flow
- ↓ SVR, SBP, PCWP, PAP, coronary vascular resistance, myocardial oxygen consumption

Fact 223:

How many lumens does a **pulmonary artery catheter** have?

Four lumens: Proximal, distal, inflation and thermistor lumen

Fact 224:

What is meant if a test has a **sensitivity** of 90%?

90% of positive tests are true positives.

Fact 225:

What cardiac output study findings would you typically expect in someone with **hypovolaemic shock**?

↓ Stroke volume
↓ Cardiac output
↓ Filling pressures (CVP and PCWP)
↑ HR
↑ SVR

Fact 226:

What critical investigations must be conducted for a patient with **invasive candidemia**, and what is the recommended treatment approach?

The majority of invasive fungal infections are caused by Candida albicans. The critical investigations include:

1. Ophthalmology evaluation for endophthalmitis, which can lead to irreversible vision loss
2. Echocardiogram to assess for fungal balls or abscesses
3. Renal imaging to check for pyelonephritis, fungal balls or abscesses in individuals with candiduria

Treatment for confirmed/suspected candidaemia is:

- *Non-neutropenic patients*: Fluconazole or an echinocandin (e.g. caspofungin or anidulafungin). IV catheters should be removed in these patients.
- *Neutropenic patients*: Echinocandins. There is less evidence of benefit for removing IV catheters in these patients, as they are more likely to have an alternative source of candidaemia.

Fact 227:

Which vitamin deficiency is a rare cause of **alcohol-related heart failure**?

Thiamine (Vitamin B1) deficiency

Fact 228:

Which phenomenon within the large bowel wall leads to the appearance of the **'thumbprint' sign** on imaging?

Oedema

This sign indicates bowel wall thickening. Causes include infective, ischaemic and inflammatory colitis

Fact 229:

Why is intravenous fluid administration important during an RSI in someone with **severe asthma**?

To avoid hypotension

Gas trapping and ↑ intrathoracic pressure → ↓ venous return → ↓ preload → ↓ CO

Fact 230:

When should you start a **beta blocker** in heart failure?

In stable disease as it may cause decompensation in acute disease.

Beta-blockers ↓ mortality in heart failure.

Fact 231:

What is the **blood flow** through the carotid artery if someone has a 75% reduction in the radius of the left internal carotid artery, assuming that the blood flow is 400 mL/min prior to the occlusion?

- Blood flow (Q) is inversely proportional to the resistance of the artery ($Q = \Delta P/R$)
- Resistance is inversely proportional to the radius raised to the fourth power (Poiseuille equation: $R = 8\,\eta L/\pi r^4$)
- As the radius has ↓ by 75%, the radius has ↓ to one-quarter of its original size. Therefore, using Poiseuille equation, the resistance has ↑ by $1/(1/4)^4$ or 256-fold.
- If the resistance has ↑ 256-fold, using $Q = \Delta P/R$, flow has ↓ to 1/256, or 0.39% of the original value.
- Flow is therefore 0.39% × 400 mL/min = **1.56 mL/min.**

This is a dramatic ↓ in blood flow to the brain, because of relationship between resistance and vessel radius.

Fact 232:

What is the recommended duration for isolating an inpatient with **rifampicin-sensitive active pulmonary tuberculosis** in a side room?

≥ 2 weeks from starting standard treatment

Fact 233:

If someone is stabbed through to the left atrium, which **coronary artery** is most likely to be affected?

Left coronary artery

The left atrium is supplied by the left coronary artery and its major branch, the left circumflex artery.

Fact 234:

How many ports and balloons does a **Linton–Nachlas tube** have in managing an upper GI bleed?

- Two ports: Gastric suction port and balloon inflation port
- One single 500–600 mL gastric balloon

Fact 235:

What happens to the y-descent in the JVP waveform in **constrictive pericarditis**?

The y-descent is exaggerated.

This is called Friedrich's sign.

Fact 236:

What might you see on an ECG in **propofol infusion syndrome (PRIS)**?

- Bradycardias leading to asystole
- Arrhythmias: AF, VT, SVT, bundle branch block
- Brugada-like changes: Coved ST-elevation in V_{1-3}

Linked to doses > 4 mg/kg/hr for >48 hours, although PRIS has been reported with doses as low as 1.9 mg/kg/hr.

Fact 237:

What urinary acid–base changes are classically seen in **gastric outlet obstruction**?

- An initial ↑ in urine pH due to renal bicarbonate loss.
- Later, a 'paradoxical aciduria' arises as hydrogen ions are swapped for sodium ions to preserve circulating volume.

Fact 238:

Is it crucial to evaluate the extent and size of a burn during the **primary survey**?

No – this is done as part of the secondary survey.

Fact 239:

If electrical cardioversion fails to effectively treat **atrial fibrillation** with adverse signs, what is the next course of action in management?

Give amiodarone 300 mg IV followed by an infusion of 900 mg over 24 hours

Further electrical cardioversion may be required.

Electrolytes such as potassium, calcium and magnesium should be optimised.

Other agents for rate control, e.g. digoxin or beta blockers, may be considered as second-line therapy.

Fact 240:

Why is lying supine in a **high spinal cord injury** important?

Improves respiratory function

In this position, the diaphragm has greater excursion in inspiration as it is pushed into the chest by the abdominal contents which act as a fulcrum.

Fact 241:

Why is hyperventilation harmful in **traumatic brain injury**?

$\downarrow pCO_2 \rightarrow$ cerebral vasoconstriction $\rightarrow \downarrow$ blood supply to ischaemic penumbra

---

Fact 242:

What is the difference between **epidemic**, **endemic** and **pandemic** in epidemiology?

- *Epidemic (outbreak)*: An $\uparrow$ in disease cases surpassing the anticipated levels during a specific timeframe within a defined population
- *Endemic*: The ongoing, typical or anticipated prevalence of disease within a specific population
- *Pandemic*: Encompasses epidemics that impact a substantial number of individuals across numerous countries, continents or regions

---

Fact 243:

Why is renal dysfunction common in **multiple myeloma**?

Kidney injury is common in multiple myeloma and typically has multiple causes, including dehydration, hypercalcaemia, and the deposition of Bence–Jones proteins, which can damage the renal tubules.

Fact 244:

What are examples of nebulisers used in **burn** patients?

- Bronchodilators like salbutamol relax bronchial muscle, $\uparrow$ mucociliary clearance, $\downarrow$ airflow resistance and $\uparrow$ dynamic compliance.
- Nebulised N-acetylcysteine and heparin, in conjunction with mechanical interventions like chest physiotherapy, airway suctioning and bronchoscopy, assist in airway clearance.

Fact 245:

Which **extinguishers** should not be used on electrical fires?

Water and foam extinguishers should not be used.

Fact 246:

What should the core temperature be for the diagnosis of **death** using neurological criteria?

>34°C

Fact 247:

Why may persistent hypotension occur immediately following removal of a **phaeochromocytoma**?

- ↓ Catecholamines as phaeochromocytoma has been removed.
- Hypovolaemia from blood loss.
- Residual α/β-blockade from treating hypertension prior to surgery.

Fact 248:

Which part of the **aorta** is most at risk from damage during blunt trauma?

Proximal descending aorta – at the site of the ligamentum arteriosum, distal to the origin of the left subclavian artery. The aorta is fixed to the chest wall here, whereas the mediastinum is relatively free to move. Rapid deceleration causes tears at this transition point.

Other mechanisms of traumatic aortic injury (TAI):

- *Water hammer*: Abdominal compression occludes the abdominal aorta, causing a huge ↑ in intra-aortic pressure and the possibility of an intimal tear.
- *Osseous pinch*: The aortic arch is crushed between the sternum and vertebral column.

Fact 249:

Why do **palmar erythema** and **spider naevi** develop in pregnancy?

↑ Oestrogen production

Fact 250:

What IV medications are viable options for managing haemodynamically stable **ventricular tachycardia**?

Flecainide
Lignocaine
Amiodarone
Propafenone

Fact 251:

Which metabolite of **codeine** is response for low GCS in someone with renal dysfunction?

Morphine-6 glucuronide

This is the active metabolite that undergoes renal excretion and can accumulate.

Fact 252:

What is the underlying pathophysiology of **limb compartment syndrome**?

↑ Pressure in fascia-bound compartment → compression of nerves and blood vessels → risk of limb-threatening necrosis especially at pressures > 30–40 mmHg

The forearm (volar compartment) and leg (anterior compartment) are more likely to develop compartment syndrome.

Causes include:

- Fractures
- *Coagulopathy*: Bleeding into compartments
- *Others*: Burns, seizures, crush injuries, prolonged or excessive exertion, long periods of immobilisation and extravasation of intravenous substances

Fact 253:

How does heparin cause **type 2 heparin-induced thrombocytopaenia (HIT)**?

Heparin binds to platelet factor 4 (PF4). The heparin–PF4 complex is immunogenic, leading to the production of HIT IgG antibodies. The heparin–PF4–IgG complex binds to platelets, causing platelet activation and subsequent removal by the reticuloendothelial system.

Fact 254:

What does the **α-angle** on a thromboelastogram measure?

The speed of solid clot formation (the rapidity of fibrinogen build-up and cross-linking)

Fact 255:

What are the three grades of **hypertension**?

Grade 1	SBP ≥ 140	OR	DBP ≥ 90
Grade 2	SBP ≥ 160	OR	DBP ≥ 100
Grade 3	SBP ≥ 180	OR	DBP ≥ 110

Fact 256:

What is **capnography** used for in critical care?

- To confirm tracheal tube placement
- To confirm the presence and effectiveness of ventilation, including the presence of bronchospasm
- To identify ↓ cardiac output states

Fact 257:

What are some coagulation abnormalities found in **disseminated intravascular coagulation**?

Increased	Decreased
APTT	Platelets
PT/INR	Protein C
Fibrinogen Degradation Products (FDPs)	Fibrinogen
D-Dimer	Antithrombin

Fact 258:

Which benzodiazepine would you use to treat alcohol withdrawal in someone with **severe liver dysfunction?**

Short/intermediate acting, e.g. lorazepam or oxazepam

This is because long-acting drugs, such as diazepam or chlordiazepoxide, tend to accumulate in individuals with liver disease. This occurs because of their dependence on demethylation/hydroxylation pathways, their prolonged half-lives (which can extend for days), and the presence of active metabolites.

The benzodiazepine equivalents for 5 mg diazepam are:

- Lorazepam: 1 mg
- Oxazepam: 15 mg
- Chlordiazepoxide: 25 mg

Fact 259:

What criteria must be met to thrombolyse someone with an **acute ischaemic stroke**?

- Within 4.5 hours of symptom onset (thrombolysis window)
- No acute intracranial haemorrhage on imaging
- BP < 185/110 (NICE guidelines)
- No contraindications to thrombolysis, e.g. high bleeding risk, significant hypo/hyperglycaemia, seizures at symptom onset, rapid symptom improvement, or severe pre-existing dependency.

Fact 260:

What is the suggested rate of **hypothermia** correction, and what are the latest guidelines for post-ROSC temperature management following a cardiac arrest?

- Correction rate of ≤0.5°C per hour to avoid localised temperature differences that can lead to cerebral hypoxia and impaired cerebrovascular reactivity.
- *Post-ROSC*: Aim for normothermia and actively prevent fever (temperature > 37.7°C). If a cooling device is being used to achieve this, aim for a target of 37.5°C (recommended particularly after the TTM2 2021 trial).

Fact 261:

What are the features of **gamma-hydroxybutyrate (GHB) toxicity**?

GHB, derived from GABA, initially induces euphoria, followed by swift CNS and respiratory depression, before rapid metabolism and recovery. Alcohol dehydrogenase mediates its metabolism, which is hindered by concurrent alcohol intoxication.

Some features of toxicity include:
↓ Temperature (hypothermia)
↓ HR (bradycardia)
↓ RR (bradyphrenia)
↓ GCS
Emesis

May require intubation to protect the airway and normalise gas exchange for a short period of time; the effects wear off after several hours.

Fact 262:

Why is **pre-oxygenation** in the sitting position particularly important in older people?

Preoxygenation is improved in the sitting position because as age increases, the closing capacity approaches or even exceeds the tidal volume. This can lead to small airway closure particularly when supine. Sitting up helps to reduce this effect, making pre-oxygenation more efficient by allowing better lung expansion and gas exchange.

Fact 263:

What is the most common organism implicated in **spontaneous bacterial peritonitis (SBP)**?

Escherichia coli

Patients with cirrhosis have ↑ intestinal permeability and ↓ immunological function which ↑ the risk of bacterial translocation and/or haematogenous spread.

A polymorphonuclear leukocyte (PMN) count > 250 cells/μL on ascitic fluid analysis is diagnostic.

Fact 264:

Why may **Wolf–Parkinson–White Syndrome** mimic a myocardial infarction on ECG?

Type A	Type B
Can mimic a posterior MI	Can mimic an inferior MI
Left sided accessory fibres	Right sided accessory fibres
Right axis deviation	Left axis deviation
Dominant R wave in V1	Non-dominant R wave in V1

Fact 265:

What is the pathophysiology of **Eisenmenger syndrome** and why are patients cyanotic?

Long-standing left-to-right shunts (e.g. due to VSDs, ASDs or PDAs) cause remodelling of the pulmonary vasculature:

Right	⬅	Left

Overtime, this leads to an ↑ pulmonary vascular resistance and shunt reversal. The new right-to-left shunt causes deoxygenated blood to enter the systemic circulation. This presents as central cyanosis:

Right	➡	Left

Fact 266:

What are some possible causes of artefact on an **EEG**?

- *Patient*: Shivering, tremors, ocular movement
- *Staff*: Suctioning, blood sampling, mouth care
- *Equipment*: Extracorporeal circuits (RRT, ECMO), infusion devices, ventilators, pressure-changing mattresses

Fact 267:

What method of **anaesthesia** is recommended for a C-section in someone with pre-eclampsia?

Neuraxial anaesthesia

Pre-eclampsia can make laryngoscopy difficult due to facial/tongue oedema. If GA is being considered, short-acting opiates like remifentanil, alfentanil or fentanyl can mitigate the pressor response during intubation. Failing to do so may result in ↑ BP, potentially leading to cerebral complications such as intracerebral bleeding.

Fact 268:

Why is doing an **awake fibreoptic intubation** risky in someone with impending upper airway obstruction?

↑ Risk of complete obstruction (the 'cork in bottle' effect)

Fact 269:

What is the ideal site of a **percutaneous tracheostomy**?

Between second and third tracheal rings

Fact 270:

What is the most likely diagnosis if someone develops a painful left-sided **ophthalmoplegia** with proptosis, chemosis and reduced visual acuity following a recent bout of sinusitis?

Cavernous sinus thrombosis – this is associated with palsies of cranial nerves 3, 4, 5 and 6.

The location of the cavernous sinuses and their extensive venous connections make them vulnerable to septic thrombi from infected sinuses, e.g. ethmoid or sphenoid sinuses. A CT-venogram may show enlargement or expansion of the cavernous sinuses with filling defects.

Fact 271:

What happens to **2,3-DPG** in stored blood?

↓ 2,3 DPG → ↑ affinity for oxygen
→ ↓ tissue O_2 delivery

Fact 272:

When do you give a PPI in **non-variceal GI bleeding** according to NICE?

Should not be offered pre-endoscopy. Give post-endoscopy if stigmata seen of recent haemorrhage.

Fact 273:

What is the pathophysiology of **ischaemic hepatitis** as a result of shock?

Shock → hypotension → ↓ hepatic perfusion → cellular hypoxia → centrilobular necrosis → acute transaminitis

Fact 274:

Why is routine carotid Doppler assessment not performed in those who have had a **posterior circulation stroke**?

The posterior circulation is usually supplied by the vertebrobasilar arterial system.

Fact 275:

What is the commonest cause of a massive **lower GI bleed**?

Diverticulosis
LGIB bleeding is bleeding distal to the ligament of Trietz.

Fact 276:

What are the standard indications for surgery in **infective endocarditis**?

Prosthetic valve infection
Embolisation – recurrent systemic embolisation
Large mobile vegetations
Valve dysfunction (severe)
Invasion beyond the valve leaflets
Sepsis that persists despite antibiotics
Severe heart failure

Fact 277:

What are some secondary causes of a **shortened QT interval** on an ECG?

- Hypercalcaemia, hyperkalaemia, hyperthermia
- Acidosis
- Digoxin
- Effect of catecholamines

Fact 278:

Which type of prosthetic valve is at a higher risk of developing a **thrombotic complication**: aortic or mitral?

Mitral valve > aortic valve

Fact 279:

When may you see a **high free T4** and **high TSH**?

- Pituitary TSH-secreting tumour
- Non-compliance with therapy in primary hypothyroidism (erratic dosing before clinic)

Fact 280:

Once brain-stem reflexes are confirmed to be absent, what are the fundamental principles of the **apnoea test** during brainstem death testing?

- Pre-oxygenation
- ↓ Minute ventilation to achieve:
  o $PaCO_2 \geq 6.0$ kPa (in patients with chronic CO_2 retention, aim for starting $PaCO_2 > 6.5$ kPa)
  o pH < 7.4
- Disconnect from the ventilator for 5 minutes while monitoring for respiratory effort (CPAP with oxygen insufflation can be given to prevent hypoxaemia).
- A positive test indicates an ↑ in $PaCO_2$ > 0.5 kPa from the initial value during apnoea.
- Ensure oxygenation and cardiovascular stability are maintained throughout the procedure.

Fact 281:

What are the NICE guidelines for systolic blood pressure management in an **acute haemorrhagic stroke (spontaneous intracerebral haemorrhage)**?

Target SBP 130–140 mmHg within 1 hour of starting treatment and maintain this blood pressure target for at least seven days.

Fact 282:

Why is it important to be cautious when replacing calcium in cases of **tumour lysis syndrome**?

Giving calcium in the presence of persistent hyperphosphataemia can exacerbate the production and deposition of calcium phosphate into tissues.

Fact 283:

What illuminates the distal camera of a single-use **bronchoscope**?

A light-emitting diode

Fact 284:

Which toxic metabolite in **methanol ingestion** is responsible for developing blindness?

Formic acid – causes retinal and optic nerve toxicity

Treatment is aimed at:

* Eliminating formate (alkaline diuresis or HD)
* Correcting acidosis with IV bicarbonate
* Preventing metabolism of methanol to formic acid by administering fomepizole (or IV ethanol)

Fact 285:

What is meant by 'dose' of **continuous haemofiltration**?

The volume of blood 'purified' per unit time. Clinically this is the effluent flow rate, e.g. 25–35 mL/kg/hr.

Fact 286:

What happens to the **dicrotic notch** of an arterial waveform in a vasodilated state?

Downwards shift

Fact 287:

What makes **ceftazidime** a useful empirical treatment for productive yellow sputum in someone with cystic fibrosis?

It adequately covers Pseudomonas (often colonised).

CF is an autosomal recessive condition (commonest gene ΔF508) where there is a defect in the Na^+/Cl^- transporter. This results in features such as recurrent LRTIs, malabsorption and infertility.

Fact 288:

Why may treatment with loop or thiazide diuretics increase the risk of **digoxin toxicity**?

They cause hypokalemia.

Digoxin competes with K^+ to bind to the Na^+/K^+-ATPase. In hypokalemia, digoxin will have less competitive inhibition from K^+ making toxicity more likely.

Fact 289:

What do you see on repetitive nerve stimulation in **botulism**?

Repetitive nerve stimulation shows incremental responses.

Fact 290:

Which classes of **antiarrhythmic drugs** in the Vaughan Williams classification should be avoided in someone with a prolonged QT?

Class I and Class 3 antiarrhythmic drugs

Fact 291:

What is the role of **reverse transcriptase (RT)** in HIV infection?

HIV uses RT to convert its RNA into viral DNA, a process called reverse transcription.

This DNA is then integrated into the host cell's genome.

Fact 292:

What may lumbar distraction fractures and anterior pelvic fractures suggest about **visceral damage** in trauma?

* *Lumbar distraction fractures*: Bowel injury
* *Anterior pelvic fractures*: Bladder/ urethral injuries

Fact 293:

What is the difference between **CRASH-1, -2 and -3**?

- CRASH-1: No benefit of giving methylprednisolone in TBI
- CRASH-2: Early administration of tranexamic acid (TXA) in trauma patients with, or at risk of, haemorrhage significantly ↓ mortality
- CRASH-3: TXA within 3 hours of TBI did not significantly affect mortality, but subgroup analysis showed ↓ mortality in patients with mild to moderate TBI (GCS 9–15).

Fact 294:

What is the gold-standard test for diagnosing an 18-year-old who presents with a two-week history of tonsillar hypertrophy, bilateral cervical lymphadenopathy, splenomegaly, low grade pyrexia, deranged liver function tests and Downey cells on blood film?

A mononuclear spot (heterophile antibody test)

This is infectious mononucleosis (glandular fever) caused by Epstein–Barr virus infection. The ↑ lymphocyte count in infectious mononucleosis results from ↑ circulating activated T cells, often referred to as Downey cells due to their atypical appearance in the peripheral blood. Supportive care is typically recommended, and individuals should avoid contact sports to ↓ the risk of splenic rupture.

Fact 295:

How do you generally classify **anticoagulants**?

Parenteral	**Direct thrombin inhibitor**	Argabatran Bivalirudin Hirudin
	Indirect thrombin inhibitor	Heparins: UFH, LMWH Fondaparinux Danaparoid
Oral	**Coumarin derivative**	Warfarin
	Direct factor Xa inhibitor	Rivaro**Xa**ban Api**Xa**ban Edo**Xa**ban
	Direct thrombin inhibitor	Dabigatran

Fact 296:

Which second messenger does **cholera toxin** stimulate?

cAMP

This leads to the activation of luminal sodium pumps and secretory diarrhoea.

Fact 297:

How can you rapidly induce **hypothermia** in a patient?

- Ice water bodily immersion
- Extracorporeal heat exchange
- Rapid infusion of cold intravenous fluid
- Central venous cooling catheter

Methods such as cold air blankets, bladder irrigation and gastric lavage are comparatively slower.

Fact 298:

What is the most likely diagnosis if someone exhibits symptoms of a **pseudobulbar palsy** and **internuclear ophthalmoplegia (INO)**, coupled with a slightly elevated CSF protein, normal CSF glucose and the presence of CSF oligoclonal bands?

Multiple sclerosis – a relapsing and remitting course is most common.

Oligoclonal bands in cerebrospinal fluid indicate ↑ IgG production by plasma cells and are found in approximately 85% of MS cases. However, they are not exclusive to MS and can also be associated with conditions such as SLE, neurosarcoidosis, CNS lymphoma and subacute sclerosing panencephalitis.

Fact 299:

What are the **anatomical landmarks** for needle decompression in a tension pneumothorax (PTX) and for pericardiocentesis?

- Needle decompression in tension PTX: Cannula in the second intercostal space in the mid-clavicular line.
- Pericardiocentesis: The point of needle insertion is immediately below and to the left of the xiphisternum, between the xiphisternum and the left costal margin.

Fact 300:

What is the most likely unifying diagnosis if someone presents with abdominal pain, lethargy, confusion and hypercalcaemia (4.5 mmol/L) with CT features of **necrotising pancreatitis**?

Primary hyperparathyroidism causing a hypercalcaemic crisis

Primary hyperparathyroidism is the most common cause of hypercalcaemia, and hypercalcaemia is a cause of acute pancreatitis.

Fact 301:

What does **jugular bulb oxygen saturation ($S_{jv}O_2$)** represent, and what are the typical ranges?

$S_{jv}O_2$ provides a global measure of brain oxygen consumption. The normal range is 55–75%. A fibre-optic catheter is placed in the jugular bulb on the ipsilateral side of an injury.

$S_{jv}O_2 < 55\%$	$S_{jv}O_2 > 75\%$
May indicate ischaemia because of either: • ↓ Oxygen delivery • ↑ Oxygen demand	May indicate hyperaemia or cell death because of either: • ↑ Oxygen delivery • ↓ Oxygen demand (dead brain tissue does not extract oxygen)

Fact 302:

Which valves are most commonly affected by **infective endocarditis (IE)**?

In decreasing order of frequency:

- Mitral valve
- Aortic valve
- Combined mitral and aortic valve
- Tricuspid valve
- Pulmonary valve – rare

Therefore, left-sided IE is more common than right-sided IE.

Fact 303:

What happens to **thyroid hormone synthesis** in pregnancy?

- Most T4 and T3 circulates bound to thyroxine-binding globulin (TBG). Only free thyroid hormones are physiologically active.
- During pregnancy, ↑ oestrogen inhibits hepatic breakdown of TBG → ↑ TBG levels.
- ↑ TBG → more bound T3/4 → ↓ free hormone → ↑ synthesis and secretion of thyroid hormones through negative feedback.

As a consequence, ↑ total T4/T3, but normal levels of free thyroid hormones (clinically euthyroid).

Fact 304:

In someone with who has had a burn, does a normal serum lactate exclude **significant cyanide toxicity**?

Yes

In cyanide toxicity, oxidative phosphorylation is inhibited.

A lactate > 10 mmol/L and a ↓ AV oxygen difference is strongly suggestive of significant toxicity.

Fact 305:

What is the most common type of **fire** in ICU, which extinguisher is best for it, and how should such fires be handled?

- *Most common fire*: Electrical fire
- *Fire extinguisher*: CO_2 extinguishers
- Managing a fire on ICU:

R	**R**escue	Remove patients and staff from immediate danger
A	**A**larm	Raise fire alarm
C	**C**ontain	Turn off oxygen outlets, close doors and windows
E	**E**xtinguish	Only attempt if fire is small, otherwise leave it alone and evacuate
R	**R**elocate	Horizontal, vertical or external evacuation

Fact 306:

What are some urinary abnormalities present in **drug-induced acute interstitial nephritis (DI-AIN)**?

Eosinophiluria, pyuria and white blood cell casts

DI-AIN accounts for 20% of unexplained AKI cases, commonly triggered by antibiotics, NSAIDs and PPIs. The classic symptoms of rash, fever and eosinophilia appear in fewer than 10% of patients shortly after starting the offending drug.

Fact 307:

Is the incidence of **refeeding syndrome** significantly different between enteral and parenteral feeding methods?

Nope

Fact 308:

How would you manage a patient with fever, confusion and **seizures**, featuring elevated CSF protein, normal CSF glucose and a high CSF lymphocyte count?

Aciclovir 10 mg/kg TDS for viral encephalitis – this is a nucleoside analogue which inhibits viral DNA replication.

Common causes of viral encephalitis include HSV types 1 and 2, varicella zoster and enteroviruses.

If bacterial meningitis is also suspected, add antibiotics and steroids:

- Ceftriaxone or cefotaxime 2 g QDS +/– ampicillin for suspected listeria
- Dexamethasone, particularly if pneumococcal meningitis is suspected

Fact 309:

What is the difference between **donor warm ischaemic time (DWIT), graft cold ischaemic time (CIT)** and **graft warm ischaemic time (WIT)** in the context of organ donation following cardiac death?

- *DWIT*: The period between life support withdrawal and starting cold organ preservation, which includes confirming cardiopulmonary arrest and a recommended 5-minute wait to prevent auto-resuscitation
- *CIT*: The time from beginning in vivo cold organ preservation to taking the graft out of 4°C storage
- *WIT*: The duration between removing the graft from cold storage and re-establishing graft perfusion

Fact 310:

What **glucose level** do you target in critically ill patients?

Glucose < 10 mmol/L (NICE-SUGAR protocol)

The risk of mortality increases with the severity and duration of dysglycaemia in a dose-dependent manner. However, tight glucose control is not advantageous and leads to a higher risk of complications due to hypoglycaemia.

Fact 311:

What is the expected discrepancy between the end-tidal carbon dioxide and arterial partial pressure of **carbon dioxide**, and what accounts for this difference?

- $ETCO_2$ is typically 0.5–1 kPa less than $PaCO_2$.
- The reason for this disparity is the influence of alveolar dead space ventilation on the exhaled gas composition.

An abrupt ↑ in dead space, e.g. PE, can widen this gap:

- Acute PE → ↓ pulmonary blood flow → ↑ dead space (lung ventilated but not perfused) → ↑ gap between $PaCO_2$ and $ETCO_2$

Fact 312:

Which agent would you choose to enhance systemic vascular tone in someone with **pulmonary hypertension**?

Vasopressin

In cases of pulmonary hypertension or right ventricular dysfunction, vasopressin selectively increases systemic vascular tone without elevating pulmonary vascular resistance and right ventricular afterload.

Fact 313:

What are some potential adverse effects of **colloids**?

Anaphylaxis, coagulopathy and acute kidney injury

Fact 314:

What are some indications for a **laparotomy** in trauma?

- Major injuries detected through bedside tests like direct peritoneal lavage or FAST scan
- Penetrating wounds that need exploration
- CT scans with contrast revealing visceral injuries like a ruptured bowel or bladder
- New onset of bleeding from orifices

Fact 315:

What are some possible options for cannulation to enable **VV-ECMO**?

Outflow cannula	Inflow cannula
Femoral vein	Internal jugular vein
Internal jugular vein	Femoral vein
Femoral vein	Femoral vein
Single (dual-lumen) cannula	

Fact 316:

What is **calcitonin** and how does it work?

Calcitonin is a polypeptide hormone secreted by the parafollicular cells of the thyroid gland:

- Inhibits calcium absorption by the intestine and renal tubules
- Inhibits osteoclastic activity
- Inhibits phosphate reabsorption by the renal tubules

Fact 317:

What is **Transfusion-Related Lung Injury (TRALI)**?

- A clinical syndrome which presents as acute hypoxia with non-cardiogenic pulmonary oedema within 6 hours of an allogeneic blood transfusion, often accompanied by hypotension and fever.
- It can occur with all blood products but does occur more frequently with products containing > 60 mL of plasma (e.g. FFP and platelets).
- TRALI is mediated by both immune and non-immune mechanisms. Immune mechanisms involve products which contain antibodies against human leukocyte antigens (HLAs) or human neutrophil antigens (HNAs).
- Treatment is supportive, including respiratory support for hypoxia.

Fact 318:

Which patient groups may benefit from a **tracheostomy tube** with an adjustable flange?

- Obese patients with a large neck
- Anatomical abnormalities, e.g. mediastinal masses or burns where the distance to the trachea is increased
- Low-lying tracheostomy stomas

The adjustable flange means that the tracheostomy tube can be adjusted to the desired length.

Fact 319:

What is the serum-ascites albumin gradient (SAAG) in **Budd–Chiari syndrome**?

SAAG >11 g/L

Budd–Chiari causes transudative ascites with a low protein content (<30 g/L). The typical triad is abdominal pain, hepatomegaly and ascites. It occurs due to thrombotic or non-thrombotic obstruction of hepatic venous flow. Doppler US has a good sensitivity and specificity, but the gold standard is hepatic venography.

Treatment options include:

- Treat ascites: Diuretics, Na^+ restriction, drainage
- Anticoagulation
- ↓ Venous pressure, e.g. portosystemic shunt

Fact 320:

What are the meanings of the terms **'false negative'** and **'false positive'** in a randomised controlled trial?

- *Type 2 or β-error (False negative)*: Incorrectly accepting the null hypothesis when a difference actually exists between the two groups.
- *Type 1 or α-error (False positive)*: Incorrectly rejecting the null hypothesis when no difference is present between the two groups.

(*Null hypothesis*: The two groups being studied are not different.)

Fact 321:

What are some complications of using **transvenous pacing wires** to manage bradycardia?

During insertion of wires	During use of wires
• Accidental arterial puncture • Bleeding • Pneumothorax • Air embolus • Arrhythmias	• Failure to pace/capture • Wire displacement • Venous thrombosis • Infection
Cardiac perforation and tamponade	

Fact 322:

What is the sequence for evacuating patients in the event of a **fire** in the intensive care unit?

- Begin with patients closest to the fire, provided it's safe to do so
- Then, prioritise moving the more stable patients before those who are less stable
- Finally, evacuate patients located in side rooms

Fact 323:

How might the risk of **refeeding syndrome** be reduced?

- Correcting K^+, PO_4^{3-}, Mg^{2+} prior to feeding
- Vitamin supplementation with IV thiamine
- Starting feeds at ≤ 50% of calculated requirements for 24–48 hours. Gradually ↑ to full requirements by day 7.
- Frequent monitoring and correction of electrolytes. If disturbances do occur, a ↓ rate may be required for longer to ensure time for adequate replacement.

Fact 324:

In which lobes of the brain are **abscesses** most frequently located?

Frontal and temporal lobes

Fact 325:

What are the two types of **mesenteric ischaemia** and what are the risk factors for developing them?

Arterial	Venous
Increased age (>70)	Previous VTE, e.g. PE/DVT
Atrial fibrillation	Portal hypertension
Cardiovascular disease, e.g. ischaemic heart disease, stroke	Pancreatitis or pancreatic cancer
Previous arterial emboli	Hypercoagulable states

Patients typically experience intense abdominal pain, disproportionate to examination findings. Other features include nausea, vomiting and bloody diarrhoea. Bloods may show ↑ WCC and fluid-resistant lactic acidosis. Preferred diagnostics are contrast CT or exploratory laparotomy. 'Damage-control surgery' is the treatment. In cases without peritonitis or perforation, options like embolectomy, local thrombolysis or stenting for mesenteric arterial occlusion may be considered.

Fact 326:

What the reference point for **ICP monitoring**?

Foramen of Munroe – external auditory meatus

Fact 327:

Why may a **pneumothorax** develop in someone with a Staphylococcus infection?

Staphylococcus may cause lung cavitation.

Fact 328:

How does **St. John's Wort** cause serotonin syndrome?

It is both a mild SSRI and cP450 enzyme inducer.

There is potential for the development of serotonin syndrome when other serotonergic drugs are given in combination, e.g. fentanyl or tramadol.

Fact 329:

What are the primary reasons for recommending **cardiac pacing**?

1. Bradycardia due to nodal dysfunction
2. Arrhythmia management, e.g. overdrive pacing
3. Cardiovascular optimisation, e.g. resynchronisation
4. Special cases, e.g. heart transplant

Fact 330:

Why do **midazolam** and **propofol** need dose adjustment in cirrhosis?

- Midazolam is metabolised by CTP3A4. Metabolism is flow-dependent. In cirrhosis, there is ↓ blood flow through the cirrhotic liver. It accumulates and should therefore be given in ↓ dose.
- Propofol is conjugated in the liver with glucuronides and sulphates before excretion in the urine. It therefore requires a ↓ dose in hepatic impairment.

Fact 331:

What is the effect of **adenosine** on the coronary arteries?

Coronary dilator and can cause coronary steal

Fact 332:

Why is a **Clark electrode** appropriate to measure the partial pressure of oxygen in an ABG sample?

Oxygen is paramagnetic and is attracted to an external magnetic field.

Fact 333:

How can **VV-ECMO** improve haemodynamic status?

- ↑ Venous return → ↑ cardiac output
- Rest ventilation → ↓ RV afterload → ↑ RV function

Fact 334:

What are the seven key diagnostic criteria for **syndrome of inappropriate antidiuretic hormone (SIADH)**?

(1) Hyponatraemia < 130mM, **(2)** low plasma osmolality < 275 mOsm, **(3)** high urine osmolality > 100 mOsm, **(4)** clinical euvolaemia and **(5)** continued natriuresis > 40 mM in the presence of **(6)** normal thyroid and adrenal function and **(7)** without recent use of diuretics.

Fact 335:

Apart from increasing the FiO_2 and considering recruitment manoeuvres, what should be the next step to optimise gas exchange in a sedated and paralysed person with **ARDS secondary to acute pancreatitis** who has an SpO_2 of 85% on FiO_2 0.85 with a plateau pressure of 29, PEEP 15, and I:E 1:1?

Prone positioning

Fact 336:

Which autoantibodies are associated with **myasthenia gravis,** and what are some of its clinical associations?

Autoantibodies	Clinical associations

• Post-synaptic nicotinic AChR (80%)
 • Post-synaptic muscle-specific kinase (MuSK) (10%)
 • Seronegative disease (10%)
	• Thymus pathology (75%)
	   o Hyperplasia (85%)
	   o Thymoma (15%)
	 • Other autoimmune diseases, e.g. hypothyroidism, SLE, rheumatoid arthritis

Fact 337:

How does a **venturi mask** provide a fixed FiO_2?

- *Bernoulli effect*: As oxygen flows through the constriction in the nozzle, the generation of sub-atmospheric pressure causes ambient air to be entrained.
- The degree of entrainment is controlled by the size of the nozzle aperture, the flow of oxygen and the size of vents through which air is entrained.
- This is independent of the minute ventilation.
- Through this process, a fixed FiO_2 is delivered (venturi masks are fixed-performance devices).

Fact 338:

What are some causes of a high and low **CSF protein**?

↓ CSF protein	↑ CSF protein
• Chronic CSF leak • Repeated lumbar punctures • Water intoxication	**S**eizures **I**nfection, e.g. meningitis, abscesses **G**uillain-Barré syndrome **H**aemorrhage **T**umours **E**levated serum protein, e.g. myeloma **D**emyelination, e.g. multiple sclerosis

↑ CSF protein is extremely non-specific. The normal range varies and is around 0.2–0.4 g/L.

Fact 339:

Which spinal tracts are predominantly affected in **anterior spinal artery (ASA) infarction**?

The ASA supplies the anterior ⅔ of the cord. Infarction affects:

- Corticospinal – paralysis below the level of the lesion
- Spinothalamic – loss of pain and temperature sensation at and below the level of the lesion

Proprioception and vibratory sensation are preserved, as these are on the dorsal side of the cord.

Fact 340:

Which coronary arteries are most commonly implicated in anterior, inferior, lateral and posterior **STEMI**?

Infarct	ECG changes	ECG leads	Most common artery involved
Anterior	ST elevation	V_1, V_2, V_3, V_4	Left anterior descending
Inferior	ST elevation	II, III, aVF	Right coronary artery
Lateral	ST elevation	I, aVL, V_5, V_6	Left circumflex
Posterior	ST depression, Tall R wave	V_1, V_2	Right coronary artery

Fact 341:

What are commonest **adverse events** in ICU?

- First: Line, drain and catheter dislodgement
- Second: Medication errors (administration/prescription)
- Third: Equipment failure

Fact 342:

Do steroids work in **Guillain–Barré syndrome (GBS)**?

No – treatment is with plasmapheresis or IVIg.

Fact 343:

How does **glucagon** work in managing refractory bradycardia and hypotension in a β-blocker overdose?

- Functions as an inotrope and chronotrope independent of β-receptors.
- It bypasses β-receptors through its action on cardiac glucagon receptors.
- These receptors are coupled to Gs proteins which ↑ cAMP.

Fact 344:

Which A-line waveform characteristic provides the most information about myocardial **contractility**?

The slope of the upstroke represented by Δpressure/Δtime

Fact 345:

Which measure on a resting transthoracic echocardiogram correlates with **systolic pulmonary artery pressure**?

Peak tricuspid regurgitation velocity

Fact 346:

When would you use a **'scoop & run' technique** for inter-hospital transfer?

When the pressing nature of the situation and the immediate need for definitive care restrict the time available for stabilisation prior to transfer. This is generally considered an uncommon event.

Fact 347:

What is the relationship between changes in the heart rate and the **QT interval**?

Inverse relationship

Fact 348:

Who can legally perform **brainstem testing** in an adult?

- Two qualified doctors (at least one of them is a consultant)
- Each should have ≥ 5 years of full registration.
- Each should be competent in conducting and interpretating results.

Fact 349:

What are some general effects of **morbid obesity** on the respiratory system?

Work of breathing	↑	Expiratory reserve volume	↓
FEV_1/FVC ratio			
Airway resistance		• Vital capacity • Total lung capacity • Functional residual capacity	
O_2 consumption and CO_2 production (↑ metabolically active tissues)			
Pulmonary artery pressure		Respiratory compliance (↑ chest/abdominal wall mass)	
CO_2 retention			

Fact 350:

Is it safe to use **propofol** for induction in someone with a confirmed egg protein allergy?

Yes

Propofol contains purified egg phosphatide, also known as lecithin, which is not recognised as an allergen. Those allergic to eggs typically react to specific egg proteins like ovoalbumin, ovomucoid and conalbumin.

Fact 351:

What do the labels A, B, C and D on the CVP waveform represent?

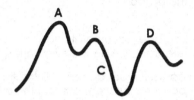

A	A-wave	Atrial contraction
B	C-wave	Doming of tricuspid valve into right atrium
C	X-decent	Atrial relaxation
D	V-wave	Atrial filling before tricuspid valve opening

Fact 352:

What is the role of the **ROSIER** and **NIHSS** scores in an acute stroke?

- *ROSIER*: Enables medical staff to differentiate between patients with stroke and stroke mimics (sensitivity of 93%)
- *NIHSS*: Quantifies the impairment caused by a stroke. Eleven items are scored, and total scores range from 0 (no stroke) to 42 (severe stroke).

Fact 353:

What is the reversal agent for **rocuronium** and **vecuronium**?

Sugammadex – a gamma cyclodextrin that encapsulates the NBMA. Rocuronium is an aminosteroid developed from vecuronium.

Fact 354:

What is the most likely diagnosis if someone with hypocalaemia, tetany and a prolonged QT interval develops features of **stridor**?

↓ Calcium → ↑ laryngeal muscle contraction → laryngospasm

Fact 355:

What are some causes of **unilateral hilar opacification** on a CXR?

- **S**arcoidosis
- **I**nfection, e.g. tuberculosis, fungal, viral
- **M**alignancy, e.g. lymphoma, bronchial carcinoma, metastases

Fact 356:

What is the difference between **'primary'** and **'secondary' outcomes** of a trial?

- The primary outcome is the difference or change that the trial is designed to look for.
- Other differences between the groups may also be found. These are secondary outcomes.

Fact 357:

Why are the following ventilatory settings appropriate in someone who has just been intubated with a large ETT for **life-threatening asthma**: VT = 400 mL, RR =10, I:E = 1:4?

To avoid dynamic hyperinflation and barotrauma

- A large ETT ↑ gas flow (flow is proportional to r^4) and ↓ risk of tube occlusion by thick secretions
- Controlled hypoventilation and respiratory acidosis minimise hyperinflation and barotrauma.
- Prolonged expiratory time allows for more complete expiration to ↓ gas trapping.
- PEEP use is debated; initially, it may worsen hyperinflation. Some recommend setting external PEEP at no more than 80% of measured intrinsic PEEP.

Fact 358:

What error may arise in estimating **cardiac output** via a pulmonary artery catheter in cases of atrial fibrillation or tricuspid regurgitation?

Cardiac output is underestimated.

Fact 359:

Why might distended neck veins be absent in cases of **cardiac tamponade** following trauma?

Concurrent hypovolemia may exist, for example due to bleeding from other sites.

Fact 360:

How does **Ringer's lactate** (RL) compare to normal saline (NS) in the management of acute pancreatitis (AP)?

- RL *may* be associated with ↓ SIRS compared to NS, but evidence varies.
- RL *may* ↓ the need for ICU admission in adults with mild AP and shorten the length of hospitalisation in adults and children with AP.
- Resuscitation with RL *seems* to ↓ the development of moderately severe or severe pancreatitis.

Fact 361:

Which pathologies cause **ICU associated weakness (ICUAW)**?

- Critical illness polyneuropathy
- Critical illness myopathy
- Critical illness neuromyopathy

ICUAW is defined as weakness in which the cause can be attributed solely to critical illness. It manifests as symmetric, widespread weakness affecting the lower motor neurons in the limbs and respiratory muscles, while sparing the facial, ocular and cranial nerves.

Fact 362:

How do you insert an **intra-aortic balloon pump (IABP),** and where should the distal end of the balloon lie?

- Retrograde via femoral artery
- Anterogradely via subclavian artery

In both cases, it is advanced until the tip of the balloon is about 2 cm distal to the origin of the left subclavian artery.

The distal end of the balloon must lie above the renal arteries (to avoid compromised renal flow).

Fact 363:

According to KDIGO criteria, which stage of **acute kidney injury (AKI)** is present if a 63 kg female excretes 150 mL of urine in 6 hours and her creatinine level has increased from a baseline of 84 µmol/L to 148 µmol/L?

Stage 1

KDIGO criteria for AKI		
Stage	**Serum creatinine**	**Urine output**
STAGE 1	1.5–1.9 times baseline OR ≥ 26.5 µmol/L increase	<0.5 mL/kg/hr for 6–12 hours
STAGE 2	2.0–2.9 times baseline	<0.5 mL/kg/hr for ≥ 12 hours
STAGE 3	3.0 times baseline OR ≥ 353.6 µmol/L OR Commencement of renal replacement therapy OR eGFR < 35 (in patients <18 years)	<0.3 mL/kg/hr for ≥ 24 hours OR Anuria for ≥ 12 hours

---

Fact 364:

What is the most sensitive indicator of impending acute hepatic failure in **paracetamol toxicity**?

Prothrombin time

Fact 365:

According to Brain Trauma Foundation (BTF), what should be the target SBP and CPP after **traumatic brain injury**?

Age	5–49 years	50–69 years	>69 years
SBP target	≥110	≥100	≥110
CPP target	60–70 mmHg		

Fact 366:

Which life-threatening chest injuries should be identified on **primary survey**?

- Tension or open pneumothorax
- Flail chest with pulmonary contusion
- Massive haemothorax
- Cardiac tamponade

Fact 367:

How should the measured **calcium concentration** be corrected for changes in the concentration of albumin?

$$\text{Corrected calcium} = \text{Measured calcium} + 0.02 \times (40 - [\text{albumin}] \, (g/L))$$

Fact 368:

How do you eliminate a significant **air leak** in a one-year-old who was intubated with a sized 4.0 uncuffed ETT?

Reintubate – with either a larger uncuffed tube or with the same-sized cuffed tube

Uncuffed tubes are used to ↓ risk of subglottic oedema.

Fact 369:

Why is **atropine** unlikely to work in managing complete heart block following an anterior myocardial infarction?

In an anterior MI, the occlusion occurs in a branch of the left anterior descending artery which affects the infranodal conducting system. Therefore, removing the vagal tone on the SA and AV nodes with atropine is unlikely to resolve bradycardia related to complete heart block.

Fact 370:

What significant complication may the administration of **rectal NSAIDs** prevent in someone having an ERCP?

Post-ERCP pancreatitis

Fact 371:

What are some features of a **mitral valve** area of <1 cm²?

A mitral valve area of <1 cm² is considered severe mitral stenosis.

Features include:

- Loud S1, opening snap and a mid-diastolic rumbling murmur
- ↑ LA pressure → ↑ valve gradient → development of atrial fibrillation, ↑ risk of systemic thromboembolism
- Pulmonary venous congestion → ↓ lung compliance, haemoptysis and dyspnoea
- ↑ Pulmonary pressures → pulmonary hypertension → ↑ RV dilatation and tricuspid regurgitation (which may then develop into RVH and right heart failure)
- ECG: atrial fibrillation and P-mitrale
- CXR: pulmonary vascular congestion and LA enlargement

Fact 372:

How do you define **drowning**?

Drowning occurs when submersion or immersion in a liquid medium leads to primary respiratory impairment:

- *Immersion*: Water splashes over the face
- *Submersion*: Airway goes below the surface

Fact 373:

How do you treat **severe symptomatic Na⁺ 120 mmol/L** of indeterminate onset?

- Give 150 mL of 3% hypertonic NaCl IV over 20 minutes.
- Then check Na⁺ level.
- Continue giving 3% hypertonic saline in 150 mL aliquots with the goal of increasing Na⁺ by 5 mmol/L to improve symptoms and limit further brain injury.
- Once the target is reached, transition to a slow IV infusion of 0.9% NaCl.
- Treat the underlying cause.
- Check Na⁺ levels at 6, 12, 24, 48 hours.
- Ensure that Na⁺ changes are restricted to a maximum of 10 mmol/L in the initial 24 hours and 8 mmol/L in each subsequent 24 hours to reduce the risk of osmotic demyelination syndrome.

Fact 374:

Why would **milirinone** be appropriate to start in a post-CABG patient who is oliguric, has a lactate of 6.5 mmol/L, has no evidence of tamponade on echocardiography and has the following cardiac output studies: HR = 115 bpm, BP = 131/78 mmHg, CVP = 19 mmHg, CI = 1.9 L/min/m², PAWP = 24 mmHg, and SVRI = 2,800 dynes/s/cm⁵/m²?

This is cardiogenic shock with signs of end-organ hypoperfusion. Starting an inodilator is appropriate.

Milirinone is a PDE3 inhibitor in cardiac myocytes and in vascular smooth muscle:

- ↑ Inotropy and ↑ lusitropy → ↑ cardiac output
- ↓ SVR (vasodilatation) → ↓ afterload
- ↓ Venous capacitance → ↓ preload

Fact 375:

If someone is unable to receive enteral metronidazole for *Clostridium difficile* due to high NG aspirates, which option would you switch to: IV metronidazole or IV vancomycin?

IV metronidazole

IV vancomycin is ineffective as it does not penetrate the large bowel in sufficient doses.

Fact 376:

What are the disadvantages of **veno-arterial (VA) ECMO** when compared to veno-venous (VV) ECMO?

- Risks of arterial cannulation, e.g. injury, dissection, pseudoaneurysm, bleeding
- Risk of arterial embolisation
- Potential for impaired pulmonary, coronary and cerebral perfusion
- ↑ Left ventricular afterload

Fact 377:

When do you get hypotension and bradycardia in a **spinal cord injury**?

- Bradycardia with lesions above T1
- Hypotension with lesions above T6

Fact 378:

What primary outcome distinctions emerged from the **EPaNIC trial (2011)** when comparing early (day 3) to late (day 8) parenteral nutrition in critically ill adults?

Patients given late PN had a ↓ ICU LOS, ↑ incidence of hypoglycaemia, ↑ likelihood of ICU discharge within eight days and no difference in hospital or 90-day mortality.

Fact 379:

How does the triad of clinical features differ between **Miller Fisher syndrome** and **Wernicke encephalopathy**?

Miller Fisher syndrome	Wernicke encephalopathy
A varient of Guillain–Barré often associated with anti-GQ1b antibodies	CNS lesions following the exhaustion of vitamin B reserves (especially thiamine, Vitamin B1)
Ophthalmoplegia Ataxia	
Areflexia	Confusion

Fact 380:

What is meant by the term **'study power'** and what factors determine its value?

- The study power is a measure of its ability to find a statistically significant difference. This is the probability of rejecting the null hypothesis when it is false.
- It is calculated during the planning phase. It depends on the actual difference between the groups, the level at which a difference is considered 'significant' (the p-value) and the number of subjects in the study.

Fact 381:

How do the electrophysiological findings differ between **critical illness polyneuropathy (CIP)** and **critical illness myopathy** (CIM)?

		CIP	CIM
Similarities	CMAP (compound muscle action potential) amplitude	↓	
	Nerve conduction velocity	Normal	
	Repetitive nerve stimulation	Absence of decremental response	
	EMG at rest	Spontaneous fibrillation potentials	
Differences	CMAP duration	Normal	↑
	SNAP (sensory nerve action potential) amplitude	↓	Normal
	Motor unit potential voluntary muscle activation	Long duration, high amplitude	Short duration, low amplitude
	Direct muscle stimulation	Normal excitability	↓ Excitability

---

Fact 382:

What are some examples of pancreatic and peripancreatic collections that can occur in **acute pancreatitis**?

Homogenous		Heterogenous	
Acute peripancreatic fluid collection	**Pancreatic pseudocyst**	**Acute necrotic collection**	**Walled-off necrosis**
Confined by normal tissue planes\n\nUsually resolves spontaneously	Encapsulated\n\nOccurs > 4 weeks after the onset of symptoms	Occurs in the presence of necrosis\n\nAbsent wall	Intrapancreatic and/or extrapancreatic\n\nOccurs > 4 weeks after the onset of symptoms

Fact 383:

In critical care, what are some scenarios that might necessitate the use of a **double-lumen tube (DLT)**?

- **L**avage of one lung
- **I**solation of one lung to protect it from contamination, soiling or high pressures
- **M**assive pulmonary haemorrhage
- **B**ronchopleural fistula

Fact 384:

What are some pre-hepatic causes of **jaundice**?

Increased bilirubin production	Impaired conjugation	Impaired liver bilirubin uptake	Physiological neonatal jaundice
Haemolysis (hereditary and acquired) Haematoma resorption	Crigler–Najjar syndrome	Gilbert syndrome	A mixture of increased bilirubin production and immature glucuronyl transferase enzymes

Pre-hepatic jaundice causes ↑ unconjugated bilirubin.

Fact 385:

What variables would you need to prescribe when commencing **renal replacement therapy**?

- RRT dose (effluent rate), e.g. 25–35 mL/kg/hr
- Rate at which blood is drawn from the patient, e.g. 200–300 mL/min
- Fluid balance target, e.g. negative 1 L or neutral balance in 24 hours
- Anticoagulation prescription, e.g. citrate, unfractionated heparin, argatroban

Fact 386:

What abnormal features might a transthoracic echocardiogram show that would support a diagnosis of a **pulmonary embolism**?

- ↑ Pulmonary artery pressures
- RV dilation +/– failure
- McConnell's sign: RV dysfunction with akinesia of the mid-free wall but normal motion at the apex
- Direct visualisation of the thrombus in the PA

Fact 387:

How do you calculate the **oxygen index (OI)**?

$$OI = (FiO_2 \times 100 \times mean\ airway\ pressure) / PaO_2$$

Fact 388:

What pharmacological therapy would you use to manage an **ischaemic stroke** after thrombolysis?

- Aspirin 300 mg for two weeks
- After two weeks, this is changed to clopidogrel or to an anticoagulant if found to be in atrial fibrillation

Fact 389:

Why is the APTT prolonged in the hypercoagulable state of **antiphospholipid syndrome**?

- Antiphospholipid antibodies, notably lupus anticoagulant, inhibit phospholipid-dependent processes within the intrinsic clotting pathway.
- This causes a paradoxical ↑ in the APTT

Fact 390:

What is the **Critical Care Pain Observational Tool**?

A validated and reproducible tool for assessing pain in ICU on an 8-point scale. It assesses pain in both intubated or sedated patients, considering facial expressions, muscle tension, movements, and compliance with ventilated breaths for intubated individuals, or vocalised pain for non-intubated patients.

Fact 391:

In normal physiology, when someone has **hypovolemic hypernatremia**, what should the urine osmolality be?

Much higher than the serum osmolality, often exceeding 800 mOsm/kg H_2O. This indicates that the kidneys are effectively concentrating urine to conserve water.

Fact 392:

How do you treat an **oculogyric crisis** in someone who takes a typical neuroleptic?

Procyclidine or benztropine

An acute dystonic reaction may manifest with conventional neuroleptics like haloperidol or chlorpromazine, though it is less frequent when using newer neuroleptics such as olanzapine or clozapine.

Fact 393:

Which condition, known for causing **proximal muscle weakness**, autonomic dysfunction and the absence of deep tendon reflexes, shows an improvement in muscle weakness when repetitive movements are performed?

Lambert–Eaton myasthenic syndrome

This is typically a paraneoplastic phenomenon associated with small cell lung cancer. There are presynaptic autoantibodies to voltage-gated calcium channels at the neuro-muscular junction.

Fact 394:

According to the Brain Trauma Foundation (BTF) guidelines, which patients with **traumatic brain injury** should receive ICP monitoring?

* Any moderate-to-severe TBI (GCS < 12) who cannot be serially neurologically assessed, e.g. if sedated
* Any severe TBI (GCS < 8) with an abnormal CT head scan
* Any severe TBI (GCS < 8) with a normal CT head scan if two of the following are present:
  o   Age > 40 years
  o   SBP < 90
  o   Abnormal motor posturing

Fact 395:

What does a **Recognition of Stroke in the Emergency Room (ROSIER) score** > 0 and ≤ 0 suggest?

The ROSIER score distinguishes between acute stroke and stroke mimics:

ROSIER score	Interpretation
>0	Stroke possible
≤0	Stroke unlikely

Fact 396:

Which feeding options can be considered in someone with high nasogastric tube aspirates following a **Hartmann's procedure**?

* Naso-jejunal feeding
* Intravenous/parenteral nutrition

Fact 397:

Can **acute renal failure** be diagnosed on urine output alone?

Yes – according to both the RIFLE and KDIGO criteria

Fact 398:

What statistical test is employed to estimate the **survival function** from lifetime data?

Kaplan–Meier estimator

This non-parametric statistic is employed to quantify the proportion of patients surviving for a specific duration, such as after receiving treatment or post-diagnosis.

Fact 399:

What is the difference between acute and chronic **hyponatraemia**?

Acute is a fall in <48 hours and chronic is a fall >48 hours

Fact 400:

Why is **hand-washing** superior to alcohol-based rub?

Alcohol-based rub is not effective against all micro-organisms, e.g. viruses (such as norovirus) and spore-forming micro-organisms (such as *Clostridium difficile*)

Fact 401:

Why would someone develop breathlessness, flushing and tachycardia 15 minutes after starting **N-acetylcysteine (NAC)** for a paracetamol overdose?

Anaphylactoid reaction to NAC

Substantial evidence suggests that NAC infusions can induce histamine release, primarily associated with the infusion rate.

Fact 402:

What is first-line treatment for **extended-spectrum β-lactamase-producing Enterobacteriaceae (ESBLs)** infections?

Carbapenems – have good in vitro and in vivo effect against ESBL producers

Fact 403:

What is the '**sniffing the morning air**' position?

Lower C-spine flexion + atlanto-occipital extension

Fact 404:

In cardiopulmonary testing, which **anaerobic threshold** is associated with significantly poorer outcomes?

Anaerobic threshold <11 mL/kg/min

This marks the juncture at which anaerobic glycolysis starts to complement aerobic metabolism, reflecting a patient's capacity to manage the additional metabolic requirements associated with surgery.

Fact 405:

Why does the **actual base excess** differ from **standard base excess**?

Base excess is the amount of strong acid required to return pH of 1 L of blood to 7.40 at a $PaCO_2$ 5.3 kPa and temperature 37°C.

Two types of base excess can be distinguished:

- Actual base excess is that present in the blood (intravascular component only)
- Standard base excess is the base excess corrected to an Hb 50 g/L. This adjustment provides a more accurate reflection of the overall acid–base balance in the body. Hb acts as a buffer in the blood but not in the interstitial space, so measuring BE at the patient's Hb (assuming >50 g/L) tends to overestimate the degree of buffering. Standard base excess is defined in terms of 1 L of extracellular fluid.

Fact 406:

What are the characteristic ECG changes in acute **pericarditis**?

- ST elevation and PR depression in most leads
- Reciprocal ST depression and PR elevation in aVR and V_1

Fact 407:

Why should **suxamethonium** be avoided from 24 hours up to one year following a significant burn injury?

- There is proliferation of extra-junctional Ach receptors
- There is an ↑ risk of significant hyperkalaemia if suxamethonium is used during this period

Fact 408:

What are some management principles in **serotonin syndrome**?

- Stop serotonergic agents and interacting drugs, e.g. SSRIs, MAOi, pethidine, fentanyl, tramadol
- Treatment is supportive in mild cases.
- Use benzodiazepines for hypertension, agitation and tachycardia.
- Consider serotonin antagonists, e.g. cyproheptadine, olanzapine or chlorpromazine with specialist input.
- Lipid emulsion has been used as a 'lipid sink' for lipophilic drugs, but its efficacy in serotonin syndrome is not well-estimated
- Severe hyperthermia and/or rigidity requires anaesthesia, intubation and paralysis.

Fact 409:

How would you treat someone for *Pneumocystis jirovecii* **pneumonia (PJP)** with a PaO_2 of 7.3 kPa if they are intolerant to co-trimoxazole?

- *Second-line treatment for PJP:* Clindamycin + primaquine
- *Prednisolone:* Corticosteroids ↓ mortality and lung damage if PaO_2 < 9.3 kPa on air

Other second-line agents include dapsone or pentamidine.

Fact 410:

What is **Hy's law** in drug-induced liver injury (DILI)?

In patients with DILI, the presence of hepatocellular injury (↑ ALT/AST > 3 × ULN) and jaundice (↑ bilirubin > 2 × ULN) confers an ↑ mortality rate.

Fact 411:

Which groups are at risk for complicated disease with **influenza H1N1**?

- Chronic disease
- Immunosuppressed, including pregnancy
- Age > 65 years
- BMI ≥ 40 kg/m²

Fact 412:

In the absence of metabolic acidosis, when would you consider giving **hypertonic 8.4% sodium bicarbonate** in a tricyclic antidepressant overdose to target pH 7.50–7.55?

- Arrhythmias
- Seizures
- QRS > 100 ms → ↑ risk of seizures
- QTc > 430 ms → ↑ risk of arrhythmias (VT/VF)
- Hypotension not due to hypovolaemia

Fact 413:

When should you consider invasive ventilation in **myasthenia gravis** using the '20/30' rule?

- VC < 20 mL/kg
- Negative inspiratory force < 30 cmH$_2$O

Fact 414:

At approximately which temperature is the **shivering reflex** obtunded?

The shivering reflex is obtunded at <33.5°C

Fact 415:

What body temperature changes can occur with a **blood transfusion**?

- *Hypothermia*: Red cells are stored at 4°C
- *Hyperthermia*: Transfusion reactions, allergic reactions, TRALI or transfusion-related infection (e.g. Gram-negative bacteria like *Pseudomonas proliferate* at 4°C)

Fact 416:

What did the **TOMAHAWK study (2021)** show regarding the use of immediate versus delayed angiography in patients without ST-segment elevation who have had an out-of-hospital cardiac arrest?

No difference in 30-day mortality between the use of immediate versus delayed/selective angiography in patients without ST-segment elevation

Fact 417:

Which haematological abnormalities may arise with **hypophosphataemia**?

Haemolytic anaemia, leukocyte dysfunction and platelet dysfunction

Fact 418:

What IV **aminophylline** dosage is appropriate for severe, life-threatening asthma in a patient who hasn't been taking oral theophylline and hasn't responded well to initial treatment?

- 5 mg/kg loading over 20 minutes
- Followed by an infusion of 0.5 mg/kg/hr

Fact 419:

Why can giving aspirin to someone presenting with **thyroid storm** make the clinical picture even worse?

Thyroid storm occurs when the thyroid gland releases too many thyroid hormones. This results in a hypermetabolic state, e.g. hyperpyrexia and tachyarrhythmias.

Most T3 and T4 are bound to plasma proteins. When bound to these proteins, they are inactive. Only unbound (free) T3 and T4 are active. Aspirin competes for binding sites on these plasma proteins.

If aspirin is given to someone with thyroid storm, it will displace T3/T4 from these plasma proteins. This means that there will be more circulating free T3/T4. More free T3/T4 will worsen the hypermetabolic state.

Fact 420:

How do you classify microalbuminuria and macroalbuminuria in **diabetic nephropathy**?

	Spot collection (µg/mg creatinine)	24-hour collection (mg/24 hours)
Normal	<30	
Microalbuminuria	30–300	
Macroalbuminuria	>300	

Fact 421:

What are the distinctions between the application of the Wallace Rule of Nines for assessing the extent of **skin burns** in adults and children?

	Adult (%)	Child (%)
Head	9	18
Anterior torso	18	
Back	18	
Right arm	9	
Left arm	9	
Right leg	18	13.5
Left leg	18	13.5
Perineum	1	

Fact 422:

What are some pharmacological therapies that reduce the risk of hospitalisation/death in **heart failure with reduced ejection fraction (HFrEF)**?

SGLT-2 inhibitors, e.g. dapagliflozin, empagliflozin
ACE-inhibitors/Angiotensin Receptor Blockers
Mineralocorticoid antagonists, e.g. eplerenone, spironolactone
Beta blockers, e.g. bisoprolol
Angiotensin receptor–neprilysin inhibitors (ARNIs), e.g. sacubitril/valsartan

Fact 423:

What are some causes of **hypervolaemic hyponatraemia**?

Urinary sodium > 20 mEq/L	Urinary sodium < 20 mEq/L
Renal failure	**Other failures**
Acute kidney injury Chronic kidney disease	Nephrotic syndrome Cirrhosis Heart failure

Fact 424:

Which structure will a thrombus go through first if it is currently in the **left gonadal vein**?

Left renal vein–the left gonadal vein drains into the left renal vein

However, if the thrombus was in the right gonadal vein, the thrombus would make its way to the IVC because the right gonadal vein drains directly into the IVC.

Fact 425:

Which diagnosis is most likely it someone has **flash pulmonary oedema**, refractory hypertension, a raised creatinine after starting an ACE inhibitor and a discrepancy in kidney size on ultrasound?

Renal artery stenosis

Fact 426:

Why are children more susceptible to developing **propofol infusion syndrome (PRIS)**?

Children have relatively ↓ glycogen storage and ↑ dependence on fat metabolism

Fact 427:

Which **clotting factors** are implicated in the extrinsic pathway, intrinsic pathway and the common pathway, and which are vitamin K dependent?

Intrinsic pathway	↑ APTT	Factors 8, 9,11,12
Extrinsic pathway	↑ PT	Factor 7
Common pathway	↑ APTT and ↑ PT	Factors 2, 5, 10
Vitamin K dependent	Factors 2, 7, 9, 10	

Fact 428:

What are some endocrine features of **myotonic dystrophy**?

- Male hypogonadism and female reproductive dysfunction
- Insulin resistance → ↑ risk of diabetes
- ↑ PTH levels, ↑ risk for vitamin D deficiency
- Benign and malignant thyroid nodules

It is inherited in an autosomal dominant pattern

Fact 429:

What are the four elements of the **Murray Lung Injury score** when referring someone for VV-ECMO in ARDS?

- CXR quadrants involved
- Compliance
- PEEP
- P/F ratio

Each element is graded on a scale from 0 to 4, where 4 represents the most severe dysfunction. The sum of these scores is then divided by 4 to yield a final score.

Inclusion criteria for VV-ECMO include:

- Severe respiratory failure that may be reversible
- Murray Lung Injury Score ≥ 3
- Uncompensated hypercapnia with a pH ≤ 7.20 on optimal management including prone positioning and LPV

Fact 430:

What are the '**adverse signs**' in an arrythmia?

- *Shock*: SBP < 90 mmHg
- *Syncope*: Transient loss of consciousness due to ↓ global blood flow
- *Myocardial ischaemia*: Ischaemic chest pain or ECG changes
- *Heart failure*: Pulmonary oedema +/− ↑ JVP

Fact 431:

Which two cardiac valves are commonly affected in **carcinoid syndrome**?

Carcinoid usually causes right heart valve diseases:

- Tricuspid valve (usually tricuspid regurgitation)
- Pulmonary valve (usually pulmonary stenosis)

Carcinoid tumours are neuroendocrine tumours which paroxysmally release hormones, such as serotonin, which may result in flushing, diarrhoea, abdominal cramping, peripheral oedema and wheeze. Surgery can cure isolated lesions, but there's no effective cure for metastatic cases. Somatostatin analogues, such as octreotide, can ↓ hormone secretion in these cases.

Fact 432:

What type of **visual field defect** do you get with lesions of the optic chiasm, optic radiation and optic nerve?

- *Optic chiasm*: Bitemporal hemianopia
- *Optic radiation*: Homonymous hemianopia
- *Optic nerve*:
  - o Partial retinal or optic nerve damage: Scotoma
  - o Complete optic nerve injury: Monocular visual loss

Fact 433:

When would you consider giving prednisolone in the management of **alcoholic hepatitis**?

Prednisolone is considered if Maddrey's discriminant function ≥ 32 (indicates severe hepatitis)

A typical course would involve prednisolone 40 mg for at least seven days to continue for one month. Some patients will not respond. These patients can be identified using the Lille Model after having had seven days of steroids.

The use of prednisolone is a subject of debate especially because the STOPAH trial (2015) revealed a mortality benefit that did not reach statistical significance.

Fact 434:

What is the reason for the potential inaccuracy of a **TEG** in evaluating platelet function in an individual taking antiplatelet medications?

It may not detect the impact of pharmacological inhibition

Fact 435:

How does **indapamide** work in treating hypertension?

- *Kidney*: It inhibits sodium and chloride reabsorption from the distal convoluted tubule by blocking the sodium/chloride co-transporter (symporter).
- *Vascular smooth muscle*: ↓ inward calcium currents and ↓ vascular reactivity to vasoactive substances such as noradrenaline and angiotension II. This promotes vasodilatation.

This diuretic is thiazide-like because it doesn't contain the benzothiadiazine heterocycle found in typical thiazide drugs, but it does have a sulphonamide component.

Fact 436:

What is meant by **pseudohypoxaemia (leukocyte larceny)** in leukaemic patients with extremely high white blood counts?

Spuriously ↓ PaO_2 in someone with ↑ WCC

White blood cells metabolise plasma oxygen in ABG samples producing a spuriously low oxygen tension.

Fact 437:

What are the mechanisms by which **SVR** is reduced?

- Direct ↓ in smooth muscle tone
- ↓ in α-1 activity
- ↑ in α-2 activity which ↓ noradrenaline release

Fact 438:

What are the effects of **ACE inhibitors** in pregnancy?

During the second and third trimesters, they have been associated with serious malformations, e.g. oligohydramnios, foetal and neonatal renal failure, bony malformations, limb contractures, pulmonary hypoplasia, prolonged hypotension and neonatal death.

Fact 439:

What is the effect of **propofol** on the GABA-A receptor?

↑ GABA-mediated inhibitory tone in the CNS

Propofol reduces the rate at which GABA dissociates from its receptor. This prolongs the opening of chloride channels, leading to ↑ membrane hyperpolarisation.

Fact 440:

What do you see on a blood film in **disseminated intravascular coagulation (DIC)**?

Schistocytes (fragmented red cells)

DIC results from inappropriate thrombin activation, resulting in fibrin formation, platelet/endothelial activation and fibrinolysis. It presents with bleeding, thrombosis or purpura fulminans. Causes include:

*   ↑ Tissue thromboplastin which activates the extrinsic pathway (e.g. burns, crush injury, dead foetus)
*   Endothelial damage which activates the intrinsic pathway (e.g. sepsis, vasculitis, burns)

Fact 441:

How should **Torsades de Pointes** be managed in someone who had prior treatment with fluconazole and linezolid and has a normal serum magnesium level?

Still give IV magnesium as this ↑ the chances of developing sinus rhythm

Fluconazole and linezolid both ↑ the QT interval

Fact 442:

What are some features of **MDMA toxicity**?

MDMA is an amphetamine. Features of toxicity include:

↑ Confusion (agitation and ataxia)
↑ Pupil size (mydriasis)
↑ Heart rate (tachycardia)
↑ Blood pressure (hypertension)
↑ Temperature (hyperthermia)
↑ Respiratory rate (respiratory alkalosis)
↑ Creatine kinase (rhabdomyolysis)
↓ Sodium (SIADH)
↓ Platelets (DIC)

Fact 443:

In what other situations can **pulse oximetry** yield unreliable results, apart from when abnormal haemoglobins or dyes are present?

Venous pulsation	e.g. Tricuspid regurgitation (the probe requires pulsatile flow to function)
Motion artefact	e.g. Tremors, myoclonus, shivering
Under-perfusion	e.g. Shock, use of vasopressors
Electrical interference	e.g. Use of diathermy
Physical barriers	e.g. Nail polish especially if it's blue, green or black

Fact 444:

Why may the serum bicarbonate remain low after treatment and resolution of **diabetic ketoacidosis (DKA)**?

↓ Strong ion difference

Treatment of DKA involves administration of large volumes of NaCl 0.9% which contains 154 mmol/L chloride. Excess chloride administration results in excessive chloride accumulation which impairs renal bicarbonate reabsorption (hyperchloraemic metabolic acidosis).

Fact 445:

What are some causes for **red cell casts**, **white cell casts** and **hyaline casts** on urinalysis?

*   *Red cell casts*: Formed from glomerular bleeding, e.g. glomerulonephritis or nephritic syndrome.
*   *White cell casts*: Present in proliferative glomerulonephritis, acute interstitial nephritis and acute pyelonephritis.
*   *Hyaline casts*: Composed of Tamm–Horsfall glycoprotein from cells of the distal nephron. This is a common finding in healthy individuals.

Fact 446:

If someone with **permanent atrial fibrillation** experiences symptomatic syncopal pauses, what pacing mode would you choose for their single-chamber pacemaker?

VVI(R) – this mode of pacing prevents ventricular bradycardia and is primarily indicated in patients with atrial fibrillation with a slow ventricular response

- The first letter denotes pacing location: Ventricle (V).
- The second letter indicates sensing location: Ventricle (V).
- The third letter signifies function: Inhibition (I) of the pacemaker when intrinsic ventricular beats are detected (outside of refractory periods).
- The fourth letter signifies rate responsiveness (R), meaning the pacing rate adjusts according to the patient's activity level.

Fact 447:

What is the difference between **neurogenic shock** and **spinal shock** in a spinal cord injury?

- *Neurogenic shock*: Bradycardia and hypotension in a spinal cord injury due to the interruption of sympathetic outflow
- *Spinal shock*: Loss of power, sensation and reflexes below the level of the lesion

Fact 448:

What are some risk factors for developing **paracetamol toxicity**?

Cytochrome enzyme induction	Glutathione depletion
Chronic excessive alcohol consumption	Malnutrition and eating disorders
Concomitant use of enzyme-inducing drugs e.g. carbamazepine, barbiturates, rifampicin	Patients with factors which cause liver injury e.g. viral hepatitis, alcoholic hepatitis

Fact 449:

Which disorders of sodium balance may be associated with a **subarachnoid haemorrhage**?

HYPOnatraemia	HYPERnatraemia
Euvolaemic/hypervolaemic: Syndrome of inappropriate ADH (SIADH)	Cranial diabetes insipidus (DI)
Hypovolaemic: Cerebral salt-wasting syndrome (CSWS)	

Fact 450:

What are some of the causes of **bilateral hilar lymphadenopathy** on a CXR?

Sarcoidosis
Infection, e.g. TB, fungal, mycoplasma
Malignancy, e.g. lymphoma
Silicosis

Fact 451:

What are the reflex arcs involved in each brain-stem test during **brainstem death testing**?

	Test	Procedure	Afferent	Efferent
1	Pupillary reflex	Bright light shone into each eye to look for direct and consensual pupil constriction	2	3
2	Corneal reflex	Cornea is brushed looking for a blinking response	5	7
3	Response to painful stimuli	Supraorbital stimulus looking for facial grimacing	5	7
4	Vestibulo-ocular reflex	Tympanic membrane visualised. 50 mL of cold water is injected into each ear canal looking for eye nystagmus.	8	3, 4, 6
5	Gag reflex	Direct stimulation of the pharynx looking for gagging	9	10
6	Cough reflex	A suction catheter is passed down the endotracheal tube to stimulate the carina looking for a cough	10	10

Fact 452:

What is the definition of **hospital acquired pneumonia** and what are some bacteria associated with it?

An acute LRTI at least 48 hours after hospital admission and was not incubating at the time of admission. It is typically caused by aerobic Gram-negative bacilli, e.g. *P*seudomonas *aeruginosa*, *E*scherichia *coli*, **A**cinetobacter_ species and *K*lebsiella *pneumoniae*.

Fact 453:

What is the meaning of the letters **IT** or **Z79-IT**, which is written on an endotracheal tube?

Denotes that the device material has been tested in rabbit muscle to ensure tissue compatibility.

Fact 454:

What is the commonest reason for **HIV-related** ICU admissions?

Acute respiratory failure secondary to lower respiratory tract infections (including PJP pneumonia)

Fact 455:

How does **stress-related mucosal damage (SRMD)** compare with **peptic ulcer disease (PUD)**?

SRMD	PUD
Gastric fundus most affected	Gastric antrum and duodenum most affected
Painless	Painful

The exact cause of SRMD's pathophysiology remains uncertain. Hypoxia, hypoperfusion and coagulopathy are contributing factors. SRMD may advance to ulceration, leading to bleeding or perforation.

Fact 456:

What are some clinical and laboratory findings of **alcoholic hepatitis**?

Clinical findings	Laboratory findings
• Jaundice • Pyrexia • Tender hepatomegaly	• ↑ AST and ↑ ALT with AST:ALT ≥2 • ↑ Bilirubin • ↑ GGT • ↑ WCC (neutrophilia)

Fact 457:

For how long do you anticoagulate someone before and after elective DC cardioversion for **atrial fibrillation**?

Three to four weeks prior to the procedure and for four weeks after as atria take time to have full function (atrial stunning).

Fact 458:

What ECG changes may you get in an **intracranial haemorrhage**?

• Deep symmetrical T-wave inversion
• Prolonged QT interval
• Bradycardia (as part of the Cushing reflex)

Fact 459:

In cases of **megaloblastic anaemia** with deficiencies in both B12 and folate, which one should be replaced first?

B12 (B comes before F in the alphabet) – Folate replacement alone may worsen B12 deficiency, leading to subacute degeneration of the cord or damage to peripheral or optic nerves.

Fact 460:

What is the reason for a person with a **phaeochromocytoma** experiencing malignant hypertension and acute pulmonary oedema upon starting propranolol to manage episodes of palpitations?

Propranolol is a non-selective β-blocker

- *Blockade of β_2*: Blockade of β_2-mediated peripheral vasodilation means that excessive circulating catecholamines bind to α-receptors to ↑ systemic vascular resistance and blood pressure.
- *Blockade of β_1*: Blockade of β_1 impairs myocardial function. This precipitates cardiac failure in the context of a severely ↑ blood pressure.

Fact 461:

How does **intravenous immunoglobulin** work in the management of necrotising fasciitis?

It works in four main ways:

1. Induces antibodies against exotoxin
2. Neutralises superantigens
3. Inhibits the membrane attack complex (C5b-9) and complement activation
4. Facilitates opsonisation of Group A Streptococcus organisms

Fact 462:

What is meant by the 'biphasic' metabolic abnormality seen in an **aspirin overdose**?

- PHASE 1: Initial respiratory alkalosis – salicylates directly stimulate the respiratory centre
- PHASE 2: Followed by a high anion gap metabolic acidosis (HAGMA) – due to uncoupled oxidative phosphorylation

Fact 463:

What is **Glanzmann thrombasthenia**?

An autosomal recessive defect which leads to abnormalities of the GP IIb/IIIa receptor. It is most often encountered in patient populations in which there is a ↑ incidence of consanguinity.

Fact 464:

What rash is pathognomonic of a **lightning strike**?

- A 'ferning' or 'arborescent' rash
- It is also known as Lichtenberg figures

Fact 465:

What is the World Federation of Neurological Surgeons classification of **subarachnoid haemorrhages**?

Grade	GCS	Motor deficit
1	15	None
2	13–14	None
3	13–14	Present
4	7–12	Doesn't matter
5	≤6	Doesn't matter

Fact 466:

What are some of the risk factors for **ICU-acquired weakness (ICUAW)**?

Modifiable	Non-modifiable
	Disease
<ul><li>Hyperglycaemia</li><li>Drugs:<ul><li>**C**orticosteroids</li><li>**H**igh-dose vasopressors</li><li>**A**minoglycosides</li><li>**P**arenteral nutrition</li><li>**S**edation and neuromuscular blocking agents</li></ul></li><li>Immobility and bed rest</li></ul>	<ul><li>↑ Duration of mechanical ventilation</li><li>Multi-organ failure</li><li>↑ Severity of illness on admission and admission APACHE II score</li><li>Systemic inflammation and catabolic states, e.g. septic shock</li></ul>
	Patient
	<ul><li>Female sex</li><li>Older age</li><li>Premorbid obesity</li></ul>

Fact 467:

What is the difference between **encephalopathy** and **encephalitis**?

- *Encephalopathy*: Non-inflammatory diffuse brain dysfunction, e.g. intoxication, metabolic causes
- *Encephalitis*: inflammation of brain tissue. Aetiologies can be infection, e.g. HSV, or autoimmune, e.g. paraneoplastic.

Fact 468:

What changes in the CVP waveform are indicative of significant **tricuspid regurgitation**?

Enlarged V waves – these can obscure or obliterate the X decent to form a CV-wave

Fact 469:

Which organism most is most likely responsible for **bacterial meningitis** in a 34-year-old adult?

Neisseria meningitidis

Fact 470:

What are the diagnostic criteria for **neutropenic sepsis** and what is the first line treatment?

Neutrophil count ≤ 0.5 × 10^9 per litre + either:

- A temperature ≥ 38°C **or**
- Other signs or symptoms consistent with clinically significant sepsis

Beta lactam monotherapy with piperacillin with tazobactam is first line treatment.

Fact 471:

What are the endoscopic management options for **peptic ulcer bleeding**?

- Endoclip +/– adrenaline injection
- Thermal coagulation + adrenaline injection
- Fibrin/thrombin + adrenaline injection

Adrenaline should not be used as monotherapy.

Interventional radiology should be offered to unstable patients who re-bleed after endoscopic treatment, and if this is not immediately available, consider referring to surgery.

Fact 472:

How does **myasthenia gravis (MG)** differ from **botulism**?

MG	Botulism
Antibodies target nicotinic acetylcholine receptors at the neuromuscular junction, often co-occurring with autoimmune conditions like hyperthyroidism.	Inhibition of acetylcholine release at the presynaptic level by neurotoxins A, B and E, originating from ingestion or wound contamination
Initial symptoms often involve the eyes, with fatiguability being a prominent feature	Common clinical features include a flaccid descending paralysis and signs involving cranial nerves, such as diplopia and ptosis
Autonomic disturbances are typically absent, although muscarinic symptoms might arise during acetylcholinesterase inhibitor treatment	Antimuscarinic features like dry mouth, mydriasis, constipation and urinary retention are present

Fact 473:

In **neutropaenic colitis**, which regions of the intestine are usually affected?

Ileo-caecum and ascending colon

Fact 474:

What is the cellular origin of **Reed-Sternberg cells**?

Lymphoid progenitors

These cells are diagnostic for Hodgkin's lymphoma (a B-cell malignancy)

Fact 475:

What is the commonest cause of **extradural haematomas (EDH)** and why are they biconvex?

A traumatic arterial bleed between dura and cranium, e.g. a blow to the temple where the relatively thin skull overlies the anterior branch of middle meningeal artery.

EDHs are biconvex because the dura has strong attachments to the cranium along the suture lines and therefore are limited by these suture lines.

Fact 476:

What type of respiratory compliance does **bronchospasm** affect more?

Dynamic compliance > static compliance

Fact 477:

What is the rationale for plasma exchange or using caplacizumab to manage **thrombotic thrombocytopaenic purpura (TTP)**?

- TTP results from a thrombotic microangiopathy linked to deficient or ↓ ADAMTS13 protease activity, which normally cleaves von Willebrand factor (vWF) multimers from endothelial cells.
- Plasma exchange (PLEX) is employed to restore ADAMTS13 levels and eliminate inhibitory autoantibodies.
- Caplacizumab is a monoclonal antibody fragment that inhibits interactions between vWF multimers and platelets.

Fact 478:

How does pregnancy affect **asthma**, and what is the recommended approach to managing acute asthma in pregnant individuals?

Asthma can either improve, worsen or stay the same during pregnancy. Managing severe asthma doesn't differ significantly from non-pregnant patients, but early involvement of a multidisciplinary team (MDT) is advisable.

Fact 479:

How does **trimethoprim** and **daptomycin** work in treating urinary tract infections?

- Trimethoprim inhibits bacterial DNA synthesis. It binds to dihydrofolate reductase and inhibits reduction of dihydrofolic acid to tetrahydrofolic acid (THF). THF is an essential precursor in the thymidine synthesis pathway.
- Daptomycin interferes with the outer membrane of Gram-positive bacteria resulting in cell death. It can be used for UTIs caused by vancomycin-resistant enterococci (VRE).

Fact 480:

What features indicate severe and life-threatening **Clostridium difficile infection (CDI)**?

Severe	Life-threatening
Any of: • WCC > 15 × 10⁹/l • AKI: Cr > 50% of baseline • Evidence of severe colitis (clinically or radiologically) • Temperature > 38.5°C	Any of: • Hypotension or shock • Ileus (partial/ complete) • Toxic megacolon • CT evidence of severe disease

Fact 481:

How would you investigate a six-month-old baby boy who presents one day after a **fall** with a soft, swollen area on the head?

Urgent CTH and skeletal survey – the boggy swelling suggests a fracture

This scenario describes possible non-accidental injury. He should be observed, monitored and placed in a secure environment pending social service investigations.

Fact 482:

How do you locate the **L4/5 intervertebral space** anatomically for the purpose of performing a lumbar puncture?

A line drawn between the top of the iliac crests, known as the intercristal line or Tuffier line, typically intersects the spine at the L4 spinous process. Just below L4 is the L4/5 intervertebral space.

Note that this alignment can vary, especially in females or obese individuals, where the intercristal line may intersect the spine at a level higher than L4.

Fact 483:

How would you treat an 82-year-old who is admitted with a 2-hour history of **severe shortness of breath** and has the following features:

- *Examination*: Bi-basal coarse crackles
- *ECG*: AF with a rate of 155 bpm and QTc of 400 ms
- *CXR*: Pulmonary oedema

Synchronised DC shock – this is a narrow complex tachycardia with adverse features

Fact 484:

How do you grade the severity of **traumatic brain injury**?

GCS is the most widely accepted tool for grading:

Mild	Moderate	Severe
GCS 13–15	GCS 9–12	GCS < 8

Fact 485:

How is a raised D-dimer related to individuals who have **traumatic brain injury (TBI)**?

↑ D-dimer is associated with ↑ risk of progressive haemorrhagic brain injury and a potentially poorer outcome.

Fact 486:

How do you maintain duct patency in a **patent ductus arteriosus**?

Prostaglandins are utilised to maintain the patency of the ductus arteriosus until surgical ligation is performed.

Drugs that inhibit COX on the other hand will close the duct, e.g. paracetamol, indomethacin or ibuprofen.

Fact 487:

What are the main differences in fluid regimes in **HHS** compared to DKA, and why is this so?

- In HHS, there is severe dehydration and the onset is more insidious. The fluid deficit is 8–10 L in HHS compared to 3–6 L in DKA. Because of the ↑ risk of cerebral oedema in HHS, the initial fluid replacement is **slower** compared to DKA.
- Fluid alone is often sufficient to manage HHS. If osmolality doesn't significantly improve with fluids alone, then a **lower** insulin regime of 0.05 units/kg/hr can be initiated.
- **Slower** correction of hypernatraemia compared to DKA is necessary due to the ↑ risk of central pontine myelinolysis.

Fact 488:

What are the five elements of the **Child-Pugh score** to assess the prognosis of chronic liver disease?

The five elements are as follows. Each element is scored 1–3, with 3 indicating most severe derangement.

1. Ascites
2. Grade of encephalopathy
3. Serum bilirubin (µmol/L)
4. Serum albumin (g/L)
5. Prothrombin time or INR

Patients are classed as A, B or C:

Points	Class	One-year survival	Two-year survival
5–6	A	100%	85%
7–9	B	80%	60%
10–15	C	45%	35%

Fact 489:

Which four antibiotic classes are **beta-lactams**?

- Penicillins, e.g. Amoxicillin, Piperacillin
- Cephalosporins, e.g. Cefuroxime, Ceftriaxone
- Monobactams, e.g. Aztreonam
- Carbapenems, e.g. Ertapenem, meropenem

Fact 490:

What are some postulated mechanisms by which **magnesium sulphate** treats eclampsia?

- Calcium channel antagonism: ↓ Cerebral vasospasm
- ↑ Prostacyclin from vascular endothelium: Inhibits platelet aggregation
- Potential additional benefits may include protection of the blood–brain barrier, limitation of cerebral oedema and acting as a central anticonvulsant

Fact 491:

What are some causes of **deranged LFTs in pregnancy**?

Condition	Trimester
Acute liver failure	Any time
Hyperemesis gravidarum	First trimester
Intrahepatic cholestasis of pregnancy	Third trimester
HELLP (haemolysis, elevated liver enzymes, low platelets) syndrome	Second half of pregnancy to postpartum
Acute fatty liver of pregnancy (AFLP)	

Fact 492:

What are the indications for a **thoracotomy** in a trauma patient with a chest drain?

- Immediate drainage of 1,000–1,500 mL of blood from a chest drain followed by ongoing loss
- >200–250 mL/hour especially if compromised

This will enable the placement of an arterial clamp and/or the suturing of bleeding vessels.

Fact 493:

What is the most likely diagnosis if a 75-year-old man with pyrexia and **meningism**, has a lumbar puncture which shows leucocytosis, raised CSF protein 0.80 g/L, low CSF glucose 1.3 mmol/L and a Gram-positive bacillus which shows a tumbling motility pattern in wet mounts of CSF?

Listeria meningitis – this is an important cause of meningitis in the elderly, immunocompromised or pregnant

Ampicillin is used as part of Listeria treatment. Gentamicin is often added for synergy, but it may be stopped after clinical improvement.

CSF glucose levels in Listeria infection can be ↓ and this is associated with a poor prognosis.

Fact 494:

What are the clinical features and radiological signs of **necrotising enterocolitis** in premature infants?

Clinical features	Possible radiographic signs
• Feeding intolerance • ↑ Gastric residuum • Abdominal distension • Blood in stool • Hypotension	• Dilated bowel loops • Paucity of gas • A 'fixed loop' • Pneumatosis intestinalis • Portal venous gas • Pneumoperitoneum

Fact 495:

What are the principles of managing **cerebral salt-wasting syndrome (CSWS)**?

- CSWS is a form of hypotonic hyponatremia.
- It is caused by renal sodium loss following a cerebral pathology.
- Treatment is based on replacing Na^+ and water, e.g. NaCl 0.9%. If the symptoms are severe, hypertonic saline can be used.
- Fludrocortisone can be used in refractory hyponatremia.

Fact 496:

What does the **sail sign** on a chest X-ray suggest?

Left lower lobe collapse

Fact 497:

How is **chronic kidney disease (CKD)** classified?

eGFR criteria		Albuminuria criteria (MG/G)	
Grade 1	>90	A1	<30
Grade 2	60–89		
Grade 3a	45–59	A2	30–300
Grade 3b	30–44		
Grade 4	15–29	A3	>300
Grade 5	<15		

Fact 498:

What is meant by **lead-time bias**?

Occurs when two tests for a disease are compared, the new test diagnoses the disease earlier, but there is no effect on the outcome of the disease.

Fact 499:

What percentage of the body surface area is affected in **Toxic Epidermal Necrolysis (TEN)** and **Stevens–Johnson syndrome (SJS)**, and what are some drugs that are implicated?

SJS	SJS–TEN overlap	TEN
<10%	10–30%	>30%

Involves the epidermis and mucus membranes.

Causative drugs:

- **A**nticonvulsants, e.g. phenytoin, carbamazepine, valproate, lamotrigine
- **A**ntibiotics, e.g. amoxicillin, co-trimoxazole, ciprofloxacin, tetracyclines
- **A**nalgesia, e.g. paracetamol, NSAIDs
- **A**llopurinol
- **Others**: Sulphasalazine, omeprazole, diuretics, HAART, e.g. nevirapine

Treatment is to remove the offending agent and to manage as you would manage a burn, e.g. isolation, IV fluids, nutrition and dressing changes.

Fact 500:

Why may **refeeding** cause generalised weakness and failure to wean off mechanical ventilation?

The development of acute hypophosphatemia

- Hypophosphatemia causes generalised muscle weakness and myalgia.
- In the respiratory system, it causes respiratory failure, diaphragmatic weakness, failure to wean and a left shift of Hb dissociation curve.

Fact 501:

What is the most likely diagnosis if someone develops hypertension, focal seizures and a headache five days after a **left carotid endarterectomy** with no new changes on their CT-head?

Hyperperfusion syndrome

Occurs when blood flow is re-established in a region of the brain where it was previously limited, overwhelming the impaired autoregulatory mechanisms. It is more common in hypertensive patients. Management involves pharmacological intervention to prevent cerebral oedema and haemorrhagic transformation. Drugs like labetalol or clonidine are preferred over nitrates, as nitrates can cause cerebral vasodilation.

Fact 502:

How can you distinguish **pre-renal acute kidney injury** from **acute tubular necrosis (ATN)**?

	Prerenal	ATN
Pathophysiology	↓ Renal perfusion	Damage to renal tubules
Easy way to remember biochemical changes	Body retains sodium to enhance water reabsorption (↑ ADH)	Sodium leaks into the urine as renal tubules lose their absorption ability
Urinary Na⁺ (mmol/L)	<20	>40
Fractional Na⁺ excretion (%)	<1	>2
Urine osmolality (mOsm/kg)	>500	<350
Specific gravity	>1.020	<1.010
Casts	Normal or hyaline casts	Granular and epithelial cell casts
Urea:Cr ratio (mmol/L: μmol/L)	>100:1	<40:1
Urine:plasma osmolality ratio	>1.5	<1.5

Fact 503:

What are the BSE reference values for **tricuspid annular plane systolic excursion (TAPSE)**?

RV systole is predominantly in the longitudinal plane with some inward motion of the RV free wall. TAPSE reflects longitudinal function and equates well with RV ejection fraction. This makes it ideal for measuring systolic function of the RV.

- TAPSE ≥ 17 mm is normal.
- TAPSE < 10 mm is severely impaired.

Fact 504:

What is the procedure for disabling the defibrillation function of an **ICD** during an emergency?

Position a ring magnet over the pacemaker box, ensuring that the magnet stays in place to keep the defibrillator function turned off.

Fact 505:

Why may a high minute volume be required when anaesthetising someone with a **major burn**?

↑ CO_2 generation due to hypermetabolism

Fact 506:

Why is **cyclizine** an appropriate antiemetic to use in Parkinson's disease (PD)?

- H_1 and M_1 receptor antagonist
- Does not cross the BBB

Other agents like haloperidol, metoclopramide and prochlorperazine inhibit the release of dopamine and can exacerbate symptoms of PD.

Fact 507:

What is the **energy input** of 1,000 mL of 10% glucose and 500 mL of 20% lipid over 24 hours?

- 10% glucose = 100 mg/mL = 100,000 mg in 1 L (100 g)
  - o 1 g glucose yields 4 kcal
  - o Therefore, 1 L of 10% glucose will give 400 kcal
- 20% lipid = 200 mg/mL = 100,000 mg in 500 mL (100 g)
  - o 1 g fat yields 9 kcal
  - o Therefore, 20% lipid will give 900 kcal
- Total energy input: 400 kcal + 900 kcal = **1,300 kcal**

Fact 508:

What is the revised definition of **pulmonary artery hypertension**?

Mean pulmonary artery pressure > 20 mmHg as measured by right heart catheterisation

Fact 509:

What are the benefits of using a **cuffed endotracheal tube** over an uncuffed tube in a four-year-old child?

Cuffed tubes are 0.5–1.0 mm smaller than uncuffed:

- ↓ Likelihood of tube exchange
- ↓ Leak
- ↑ Performance if higher ventilatory pressures are required

Fact 510:

What would you expect to see on a V/Q scan in someone with a **pulmonary embolism**?

Persistent ventilation in a region with absent perfusion

The presence of coexisting pulmonary pathology ↓ sensitivity of this investigation.

Fact 511:

What may you see in lead aVR on an ECG in acute severe **tricyclic antidepressant poisoning**?

A dominant R-wave > 3 mm in lead aVR

Fact 512:

What are the two types of **haemolytic uraemic syndrome (HUS)**?

In HUS there is the triad of microangiopathic haemolytic anaemia (MAHA), thrombocytopenia and renal failure:

Typical (D+ HUS)	Atypical (D- HUS)
Linked to a preceding illness and the presence of bloody diarrhoea resulting from infection with a verotoxin-producing organism (such as *E. coli* 0157) or Shigella.	Attributed to genetic mutations leading to persistent, unregulated and excessive complement system activation, e.g. factor H and I deficiencies.
In most instances, treatment is supportive. Antibiotics are used in specific contexts.	Treatment typically involves eculizumab and/or plasma exchange.

Fact 513:

When is the use of **human albumin solution (HAS)** supported by the evidence?

Equivalence to 0.9% saline	• Volume resuscitation • ARDS with hypoalbuminaemia • Septic shock
Supported	↓ Mortality in spontaneous bacterial peritonitis (Sort et al. 1999)
Not supported	In TBI, has been shown to ↑ mortality (SAFE 2004 trial)

Fact 514:

What is the NHS definition of **alcohol misuse**?

Consuming alcohol on a regular basis (most weeks) at a level exceeding 14 units per week

Fact 515:

What procedure can help to manage altered lower limb neurology which develops **post-aortic dissection repair**?

CSF fluid drainage, e.g. lumbar drain to ↓ CSF pressure

↑ Spinal perfusion pressure can be achieved by ↑ MAP or ↓ CSF pressure

Fact 516:

What are the diagnostic criteria for **pre-eclampsia**?

SBP ≥ 140 mmHg or DBP ≥ 90 mmHg

+

Either Proteinuria or ≥ 1 organ dysfunction:

Proteinuria	≥ 1 Organ dysfunction	
	System	Examples of dysfunction
	Renal	Creatinine ≥ 90 μmol/L
Urinary PCR ≥30 mg/mmol or ACR ≥ 8 mg/mmol	Liver	ALT > 70 IU/L or 2 × upper limit of normal
	Neurological	Eclampsia, severe headaches, visual disturbance
	Haematological	• Platelets < 150 × 10⁹/L • DIC • Haemolysis • HELLP syndrome
	Uteroplacental dysfunction	Foetal growth restriction or abnormal umbilical artery Doppler waveform analysis

Fact 517:

Why might **supraglottic suction** be added to an endotracheal tube design?

To ↓ the risk of micro-aspiration and subsequent VAP

Fact 518:

Which **non-depolarising muscle relaxant** is most likely to cause an anaphylactic reaction?

Rocuronium

Fact 519:

What is the most likely diagnosis if someone with a short history of a dry mouth, diplopia and dysphagia then develops a **symmetrical descending weakness**, initially affecting the trunk and proximal limb muscles, which then spreads more peripherally without any sensory involvement?

Botulism

This is caused by an exotoxin released from *Clostridium botulinum*. It is characterised by a descending motor paralysis affecting primarily cranial, respiratory and autonomic nerves.

Fact 520:

How does **cocaine** cause strokes and movement disorders?

Strokes		Movement disorders
Ischaemic	**Haemorrhagic**	Accumulation of dopamine in the basal ganglia in repeated cocaine ingestion may lead to a choreoathetosis, dystonias and akathisia
Cerebral vasospasm Arterial thrombosis	Hypertensive crises especially if there are aneurysms or AV malformations	

Fact 521:

If someone with **acute severe asthma** develops progressive hypotension and tachycardia 30 minutes after being intubated, why may disconnecting the ventilator help to restore cardiovascular stability?

To allow complete passive exhalation

This deterioration coincided with mechanical ventilation; hyperinflation → ↓ venous return → ↓ cardiac output

Fact 522:

What is the most likely diagnosis if someone in her third trimester of pregnancy develops nausea, vomiting and hypertension (160/100 mmHg), along with the following abnormal blood tests:

- ↑ Bilirubin 160 µmol/L
- ↑ AST 650 IU/L
- ↑ Prothrombin time 24 seconds
- ↓ Fibrinogen 0.5 g/L
- ↓ Glucose 2.1 mmol/L

Acute fatty liver of pregnancy (AFLP)

This is caused by microvesicular fatty infiltration of hepatocytes and occurs in the third trimester. Distinguishing features of AFLP from HELLP syndrome include ↑ bilirubin, ↓ glucose and coagulopathy. In severe cases of AFLP, hepatic encephalopathy may also occur.

Definitive treatment involves delivery of the fetus, irrespective of gestational age and MDT input/care. Blood tests typically normalise within 7–10 days.

Fact 523:

What type of acid–base abnormality is associated with **diuretic use**?

Metabolic alkalosis

Fact 524:

What is meant by a **saturation gap** in carbon monoxide poisoning?

- A standard pulse oximeter measures only two wavelengths of light. It falsely interprets COHb as oxyhaemoglobin. This overestimates the true SaO_2.
- A co-oximeter uses multiple wavelengths of light. This gives the true SaO_2. The true SaO_2 will be very ↓ when compared with the SpO_2 on the pulse oximeter.
- The difference between the falsely ↑ SpO_2 and the true SaO_2 is called the 'saturation gap'.

Fact 525:

Where do the vertebral arteries unite to form the **basilar artery**?

At the base of the pons

Fact 526:

Which hormones does the **posterior pituitary** produce?

ADH and oxytocin

Fact 527:

What is the most frequent reason for persistent elevation of serum **TSH** in patients taking thyroid replacement?

Poor compliance

Changes in TSH lag behind changes in T_3/T_4 after about eight weeks of thyroid hormone replacement.

Fact 528:

How does **hydroxocobalamin** work to treat cyanide poisoning?

It combines with cyanide to form cyanocobalamin (Vitamin B12).

- Cyanocobalamin is then renally cleared.
- Cyanocobalamin may also dissociate slowly from cyanide. This allows cyanide detoxification by the mitochondrial enzyme, rhodanese.

Fact 529:

What is the **arterial supply** of the bowel?

- *Coeliac trunk*: Stomach to second part of duodenum
- *SMA*: Distal second duodenum to ⅔ transverse colon
- *IMA*: Distal third of transverse colon to rectum

Fact 530:

How can you confirm active ongoing **haemolysis** in thrombotic thrombocytopenic purpura (TTP) or HELP syndrome?

- *Blood film*: Fragments of the RBCs (schistocytes)
- ↓ Haptoglobin (this serum protein binds to free haemoglobin liberated from lysed cells)
- ↑ Reticulocyte count (immature red cells)
- ↑ LDH
- ↑ Unconjugated bilirubin (from RBC breakdown)

Fact 531:

What are some causes of a **low serum albumin**?

- Redistribution, e.g. endothelial leak/ damage
- ↓ Production, e.g. hepatic dysfunction
- ↑ Loss, e.g. renal dysfunction/nephrotic syndrome
- ↑ Catabolism (very rare)

Albumin is a single polypeptide synthesised by the liver, reflecting its synthetic activity. It's highly soluble and carries a negative charge. About 40% of albumin is found intravascularly, with the rest residing in the interstitial compartment.

Fact 532:

What significant concern may a sudden decrease in urine output suggest in someone with an **intra-aortic balloon pump (IABP)**?

Balloon displacement

Renal blood flow should ↑ by up to 25% with an IABP. A sudden ↓ in urine output may indicate balloon migration and compromise of renal blood flow.

Fact 533:

Which type of **delirium** has the highest mortality: hyperactive or hypoactive?

Hypoactive delirium

Fact 534:

What disadvantages are specific to **enteral nutrition** that do not apply to parenteral nutrition?

- Relies on a functional GI tract
- ↑ Risk of VAP
- NGT misplacement → lung feeding (a 'never event')
- Known to cause diarrhoea
- Discomfort from NG/NJ tubes

Fact 535:

How would you manage someone with **sickle cell disease (SCD)** who presents with hemiparesis and a CT-head which shows an ischaemic stroke?

Red blood cell exchange transfusion

Acute stroke in SCD is an indication for an exchange transfusion. This is required to ↓ the percentage of haemoglobin S to < 30% to ↓ symptom severity and incidence of long-term complications.

Simple red blood cell transfusions are not effective in these cases.

Fact 536:

What are some absolute contraindications to inserting an **intra-aortic balloon pump (IABP)** use?

- Severe aortic regurgitation
- Aortic dissection or aortic stents
- End-stage heart disease with no expectation of improvement

Fact 537:

Define **flail chest**, outline the benefits of rib fixation and identify a potential long-term issue post-rib fixation?

- *Flail chest*: Fractures of ≥2 adjacent ribs in ≥2 places resulting in paradoxical chest movement
- Benefits of rib fixation:
  - o ↑ Analgesia
  - o ↑ Respiratory function over time
  - o ↓ Risk of pneumonia
  - o ↓ Duration of mechanical ventilation
  - o ↓ Critical care and hospital stay
  - o ↓ Chest wall deformity
- *Long-term issue*: Chronic pain

Fact 538:

What is the gold standard to investigate for **renal artery stenosis**?

- *Invasive*: Percutaneous angiography. This also enables angioplasty if indicated.
- *Non-invasive*: MR angiography with gadolinium contrast.

Renal artery Doppler is prone to more false-negative results than angiography.

Fact 539:

What is the most likely diagnosis if someone with **atrial fibrillation** develops a sudden onset of bilateral leg weakness, areflexia and extensor plantars with a sensory level at the umbilicus?

Spinal Infarction – a sudden onset of limb weakness and altered neurology in someone with atrial fibrillation is most likely to be due to embolic phenomena

Other differentials include a tumour or bleed, and an urgent MRI is indicated to rule out a compressive lesion.

Fact 540:

What is the pathophysiology of **sickle cell disease**?

Autosomal recessive inheritance

- Point mutation on chromosome 11 at position 6.
- Valine is substituted for glutamate on the β-globin subunit of HbA to form HbS. HbS is less soluble and more viscous than HbA with a tendency to polymerise and precipitate, especially in hypoxia.
- In sickle cell disease, sickled cells break down rapidly. This results in haemolytic anaemia, microvascular occlusion, thrombosis and distal infarction.

Fact 541:

What is the most likely diagnosis if an HIV-positive man with features of **meningitis** and a normal CT-head has CSF that shows a raised protein, low glucose and a mononuclear pleocytosis with negative Gram staining and negative India ink staining?

TB meningitis

↑ Protein, glucose <60% of plasma glucose and mononuclear pleocytosis are strongly suggestive of TB meningitis.

India ink staining tests for Cryptococcus

Fact 542:

Which organism causes **tetanus**?

Clostridium tetani – anaerobic, motile, spore-forming, gram-positive rod

Its spores can be found in soil, manure and the GI tract of animals. These can infect the body through contaminated wounds.

Tetanus toxaemia is caused by a specific neurotoxin produced by *Clostridium tetani* called tetanospasmin. It is produced in an anaerobic environment, such as in necrotic tissue. This toxin inhibits the release of neurotransmitters from presynaptic GABA inhibitory neurons, leading to symptoms like skeletal muscle rigidity and spasms, as well as autonomic instability/dysfunction.

Fact 543:

What is the pathophysiology of **drowning-related lung injury**?

Initial response
• Breath-holding is the initial response to submersion/immersion. • Laryngospasm may initially protect the lower airways.
Within a minute or so
• As hypercapnia and acidosis progress, the urge to breathe becomes irresistible. • Simultaneously, as cerebral hypoxia occurs, the laryngeal muscles relax. • Consequently, water enters the lungs, resulting in aspiration.
Consequences of aspiration
a. Surfactant washout and dysfunction → **atelectasis** b. Development of an osmotic gradient across the alveolar membrane and ↑ permeability of this membrane → fluid and electrolyte shifts → widespread alveolar-capillary damage (alveolar toxicity) → **pulmonary oedema.** This process remains consistent, regardless of whether it occurs with freshwater or saltwater exposure. c. **Bronchospasm**
Outcome
All these processes result in a hypoxia, shunt formation and ↓ lung compliance → ARDS

Fact 544:

What are some cardiovascular changes that occur in **pregnancy**?

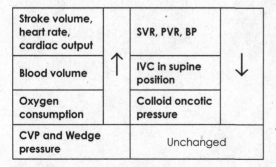

Stroke volume, heart rate, cardiac output		SVR, PVR, BP	
Blood volume	↑	IVC in supine position	↓
Oxygen consumption		Colloid oncotic pressure	
CVP and Wedge pressure		Unchanged	

Fact 545:

What are some of the indications for an exchange transfusion in **sickle cell disease**?

Multi-organ failure
Acute chest syndrome
Stroke
Hepatic sequestration (RUQ syndrome)

An exchange transfusion helps to ↑ oxygen carrying capacity and ↓ blood viscosity. It is particularly effective when the haemoglobin level is significantly high, typically > 100 g/L, which can ↑ blood viscosity.

Fact 546:

Under what circumstances might surgical drainage of a **pericardial tamponade** be favoured over pericardiocentesis?

If there is intrapericardial bleeding, clot/s within the pericardium and/or a loculated effusion.

Fact 547:

What is meant by the **Michaelis–Menten constant**?

• Michaelis–Menten kinetics is a model of enzyme kinetics.
• The Michaelis–Menten constant is the concentration of the substrate at which the enzyme is working at half its maximal rate.

Fact 548:

How common is extraocular weakness on initial presentation in **myasthenia gravis**?

Around 85%

Patients complain of diplopia, ptosis or both

Fact 549:

Which part of the **immune system** is activated if someone has a temperature of 38°C and displays flushing, breathlessness, hypotension and haemoglobinuria within 30 minutes of a red blood cell transfusion?

The classical complement pathway

This is a severe intravascular haemolytic reaction secondary to ABO incompatibility. Red cells are destroyed in the bloodstream with consequent release of haemoglobin into the circulation. The antibodies implicated (anti-A or anti-B) cause rapid activation of the complement cascade.

Fact 550:

Which agents would you use to treat a crisis of **myasthenia gravis**?

IVIg or plasmapheresis

If intubated and ventilated, pyridostigmine is generally stopped to ↓ airway secretions and to ↑ sensitivity to pyridostigmine (a brief drug holiday may ↑ responsiveness when resumed).

Long-term suppression with steroids or steroid-sparing agents, e.g. azathioprine or ciclosporin is considered later on.

Fact 551:

What is **toxic shock syndrome** and what causes it?

An acute inflammatory multisystem disorder mediated by exotoxin release from severe Gram-positive infections. Characterised by shock, rash, desquamation and fever.

Some causes include:

Group A β-haemolytic streptococcus, e.g. Streptococcus pyogenes	Staphylococcus aureus
• Burns • Necrotising fasciitis	• Menstrual products • Nasal packing • Intrauterine devices • Soft tissue infections • Pneumonia

Fact 552:

What steps are necessary when administering defibrillation to someone with a **permanent pacemaker**?

Position the defibrillator pads at a considerable distance from the pacing box (at least 8 cm away), and promptly assess the pacemaker's settings and functionality following defibrillation.

Fact 553:

What steps would you take in managing someone who ingested **ecstasy** 8 hours ago and is currently experiencing restlessness, tachycardia 140 bpm, hypertension at 185/115, hyperthermia at 40.3°C, metabolic acidosis and hyponatremia at 114 mmol/L?

- *Agitation*: Treat with benzodiazepines or butyrophenones (e.g. haloperidol).
- *Hypertension and tachycardia*: This may be helped by treating agitation. It may also require α- and β-blockade. Pure β-blockade is avoided as unopposed α-stimulation may cause a hypertensive crisis.
- Active cooling. Dantrolene has been used in this setting but its role in unclear. Dantrolene can cause hepatotoxicity which may potentiate ecstasy toxicity.
- *Hyponatraemia (may be SIADH)*: In the first instance, can cautiously give NaCl 0.9% or hypertonic saline, while investigating the cause with paired osmolalities.
- *Metabolic acidosis*: IV fluids may help if it is secondary to hypermetabolism/AKI. RRT may be needed though.

Fact 554:

How does **spironolactone** work?

It is a competitive aldosterone antagonist that is used as an oral diuretic in chronic liver and heart failure. It can cause ↓ Na+, ↑ K+ and anti-androgen effects, e.g. gynaecomastia.

Fact 555:

What is the **power** of a study if the chance of a false negative result is 20%?

- False negative is also called a type 2 error or β-error
- Type 2 error = 100 – power
- Therefore, power = 100 – 20 = **80%**

Fact 556:

What is the composition material of an **endotracheal tube**?

Polyvinyl chloride

Fact 557:

What are the criteria for direct referral to a **major trauma centre (MTC)** and bypassing the **local trauma unit (TU)**?

- If patients activate a prehospital trauma triage tool and the MTC can be reached within a 45-minutes, they should be transported directly to the MTC.
- If the patient is too unstable for direct transfer, initial stabilisation should take place at the nearest TU before considering a secondary transfer to the MTC.

Fact 558:

What is the effect of **thiopentone** on cerebral metabolic rate of oxygen ($CMRO_2$), cerebral blood flow (CBF) and intracranial pressure (ICP)?

- ↓ $CMRO_2$
- ↓ CBF
- ↓ ICP

Fact 559:

What is the first-line route of nutrition in someone with **acute pancreatitis** who is ventilated?

Enteral nutrition

PN should be reserved for intolerance to enteral feeding.

Fact 560:

How do you treat **toxic megacolon** on a background of known pseudomembranous colitis?

This is a surgical emergency

Colectomy or a de-functioning ileostomy may be performed.

Fact 561:

How do you distinguish between a transudative and exudative **pleural effusion** if the protein level is between 25 and 35 g/L?

By using Light's criteria:

	Transudate	Exudate
Protein (pleural/ serum)	≤0.5	>0.5
LDH (pleural/ serum)	≤0.6	>0.6
	Pleural LDH ≤ ⅔ upper limit of normal serum LDH	Pleural LDH > ⅔ upper limit of normal serum LDH
Some causes	• Heart failure • ↓ Albumin states (cirrhosis, nephrotic) • Hypothyroid • Peritoneal dialysis • Sarcoidosis	• Infection • Malignancy • Pancreatitis • Dressler's • Yellow nail • Boerhaave • Connective Tissue disease (RA, SLE) • Pulmonary embolism
	Meig's syndrome	

Fact 562:

Along with wound washout, debridement and human tetanus immunoglobulin, which antibiotic would you use for bacterial eradication of *Clostridium tetani*?

Metronidazole

Fact 563:

How would you manage a **retro-orbital haematoma with proptosis** in a trauma patient?

Lateral canthotomy – to decompress the orbit and release tension from the optic nerve

This is a sight-threatening condition. Retro-orbital pressure on the optic nerve can cause rapid and irreversible damage. Conscious patients will have extreme pain, visual disturbance and ophthalmoplegia. A heightened clinical suspicion is necessary for sedated patients.

Fact 564:

At what threshold should an **elevated ICP** be treated according to the Brain Trauma Foundation (BTF)?

>22 mmHg

Fact 565:

What is the physiological response to **tonsillar herniation (coning)** as the cerebellar tonsils are forced through the foreman magnum in response to raised ICP?

- ↑ ICP causes 'coning' which results in compression of the brainstem and cervical cord.
- When ICP > MAP, brain perfusion is compromised.
- This results in ↑ sympathetic discharge which causes an initial ↑ HR and ↑ MAP (vasoconstriction) to improve cerebral perfusion. This sympathetic storm ↑ myocardial oxygen demand and ↑ risk of arrhythmias. There is an ↑ risk of myocardial ischaemia and neurogenic pulmonary oedema.
- ↑ MAP → activates the aortic and carotid baroreceptors → reflex bradycardia.
- As ICP increases further, the cardio-respiratory centres within the brainstem are compressed resulting in Cushing's triad:
  - o   Irregular and ↓ respiratory patterns
  - o   Hypertension with a widened pulse pressure
  - o   Brady-arrhythmias
- This is then followed by loss of sympathetic tone resulting in marked vasodilatation, relative hypovolaemia and myocardial depression.
- Organ function rapidly deteriorates if these abnormalities are not adequately controlled.

Fact 566:

Why is **phenoxybenzamine** preferred over phentolamine in the initial treatment of a phaeochromocytoma?

- It provides irreversible α-blockade.
- It forms a covalent bond affecting calcium influx.

Fact 567:

When employing **active humidification**, what issues can arise due to condensation in the ventilation circuit tubing, and what measures can be taken to prevent it?

Issues	Prevention
• Auto-triggering • Obstruction • Infection	• Adding water traps • Adding a heated expiratory filter • Heating the circuit downstream from the humidifier

Fact 568:

What is the relationship between obesity and **acute pancreatitis**?

- ↑ Risk of acute pancreatitis
- ↑ Severity of acute pancreatitis

Fact 569:

What are the primary benefits of modifying a **continuous haemofiltration circuit** to introduce a higher volume of fluid replacement before the haemofilter (pre-dilution) compared to after (post-dilution)?

↑ Filter lifespan
↓ Blood viscosity → ↓ clotting risk

Fact 570:

Would you correct coagulopathy in **acute fulminant liver failure** when there is no evidence of bleeding?

No – coagulopathy is a useful marker of synthetic function to guide transplantation.

Correction may be considered if a procedure is needed.

Fact571:

How does an IV **propofol 1% infusion** provide a significant proportion of daily calorie intake?

Propofol 1% contains 1.1 kcal/mL of energy.

Fact 572:

What energy would you use for cardioversion to treat **supraventricular tachycardia** with adverse signs?

Synchronised DCCV: 70–120 J (biphasic)

If cardioversion is not achieved with three shocks, give amiodarone 300 mg IV before giving further shocks.

Fact 573:

What bedside clinical signs could indicate **heightened respiratory effort** in a one-year-old child?

- **S**weating
- **T**achypnoea
- **I**ntercostal and subcostal recession
- **N**asal flaring
- **G**runting

Fact 574:

Which serum potassium abnormality precipitates **digoxin toxicity**?

↓ K+ (hypokalaemia)

Hyperkalaemia occurs as a result of toxicity.

Fact 575:

What are the directly measured and derived variables from a **pulmonary artery catheter**?

Directly measured	Derived
Temperature	
Central venous pressure	
RA pressure	Cardiac Index
RV pressure	SV and SVI
PA pressure	SVR and SVRI
PA occlusion pressure	PVR and PVRI
Cardiac Output	
SvO$_2$	

Fact 576:

What equation does the National Kidney Foundation recommend using to estimate **glomerular filtration rate**?

CKD-EPI Creatinine Equation (2021)

This contains the variables of sex, age and creatinine.

Accuracy is increased when cystatin C is added as a variable, but this is not available in all laboratories.

Fact 577:

What are the four basic **ethical principles** in healthcare?

- Respect for autonomy: Can independently arrive at decisions through thoughtful consideration.
- Beneficence: Do good.
- Non-maleficence: Do no harm.
- Justice: Fairness between competing claims.

Fact 578:

What is **Takotsubo Cardiomyopathy (apical ballooning syndrome, stress-induced cardiomyopathy or 'broken heart syndrome')** and how do you treat it?

- A potentially reversible cause of acute heart failure.
- Characterised by regional LV apical or mid-ventricular systolic dysfunction.
- Thought to occur because of ↑ endogenous catecholamines following emotional or physical stress, e.g. bereavement or myocardial stunning following a SAH, sepsis, phaeochromocytoma crisis or post-ROSC.
- Angiography is required for diagnosis as ECG/TnI/TTE may resemble ACS, including a STEMI.
- Management is as with acute heart failure until ventricular function recovers.

Fact 579:

How well is **neomycin** absorbed from the GI tract?

Poorly absorbed – it can be given orally to alter gut flora in hepatic encephalopathy.

Fact 580:

Why are children particularly susceptible to **hypothermia**?

Hypothermia is more likely in children due to their high surface area-to-body mass ratio.

Fact 581:

What has most likely occurred if someone develops pulmonary oedema, a new pansystolic murmur and a low cardiac index, high SVR, raised CVP and hypotension following an **inferior myocardial infarction**?

Papillary muscle rupture leading to cardiogenic shock

- The murmur suggests underlying mitral regurgitation.
- Papillary muscle rupture is common with inferior MIs.

Fact 582:

Why is **vasopressin** first line for hypotension resistant to fluid therapy in a DBD donor?

- Restores vascular tone
- Treats diabetes insipidus which may occur
- Minimises catecholamine requirements
- Less likely to cause metabolic acidosis or pulmonary hypertension when compared to noradrenaline

The focus of management moves from patient-focused to organ optimisation. The aim is to maintain cardiac output while reducing ↓ cardiac work/myocardial oxygen. Metaraminol is not recommended first line due to the risk of developing brady-dysrhythmias.

Fact 583:

Why may a **high PEEP** ventilatory strategy be concerning in someone who is bleeding?

↑ Intrathoracic pressure → ↓ venous return → ↓ BP

Fact 584:

What are some benefits of **daily sedation holds?**

↓ Mechanical ventilation, ↓ delirium, ↓ ICU LOS

Fact 585:

What are some of the possible echocardiographic findings in **PIMS (Paediatric Inflammatory Multisystem Syndrome)**?

Occurs in children/adolescents following exposure to SARS-CoV-2. Characterised by systemic inflammation with multi-organ involvement. Echocardiographic findings vary depending on the stage of the disease and the degree of cardiac involvement. Possibilities include:

- Coronary artery abnormalities, e.g. coronary artery dilation or aneurysms (similar to Kawasaki disease)
- LV dysfunction, e.g. ↓ ejection fraction, regional wall motion abnormalities
- Valvular abnormalities, e.g. mitral regurgitation
- Pericardial effusion
- Myocarditis

Fact 586:

What is the significance of a **Reynolds number** of 2,000?

- Reynolds > 2,000 turbulent flow more likely
- Reynolds < 2,000 laminar flow more likely

Laminar flow is more efficient than turbulent flow.

Fact 587:

For how long can oxygen from a full-size E cylinder sustain a **patient transfer**, assuming a FiO_2 of 1.0 and a minute volume of 9 L/min, given that the portable ventilator consumes 1 L/min of driving gas?

68 minutes

- A size E cylinder supplies 680 L of oxygen
- The required volume is 10 L/min

Fact 588:

If someone experiences **tetany** following the administration of multiple units of packed red blood cells, what treatment is typically required?

IV calcium

Serum calcium can ↓ with rapidly transfused blood products due to the citrate preservative. Citrate binds to endogenous calcium which renders it non-functional.

Fact 589:

What are some disadvantages of using an **intraparenchymal probe** to measure intracranial pressure?

- Most cannot be recalibrated once in situ.
- They are subject to zero drift over time.
- Only measures local pressure (not entirely accurate in the presence of intracranial pressure gradients).
- Cannot drain CSF.

Fact 590:

How would you treat **staphylococcal toxic shock syndrome** in someone who just had an incision and drainage of a thigh abscess?

- β-lactam (bacteriocidal) and clindamycin/linezolid (bacteriostatic to ↓ toxin production)
- Fluids +/− vasopressors
- Source control, e.g. extensive debridement
- IVIg can be considered for toxin control in select cases

Fact 591:

Why may **RV failure** develop post pneumonectomy?

Because of ↑ pulmonary vascular resistance

Fact 592:

What is the effect of **hyperoxia** post-cardiac arrest?

Adversely influences outcome and has a significant impact on morbidity and mortality.

Fact 593:

How can the short acting cholinesterase inhibitor, **edrophonium**, help to differentiate between a myasthenic crisis and cholinergic crisis?

Myasthenic crisis	Cholinergic crisis
There is a lack of acetylcholine	There is an excess of acetylcholine
Edrophonium will make a myasthenic crisis better	Edrophonium will make a cholinergic crisis worse

---

Fact 594:

Why are **flutter valves** useful in chest drain management?

Allows for earlier mobilisation and therefore earlier discharge from hospital

---

Fact 595:

What is the **DeBakey classification** of an aortic dissection?

- Type 1: Entire aorta
- Type 2: Ascending aorta only
- Type 3: Descending aorta only
  - o 3a: Extends to diaphragm
  - o 3b: Extends beyond diaphragm

Fact 596:

What would you do next if a **unilateral pneumothorax** persists in spite of having a 12F chest drain on low-pressure suction for three days in a young and fit person?

Refer to thoracic surgery to consider pleurectomy, either via open thoracotomy or via <u>V</u>ideo <u>A</u>ssisted <u>T</u>horacoscopic <u>S</u>urgery (VATS)

Pleurectomy is recommended over pleurodesis to treat the persistent air leak because it has a lower pneumothorax recurrence rate.

Alternative options for those unfit for surgery, e.g. elderly or frail, include medical pleurodesis or insertion of a long-term Heimlich valve.

Fact 597:

What is the difference between **static and dynamic compliance**?

Static compliance	Dynamic compliance
Measured when gas flow is absent. Calculated by performing an end-inspiratory hold manoeuvre. $C_{stat} = V_T/(P_{plat} - PEEP)$ Static compliance is typically ↓ by lung parenchymal disease, e.g. ARDS. Other causes include: • Chest wall disease (kyphoscoliosis, obesity, circumferential burns) • ↑ Intra-abdominal pressure	Measured during rhythmic breathing. $C_{dyn} = V_T/(P_{Peak} - PEEP)$ P_{Peak} represents the compliance of the lung and chest wall + the pressure required to overcome airway resistance. Usually, $C_{dyn} < C_{stat}$. A large discrepancy between C_{dyn} and C_{stat} arises in the context of obstructive airway disease where ↑ pressure is required to overcome ↑ airway resistance.

Fact 598:

Where is ablation typically performed during the initial procedure for **atrial fibrillation**?

- Around the pulmonary veins
- The procedure is known as pulmonary vein isolation.

Fact 599:

What are some benefits of a **tracheostomy**?

- ↑ Comfort, ↓ sedation and ↑ communication
- Aids weaning from the ventilator
- Helps with secretion clearance
- Allows vocal cords to mobilise: Protects against aspiration and allows phonation
- ↑ Laryngeal sensation and ability to swallow: Facilitates return to oral diet and prevents further deconditioning

Fact 600:

Why shouldn't you use **midazolam** in renal impairment?

Delayed metabolism and reduced elimination lead to an ↑ accumulation of the active metabolite, α-hydroxymidazolam.

Fact 601:

What is the significance of **post-resuscitation GCS** in TBI?

- It is the most important prognostic indicator.
- The motor component is the most useful part.

Fact 602:

What is **selective decontamination of the digestive tract (SDD)?**

A strategy where oral, enteral and IV antimicrobials are used to target and eliminate potentially harmful bacteria in the GI tract while sparing beneficial bacteria. It is based on the theory that most ICU infections arise from an ↑ growth of gut flora (colonisation). It aims to control:

- Primary endogenous infection (pathogens on admission)
- Secondary endogenous infection (pathogens acquired during colonisation)
- Exogenous infection (infection without colonisation)

SDD has been shown to ↓ overall mortality and the odds ratio of lower respiratory tract infections, e.g. VAP. It is not widely used in the UK due to local microbiological variances, concerns over resistance (although not demonstrated) and the cost of training staff. NICE does not recommend it as very few studies were conducted in the UK.

Fact 603:

What happens to endogenous **vasopressin** levels in sepsis?

Endogenous levels are ↓

Fact 604:

What are the features of **subclavian steal syndrome**?

- Occurs when there is subclavian artery stenosis proximal to the origin of the vertebral artery.
- The subclavian artery steals reverse-flow blood from the vertebrobasilar arterial circulation to supply the arm during exertion.
- This results in vertebrobasilar insufficiency (posterior circulation symptoms).

Fact 605:

Why are **thiazide diuretics** not preferred over loop diuretics for maintaining diuresis in individuals at risk of tumour lysis syndrome?

Thiazide diuretics ↑ urate levels

Fact 606:

What happens to the effectiveness of **prokinetics** after 72 hours?

The effectiveness is ↓ to one-third after 72 hours.

Fact 607:

What are the four mechanisms of **hypoxia**?

Hypoxaemic hypoxia	↓ Arterial oxygen tension, e.g. • V/Q mismatch • Shunts • Alveolar hypoventilation • ↓ FiO_2
Anaemic hypoxia	Failure of oxygen carriage, e.g. • ↓ Hb • Impaired Hb, e.g. methaemoglobinaemia, CO poisoning
Stagnant hypoxia	↓ Cardiac output
Cytotoxic hypoxia	Abnormal cellular utilisation of oxygen leads to failure of aerobic respiration despite adequate oxygen delivery, e.g. cyanide poisoning

Fact 608:

What is the role for early revascularisation in **infarct-related cardiogenic shock**?

- Studies have shown a significant improvement in survival with early revascularisation in the treatment of infarct-related cardiogenic shock.
- In the vast majority of cases, this is achieved by percutaneous coronary intervention (PCI).

Fact 609:

What are some interventions that have shown a mortality benefit in **ARDS**?

- Lung protective ventilation, e.g. TVs 6 mL/kg IBW and P_{plat} < 30 cmH_2O (ARDSnet)
- Prone positioning (PROSEVA)
- Early paralysis within 48 hours (ACURASYS)
- Transfer to specialist centre for consideration of VV-ECMO (CESAR – although not all patients in the intervention group received ECMO)

Fact 610:

Why might the **acidaemia** not improve on CVVH?

- Pressures problems:
  o ↓ Access pressures, e.g. improperly positioned catheter, hypovolaemia
  o ↑ Outflow pressures, e.g. patient movement, coughing, obstructed catheter
- ↑ Demands, e.g. worsening of underlying pathology
- Errors, e.g. inadequate prescription, operator error
- Filter problems, e.g. malfunction, filter exhaustion
- Interruptions, e.g. circuit clotting, disconnections

Fact 611:

Why would adding **metolazone** to furosemide be beneficial in managing pulmonary oedema in someone who has a serum sodium of 160 mmol/L?

To promote natriuresis

Furosemide promotes diuresis but not much natriuresis. Therefore, there is more H_2O than Na^+ loss. A thiazide like metolazone can promote Na^+ loss in the distal nephron.

Fact 612:

How can CT appearances grade the severity of **acute pancreatitis**?

The Balthazar CT Severity Index grades pancreatitis radiologically (based on inflammation, collections and necrosis) with associated mortality values.

Fact 613:

What serum potassium disturbance do you get in **theophylline** overdose?

Hypokalaemia

Fact 614:

What ECG findings are typical of **right ventricular hypertrophy**?

- Right axis deviation
- Dominant R wave in V_1
- Dominant S wave in V_5 or V_6
- QRS duration < 120 ms (i.e. changes not due to RBBB)

Fact 615:

What are some risks of using **inhaled nitric oxide (iNO)** to treat pulmonary hypertension?

- Exacerbation of cardiogenic pulmonary oedema through ↑ LV preload (high dose use)
- Methaemoglobinaemia (prolonged high dose use)
- Renal impairment (prolonged high dose use)

NO stimulates ↑ cGMP in vascular smooth muscle, leading to vasodilation. The effectiveness tends to ↓ over a period of days (tachyphylaxis). The normal range is 1–80 ppm, starting at 5 ppm and up titrating by 5–10 ppm every 30 minutes.

Fact 616:

What is **anti-NMDA receptor encephalitis**?

- A treatment-responsive encephalitis associated with anti-NMDA receptor (NMDAR) antibodies. These bind to the NR1/NR2 heteromers of NMDA receptors.
- Most patients are female. Half of them have a neoplasm, most commonly an ovarian teratoma.
- It has five stages: Prodromal viral infection-like phase, psychotic phase, unresponsive phase, hyperkinetic phase and recovery phase.
- Anti NMDAR IgG antibodies detected in the CSF and/or serum are diagnostic (titres are higher in the CSF). When diagnosed, a tumour should be ruled out.
- Brain MRI may be normal, but non-specific white and grey matter T2/FLAIR signal hyperintensities may be present, especially in the hippocampus. EEG shows a delta brush pattern.
- Corticosteroids, immunoglobulin infusion (IVIg) and plasmapheresis (PLEX) are first-line therapies, with tumour removal if applicable.

Fact 617:

What is the suggested dose of **fresh frozen plasma** in the bleeding trauma patient with coagulopathy?

15–20 mL/kg

Fact 618:

What does an absent hum on auscultation in someone with a continuous non-pulsatile **LVAD** suggest?

LVAD failure

When this occurs, there is an ↑ risk of thrombosis of the LVAD itself or distal embolisation.

Fact 619:

Does hypotension secondary to a **Mobitz Type 2 block** following a myocardial infarction respond to atropine?

Not really

While atropine may be useful for sinus or junctional bradycardia, giving atropine in the setting of Mobitz type 2 can worsen the block and ↑ the risk of complete heart block or asystole.

Because of the significant risk of asystole or complete heart block, temporary cardiac pacing is indicated in the first instance. Transvenous can be performed via the femoral or internal jugular veins. Transcutaneous pacing should only be used as a holding measure in an emergency.

Fact 620:

What assumptions are made when extracting information from an **oesophageal doppler**?

- **S**troke volume: 70% of SV enters the descending aorta (SV = velocity-time integral × CSA).
- **C**ross section area (CSA): The aortic cross-sectional area remains constant throughout systole.
- **R**ed cells: All RBCs are moving at maximum velocity and flow in the descending aorta is laminar.
- **A**orta: The aorta is a uniform cylinder, the ratio ascending:descending aortic flow is fixed, and the descending aorta runs parallel to the oesophagus.
- **P**robe: The probe placement is optimal.
- **E**xtrapolation: The nomogram accurately calculates true aortic cross-sectional area.
- **D**iastole: There is no diastolic aortic blood flow.

Fact 621:

What is the significance of a narrowed pulse pressure in **haemorrhagic shock**?

- Indicates significant blood loss
- Occurs just before a significant ↓ in BP

Blood loss causes ↑ sympathetic activity and ↓ vagal tone. This results in ↑ cardiac output and ↑ SVR. BP falls when blood loss exceeds these compensatory mechanisms.

Fact 622:

What are diagnostic criteria to detect **acute kidney injury (AKI)**?

Any of the following criteria:

- ↑ Creatinine by ≥26 micromol/L within 48 hours
- ↑ Creatinine by 50% in seven days
- ↓ UO < 0.5 mL/kg/hr for >6 hours

Fact 623:

What is the target of the antibodies in **anti-GBM disease (Goodpasture's syndrome)**?

Type 4 collagen in the glomerulus and alveolar basement membranes

- This is a small vessel vasculitis which can lead to rapidly progressive glomerulonephritis and diffuse alveolar haemorrhage.
- The diagnosis is made through immunology +/− a renal biopsy.
- Treatment is with PLEX and immunosuppression.

Fact 624:

How do you diagnose **diabetes insipidus** biochemically in someone with polyuria and dehydration?

↑ Plasma osmolality
↑ Serum sodium
↓ Urine osmolality
↓ Urinary specific gravity <1.005

Note that cerebral salt wasting syndrome (CSWS), furosemide and mannitol can also cause polyuria and dehydration, but with different biochemical changes:

- CSWS and furosemide-induced diuresis: ↓ serum sodium and ↓ plasma osmolality
- Mannitol-induced diuresis: ↓ serum sodium and ↑ plasma osmolality

Fact 625:

Using the **rule of nines**, what is the TBSA involved if the entire anterior torso, face and the front of both arms are burnt in an adult?

Anterior torso = 18%

Face = 4.5% (head is 9% so face is half of this)

Right arm = 4.5% (arm is 9% so 1 side is half of this)

Left arm = 4.5% (arm is 9% so 1 side is half of this)

18% + 4.5% + 4.5% + 4.5% = **31.5% TBSA burn**

Fact 626:

What is the likely cause of the **collapse** in an individual who was found cyanotic, had a small brown bottle in their pocket, an SpO_2 of 85%, and a methaemoglobin concentration of 25%?

Ingestion of a volatile nitrite (e.g. amyl nitrite)

- Nitrites oxidise haemoglobin from its ferrous (Fe^{2+}) state to its ferric (Fe^{3+}) state, resulting in the formation of methaemoglobin (MetHb).
- MetHb does not bind oxygen, which leads to a functional anaemia. MetHb also shifts the oxygen–haemoglobin dissociation curve to the left, which results in ↓ off-loading of oxygen to tissues.
- Its absorbance closely resembles that of an SpO_2 of 85% in the absence of methaemoglobin.
- Treatment is with oxygen and methylthioninium chloride (methylene blue) as a reducing agent.

Fact 627:

Why does **fluconazole** increase the INR in someone who takes warfarin for atrial fibrillation?

Fluconazole is a strong cP450 inhibitor for which warfarin is a substrate.

Fact 628:

What systolic BP target is recommended for someone with a **subarachnoid haemorrhage**, an unprotected aneurysm and intermittent seizures?

Systolic BP < 160 mmHg

Anticonvulsants are used for to treat secondary seizures, but the use of prophylactic anticonvulsants is discouraged as it may lead to a worse outcome.

Fact 629:

According to NICE guidelines, when would you consider giving **activated charcoal** to someone with a paracetamol overdose?

One hour within ingestion of >150 mg/kg paracetamol

Paracetamol levels should be taken at ≥4 hours. If the level is above the treatment normogram, give NAC.

NAC should be given empirically if:

- Presentation ≥ 8 hours after ingestion
- Paracetamol level is not available within an 8-hour time window
- There is uncertainty as to the timing of the overdose
- Patients are unconscious

Fact 630:

What is a **Caldicott Guardian**?

- A person responsible for protecting the confidentiality of patient information and making sure it is used properly.
- All NHS organisations should have one.
- They oversee the upholding of the eight Caldicott principles to ensure proper handling and preservation of patient information. These principles also apply to the deceased, as confidentiality continues after death.

Fact 631:

What International Society on Thrombosis and Haemostasis (ISTH) score suggests a diagnosis of **disseminated intravascular coagulation (DIC)**?

The ISTH group produced a simple scoring system depending on the platelet count, prothrombin time, fibrinogen level and FDP/D-Dimer results.

A total score of ≥5 is diagnostic for DIC. A total score ≤5 is negative for DIC, but a patient could still have 'non-overt DIC' or 'early DIC' which could later evolve into frank DIC.

Fact 632:

What is the mechanism of action of **heparin** as an anticoagulant?

- Heparin binds to antithrombin III
- The heparin–antithrombin complex inactivates factor 2a (thrombin) and factor 10a
  - o Thrombin cannot convert fibrinogen to fibrin.
  - o Factor 10a cannot convert prothrombin to thrombin.

Fact 633:

What is the definition of **massive haemoptysis**?

No universally accepted definition. Examples include:

- 100 mL in one episode
- 1,000 mL in 24 hours
- Life-threatening volume due to airway obstruction or blood loss

Ninety percent occurs from the bronchial circulation (higher pressure than pulmonary circulation). Death results from asphyxiation.

There are lots of causes including bronchiectasis, tuberculosis, lung cancer and vasculitis (e.g. granulomatosis with polyangiitis). Investigations to identify the source include CXR, bronchoscopy, CT and angiography.

Fact 634:

In what situations would you opt for an **analysis of variance (ANOVA)** instead of a t-test?

ANOVA is a statistical technique that is used to check if the means of 2 or more groups are significantly different from each other. ANOVA assumes that the variable is normally distributed.

A t-test can perform a similar comparison, but it's only suitable when there are two groups. If there are more than two groups, a t-test would not be reliable.

Fact 635:

What is the most likely diagnosis if someone has dyspnoea, hypotension (80/60), distended neck veins and a harsh systolic murmur five days after an **anterior MI**, along with pulmonary venous congestion on CXR, a PA pressure of 50/23 and PA SaO$_2$ of 90%?

Ventricular septal rupture – which results in L → R shunt

- Shunt → ↑ RV volume overload → ↑ pulmonary blood flow → secondary LV volume overload
- Shunt → ↑ RV and PA oxygen saturation (mixed venous oxygen is usually around 70%)

Fact 636:

How do **organophosphates** cause their toxic effects?

Irreversibly bind to acetylcholinesterase in the synaptic clefts to prevent the breakdown of acetylcholine (Ach). This results in synaptic overstimulation:

Overstimulation of muscarinic AChRs	Overstimulation of nicotinic AChRs
Salivation **L**acrimation **U**rination **D**efecation **G**I cramps **E**mesis	• Involuntary twitching • Fasciculations • Weakness Can be misdiagnosed as a myasthenic crisis

Note that atropine competitively inhibits the effects of cholinesterase inhibitors at muscarinic, but not nicotinic cholinergic receptors.

Fact 637:

Why might an **external ventricular drain (EVD)** be indicated in an acute subarachnoid haemorrhage (SAH)?

Acute hydrocephalus occurs in about 20% of SAHs

An EVD drains CSF to ↓ intracranial pressure and is the gold standard intracranial pressure monitoring device.

Fact 638:

Which **Korotkoff sounds** are important in measuring NIBP?

The cuff is inflated until there are no sounds and then slowly deflated at about 2 mmHg/s:

- First Korotkoff sound: Indicates the SBP when blood begins to flow through the brachial artery.
- Fifth Korotkoff sound: Indicates the DBP where there is loss of all sound.

The BP cuff should be 20% wider than the arm's diameter, with its centre positioned over the brachial artery. Small cuffs overestimate BP and large cuffs underestimate BP.

When using a mercury manometer, ensure it is vertical with unobstructed tubes and vents. Aneroid gauges require regular calibration.

Fact 639:

What characteristics of an intracranial aneurysm favour neurosurgical **clipping** over coiling?

- Middle cerebral artery territory aneurysm
- Aneurysms with a broad neck
- Aneurysms in close proximity to arterial tributaries

Fact 640:

What is the **LEMON tool** for assessing difficult intubation?

L	Look	Check for facial trauma, large incisors, beard or moustache, large tongue
E	Evaluate 3–3–2	• *Inter-incisor distance:* Mouth opened adequately to allow **3** fingers between the upper and lower teeth • *Hyomental distance:* **3** finger breadths • *Thyromental distance:* **2** finger breadths
M	Mallampati	Class I, II, III, IV
O	Obstruction	Check for stridor, foreign bodies and other forms of sub- and supraglottic obstructions including tumours, abscesses, inflamed epiglottis or enlarging hematomas
N	Neck mobility	Assessed by ability to touch chin to chest and extend neck to view the ceiling

Fact 641:

How might **CMV infection** manifest in adults?

- In immunocompetent individuals, it is usually asymptomatic and seropositivity ↑ with age.
- It can mimic infectious mononucleosis like EBV.
- Reactivation can impact various systems, including Guillain–Barré syndrome (GBS), graft-versus-host disease (GvHD) and retinitis. This may happen in immunocompromised individuals (e.g. transplant recipients, HIV, SLE) or in immunocompetent individuals with critical illness.

Fact 642:

How would you initially manage someone with **sepsis** who is hypotensive (70/40) despite a noradrenaline infusion running at 0.32 mcg/kg/minute and has cool peripheries, a lactate of 7 mmol/L, $S_{cv}O2$ of 70%, CVP of 2 mmHg and a non-invasive cardiac index of 2.4 L/min/m²?

IV fluid challenge – this is septic shock.

- The cool peripheries and ↑ lactate suggest an ↑ SVR
- The ↓ CVP suggests ↓ preload which accounts for the borderline ↓ CI
- The $S_{cv}O2$ is largely normal

Fact 643:

What are some signs of **elevated ICP** on a CT scan?

- Brain parenchymal herniation
- Compression of ventricles and midline shift
- Sulci flattening/effacement
- Features of diffuse brain injury

Loss of grey/white matter differentiation is a sign of cerebral oedema and may also suggest an elevated ICP.

Fact 644:

What are some of the characteristic metabolic derangements seen in **rhabdomyolysis**?

- High anion gap metabolic acidosis (HAGMA)
- ↑ Potassium
- ↑ Uric acid
- ↑ Phosphate

Rhabdomyolysis is breakdown of skeletal muscle, e.g. due to ischaemia secondary to vascular obstruction, crush injury, sepsis, hyperthermia, cocaine and amphetamines.

Creatine kinase > 5,000 IU/L is diagnostic.

Early and aggressive fluid resuscitation is key to prevent AKI to achieve a urine output of 1–3 mL/kg/hr. A fasciotomy may be required in compartment syndrome.

Fact 645:

What is the basic pathophysiology of **oxygen toxicity**?

- Occurs when reactive oxygen species (ROS) overwhelm the body's natural antioxidant defence system.
- Continued exposure to high concentrations of oxygen results in heightened free radical production.
- It manifests in three major forms: Neurological, pulmonary and ocular.

Fact 646:

How does **tranexamic acid (TXA)** work?

Antifibrinolytic

- TXA is a synthetic reversible competitive inhibitor to the lysine receptor found on plasminogen.
- Normally plasminogen is converted to plasmin which breaks down fibrin to degradation products.
- When TXA binds to the lysine receptors, it prevents the conversion of plasminogen to plasmin. This therefore prevents the breakdown of fibrin and ultimately stabilises the fibrin matrix.

Fact 647:

Which agents may be effective against **Vancomycin-resistant Enterococcus (VRE)** and **Carbapenemase-producing Enterobacteriaceae (CPE)**?

VRE	CPE
• Linezolid • Tigecycline • Daptomycin	• Polymyxins (e.g. colistin) • Tigecycline • Fosfomycin • Aminoglycosides (e.g. gentamicin)

Fact 648:

What are the components of the modified Duke criteria for diagnosing **infective endocarditis (IE)**?

Major criteria	Minor criteria ('TRIBE')
Positive blood cultures consistent with IE Evidence of endocardial involvement on echo	**T**emperature > 38°C
	Risk factor: Known cardiac lesion, recreational drug injection
	Immunological problems, e.g. Osler's nodes, Roth's spots, glomerulonephritis
	Blood cultures that are atypical
	Embolic phenomena, e.g. Janeway lesions, arterial emboli, pulmonary infarcts

Diagnosis: 2 major, 1 major + 3 minor, or 5 minor criteria

Fact 649:

What is the **total body surface area (TBSA) burn** in a five-year-old with facial, chest and abdominal burns?

Face = 9% (rather than 4.5% in adult)

Anterior Torso = 18%

Therefore, TBSA burn = 9 + 18 = 27%

(A severe burn in a child < 10 years is ≥20% TBSA)

Fact 650:

What is the **GRACE (Global Registry of Acute Coronary Events) score** used for?

- To risk stratify in NSTEMI/unstable angina
- Determines future adverse cardiovascular events and prediction of six-month mortality

Fact 651:

How would you manage someone with a background of alcohol excess who has a self-limiting **tonic-clonic seizure** in the emergency department and now has a GCS of E3V2M4 with a blood glucose of 3.5 mmol/L?

Treat hypoglycaemia + give IV vitamin supplementation– this is likely to be an alcohol withdrawal fit

Traditional teaching advises against treating hypoglycaemia before administering thiamine to prevent precipitating Wernicke's encephalopathy. The concern is that providing glucose to hypoglycaemic alcoholics may deplete their remaining thiamine reserves. While this has been observed in prolonged TPN administration without thiamine supplementation, there are no reported cases of a single glucose bolus causing Wernicke's. Therefore, do not to delay treatment of hypoglycemia.

Fact 652:

What is the diagnostic triad of **diabetic ketoacidosis** and what are the targets of treatment?

Diagnostic triad	Targets
• Blood glucose >11.0 mmol/L	• ↓ Blood glucose by 3 mmol/L/hr
• Ketonaemia ≥ 3.0 mmol/L or ketonuria > 2+	• ↓ Ketones by 0.5 mmol/L/hr
• Bicarbonate <15.0 mmol/L +/or venous pH <7.3	• ↑ Bicarbonate by 3 mmol/L/hr

Fact 653:

In which contexts is **pulse pressure variation (PPV)** not valid as a dynamic measure of fluid responsiveness?

- Spontaneously breathing
- Presence of arrhythmias, e.g. atrial fibrillation
- ↓ Tidal volumes and lung compliance

PPV > 13% in a mechanically ventilated patient in sinus rhythm is a sensitive and specific indicator of a positive response to a fluid challenge.

Fact 654:

How would you treat a confused patient with a **corrected calcium** of 3.20 mmol/L that has not improved after 3 L of 0.9% NaCl over 24 hours?

IV bisphosphonate

The principles of managing hypercalcaemia include:

- Avoid drugs that contribute to hypercalcaemia, e.g. thiazides, lithium, vitamin D supplements
- First line: IV fluids, e.g. 1 L NaCl 0.9% every 6–8 hours. Furosemide may be used in select cases to promote urinary calcium excretion or to manage volume overload.
- Second line: If calcium remains >3 mmol/L, drugs to inhibit osteoclast-mediated bone resorption are indicated:
  o Bisphosphonates, e.g. pamidronate, zolendronic acid
  o Calcitonin when bisphosphonates don't work
- Treating the cause, e.g. chemotherapy for malignancies, steroids for sarcoidosis, surgery for primary hyperparathyroidism
- For severe refractory hypercalcaemia, haemodialysis may be required with adjustment of calcium in the dialysate.

Fact 655:

What is the best step to manage a haemodynamically unstable patient who has an **open-book pelvic fracture**?

External binder – this stabilises the fracture, ↓ volume of disrupted pelvic ring and tamponades bleeding.

This is time-critical as the primary mechanism of death within 24 hours is exsanguination.

An open-book pelvic fracture is disruption of the pelvic ring with widening of the symphysis pubis. ↑ Degree of disruption → ↑ haemorrhage from damaged vessels and cancellous bone fragments (venous > arterial bleeding).

- If stability is achieved with a pelvic binder, then further imaging may be appropriate and consideration of other injuries, e.g. spinal, bowel, bladder and urethral
- If remains unstable, rapid intervention, e.g. external pelvic fixation or angio-embolisation, along with transfusion, are recommended.

Fact 656:

What are the three most common opportunistic infections in the ICU in someone with **AIDS**?

- *Pneumocystis jirovecii* pneumonia
- Tuberculosis
- Cerebral toxoplasmosis

Fact 657:

How is **cardiac output** derived using a pulmonary artery catheter?

Using the thermodilution principle

- A cold saline bolus is injected through a port 10 cm proximal to the tip.
- A thermistor at the tip monitors the resultant change in blood temperature.
- The Stewart–Hamilton equation is applied to the resulting curve to calculate the cardiac output (CO).
- CO is inversely proportional to area under the curve.

Fact 658:

How does hypoventilation and high altitude influence the **alveolar PO₂ (P_AO_2)**?

Both lower the alveolar PO₂ according the alveolar gas equation:

$$P_AO_2 = [F_iO_2(P_{ATM} - P_{H2O})] - \frac{P_ACO_2}{Respiratory\ quotient}$$

- Hypoventilation: ↑ alveolar pCO_2
- Altitude: ↓ atmospheric pressure

Fact 659:

What is the treatment of choice for **CMV infections** that do not respond to ganciclovir?

Foscarnet – this is a reversible non-competitive inhibitor of DNA polymerase

It is used in resistant CMV or HSV infections. One of its concerning side effects is nephrotoxicity.

Fact 660:

What is **heliox (HeO_2)**?

- HeO_2 is an oxygen–helium mixture, usually supplied as a 20:80 or 30:70 percentage mixture.
- This mixture has a lower density compared to normal room air.
- The ↓ density of heliox leads to ↓ resistance to gas flow in areas where flow is turbulent.
- Turbulent flow is generally found in larger airways, while smaller airways experience laminar flow, which is determined by Reynold's number.
- Diseases which affect larger airways may ↑ resistance to turbulent flow, thereby increasing the work of breathing.
- Therefore, HeO_2 is traditionally used in upper airway obstruction or narrowing to ↓ airway resistance.

Fact 661:

When screening for **inattention** using the CAM-ICU, how many errors rule out delirium?

≤2 errors rule out delirium

The CAM-ICU assessment is as follows:

- Consider whether there is an acute fluctuation in mental status in the past 24 hours. If so, proceed to test for inattention.
- **Inattention**: 'Squeeze my hand when I say the letter "A"', e.g. SAVEAHAART. If there are 0–2 errors, this is not delirium. If there are >2 errors, then proceed to test for an altered level of consciousness with the RASS.
- **Altered level of consciousness**: If the RASS is anything other than zero, then the patient has delirium. If the RASS is 0, then proceed to test for disorganised thinking.
- **Disorganised thinking** is tested using questions or commands, e.g. 'Will a stone float on water?' and 'Are there fish in the sea?'
- If the patient makes more than one error, then they have delirium. If they make ≤ 1 errors, this is not delirium.

Fact 662:

What causes **Brown–Sequard syndrome** and what are its clinical features?

Lateral hemisection of the spinal cord, e.g. due to trauma, malignancy or multiple sclerosis

Ipsilateral	Contralateral
UMN weakness (corticospinal tract) Loss of proprioception and vibration sense (dorsal column)	Loss of pain and temperature (crossed spinothalamic tracts)

Fact 663:

What is the **Marshall classification** of traumatic brain injury (TBI)?

- A CT-derived metric to predict outcome in TBI.
- The metrics can be recalled using **'BEDS'**:
  o **B**asal cistern involvement
  o **E**vacuation of lesions
  o **D**ensity of mass lesions
  o **S**hift in midline
- There are six grades (I–VI)
- The higher the Marshall grade, the worse the outcome.

Fact 664:

What are some purposes or objectives of using **scoring systems** in critical care?

- **T**ailor treatment, e.g. eligibility for transplantation
- **R**isk of death, e.g. P-POSSUM
- **A**udit/research to compare ICU performance, e.g. ICNARC, and to match populations for clinical studies
- **P**redict survival, morbidity or mortality in populations, e.g. APACHE can be used retrospectively
- **S**everity of illness in individual patients, e.g. GCS

Fact 665:

What are some causes of **metabolic alkalosis**?

- Loss of gastric acid, e.g. prolonged vomiting, NGT aspiration/suction
- Mineralocorticoid excess, e.g. Conn's syndrome
- Glucocorticoid excess, e.g. Cushing's syndrome
- Diuretic therapy
- Severe and prolonged potassium deficiency
- Exogenous alkali, e.g. sodium bicarbonate infusion

Fact 666:

What is the commonest late complication of **tracheostomy**?

Tracheal stenosis – narrowing is most commonly at the level of the stoma or directly above it.

Infection-related chondritis or tracheal wall ischaemia → granulation tissue → weakening of the anterior and lateral walls → fibrosis and stenosis

Risk factors: Prolonged intubation prior to stoma formation, stomal site infection, older age, ↑ illness severity, oversized cannulae and excessive tube motion

May be asymptomatic until 75% narrowing. Can present with failure to wean from ventilation. Other features include cough, inability to clear secretions, dyspnoea and stridor.

Fact 667:

What is the impact of raised glucose on **serum sodium**?

↑ Glucose can give a false impression of hyponatraemia (pseudohyponatraemia).

Sodium levels can be corrected by using the following formula (all in mmol/L):

True Na⁺ = Measured Na⁺ + 2.4(glucose − 5.5)

Fact 668:

What are the benefits of **prone positioning**?

Ventilation	Perfusion
• More homogenous distribution of ventilation resulting from improved thoraco-abdominal compliance. • More uniform distribution of alveolar pressure, reducing the likelihood of vulnerable lung units collapsing during expiration. • Prevention of compression of posterior lung units by the dependent heart. • ↑ Alveolar recruitment • Better drainage of secretions	• More homogenous distribution of perfusion • In a semi-recumbent position, perfusion and atelectasis are most prominent at the lung bases, while proning shifts perfusion to better-aerated regions. • Possible ↓ in extra-vascular lung water

Fact 669:

What is meant by **afterdrop** in re-warming?

A further fall in temperature after re-warming

Rewarming → peripheral vasodilation → release of cold peripheral blood to core → drop in core temperature

Fact 670:

What is the most common complication observed following the insertion of a **pulmonary artery catheter** through the internal jugular vein?

Colonisation of the catheter with skin commensal bacteria, e.g. *Staphylococcus aureus* and *Staphylococcus epidermidis*.

Following this are complications such as carotid artery puncture and an arrhythmia which requires treatment.

Fact 671:

When is rhythm-control first line for **atrial fibrillation/flutter**?

- AF is new.
- It has a reversible cause.
- It is the primary cause of heart failure.
- It may be amenable to ablation (flutter).

Fact 672:

How does lactate correlate with survival post-**ROSC**?

Initial lactate and rate of lactate clearance correlate with survival.

Fact 673:

What pattern of weakness in the motor system would someone develop if they had **spinal cord compression** above the level of C5?

Spastic quadriparesis

There will be spasticity, brisk reflexes and upper motor neuron distribution of weakness affecting all four limbs, with extensor plantar responses.

Fact 674:

What is **Grey Turner's sign** and what causes it?

Flank bruising following retroperitoneal bleeding. It takes approximately 24–48 hours to appear.

Causes of retroperitoneal haemorrhage:

- **S**pontaneous on blood thinners
- **H**aemorrhagic pancreatitis
- **I**R, e.g. after femoral artery cannulation
- **R**uptured AAA
- **T**rauma

Fact 675

What happens to the serum calcium in **rhabdomyolysis**?

- Early: ↓ calcium (binding to phosphate in the ECF)
- Late: ↑ calcium (impaired excretion)

Fact 676:

How does **dobutamine** work, why is it useful in acute heart failure and why can it precipitate arrhythmias?

ß$_1$ agonist	• ↑ Systolic and diastolic function → ↑ CI and ↓ LVEDP • ↑ HR and AV conduction → arrhythmias, e.g. AF	
ß$_2$ agonist (mild)	↓ SVR → ↓ BP	At therapeutic doses, these effects balance each other out and have little effect on SVR
α$_1$ agonist (mild)	↑ SVR → ↑ BP	

Fact 677:

What dose of **nebulised adrenaline** can you use in the management of haemoptysis?

1 mL of 1:1,000 mixed with 4 mL of NaCl 0.9%

Fact 678:

How do you manage **thyroid storm**?

- *Supportive measures*: Cooling, electrolyte optimisation, hydration, treating the cause
- Anti-thyroid medication:
  - *Propylthiouracil*: Blocks T3/T4 production and ↓ peripheral conversion of T4 to T3. Potassium iodide or Lugol's solution is given approximately 1 hour after administration. This blocks further release of hormones from the thyroid gland.
  - Carbimazole blocks T3/T4 production and can be used instead. It is not used in the first trimester due to the risk of congenital defects.
- *Corticosteroids*: This is a glucocorticoid-deficient state and correction of thyrotoxicosis may precipitate an Addisonian crisis. They also ↓ peripheral conversion of T4 to T3.
- Beta-blockade (e.g. propranolol or metoprolol) to control sympathetic effects. They also ↓ peripheral conversion of T4 to T3.
- Dantrolene and PLEX may be considered in some cases.

Fact 679:

How can you clinically differentiate between **coma, a vegetative state (VS)** and **a minimally conscious state (MCS)** following an acute brain injury?

- *Coma*: Absent wakefulness + absent awareness
- *Vegetative state*: Wakefulness + absent awareness (secondary to bilateral cortical damage but preservation of brainstem)
- *Minimally conscious state*: Wakefulness + minimal awareness (secondary to global neuronal damage)

	Coma	VS	MCS
Eye opening		Yes	Yes
Sleep wake cycles		Yes	Yes
Visual tracking			Often
Following commands	No		
Contingent emotion		No	Inconsistent
Object recognition			
Communication			

Many will progress through stages of coma, VS and MCS before they emerge into a state of full awareness. Some, however, will remain in either a VS or MCS for the rest of their lives.

Fact 680:

What is the difference between a **full, partial and inverse agonist**?

Full agonist	Partial agonist	Inverse agonist
Binds to receptors (has affinity) and produces a maximal response (efficacy = 1)	Binds to receptors (has affinity) but produces a sub-maximal response (efficacy < 1)	Bind to receptors (has affinity) but produces the opposite effect to the endogenous agonist (efficacy = −1)
e.g. morphine acting on MOP receptors	e.g. buprenorphine acting on MOP receptors	e.g. naloxone acting on MOP receptors in morphine pre-treated tissues

Fact 681:

How does **positive pressure ventilation** affect pulmonary blood flow?

↑ Intrathoracic pressure → ↓ venous return → ↓ RV output → ↓ pulmonary blood flow

Fact 682:

How do you classify **hypothermia** based on temperature?

Mild	<35°C	Shivering absent < 32°C
Moderate	<32°C	Pupils fixed and dilated < 30°C
Severe	<28°C	VF and loss of brainstem reflexes < 28°C Asystole < 25°C

Fact 683:

Which glycoprotein changes in the **influenza** virus are responsible for epidemics and pandemics?

Influenza epidemics	Influenza pandemics
• Seasonal outbreaks • Caused by **antigen drift**–minor changes in the viral hemagglutinin (HA) and neuraminidase (NA) • Causes less severe disease in people who have been exposed to the antecedent virus	• Rapid and worldwide spread • Occurs when a Type A virus undergoes a major change (**antigen shift**) due to acquisition of new gene segments. This creates a strain to which the majority of the population do not have immunity.

Fact 684:

What is the risk of over-draining a **large pleural effusion**?

Re-expansion pulmonary oedema

Preventive strategies include limiting drainage of pleural fluid, e.g. 1.0–1.5 L at a time, and using low negative pressure for suction (≤ −10 to 20 cmH$_2$O) during thoracentesis.

Fact 685:

What are some extra-articular complications of **rheumatoid arthritis**?

- Pancarditis: Pericarditis, myocarditis and endocarditis
- Lower lobe fibrosis
- Peripheral neuropathy
- Raynaud's phenomenon
- Felty's Syndrome (presence of HLA-DR4) and ↑ risk of infection:
  - o **S**plenomegaly
  - o **A**naemia
  - o **N**eutropenia
  - o **T**hrombocytopenia
  - o **A**NA positive in 90% of patients

Fact 686:

What causes the normal **anion gap**?

Serum albumin and phosphate

- Albumin is the major unmeasured anion and contributes to most of the anion gap.
- Every 1 g/L ↓ in albumin will ↓ anion gap by 0.25 mmol/L, e.g. a high anion gap metabolic acidosis in someone with hypoalbuminaemia may appear as a normal anion gap acidosis.

Fact 687:

What are some common neurological complications of **subarachnoid haemorrhage**?

- *Hydrocephalus (≤72 hours)*: More common in severe grades, especially in those with ↑ 'blood load'
- *Rebleeding (≤72 hours)*: Highest risk immediately after the aneurysm rupture, decreasing over time. Promptly securing the aneurysm is crucial to minimise this risk.
- *Delayed cerebral ischaemia (DCI)*: Any neurological deterioration lasting > 1 hour due to ischaemia. It can result from microvascular thrombosis or cerebral vasospasm (which typically manifests between day 3 and day 10, resolving by day 21).
- Additional potential complications include haematoma formation, seizures, ↑ ICP and cerebral oedema.

Fact 688:

What are the contraindications to treatment with **adenosine** for a narrow complex tachycardia?

- Asthma (and sometimes severe COPD)
- Decompensated heart failure
- Long QT syndrome
- Second- or third-degree heart block
- Sick sinus syndrome
- Severe hypotension – should be considering DC cardioversion rather than adenosine

Fact 689:

How does a **Passy–Muir Valve (PMV)** work on a tracheostomy?

It is a one-way valve which stays closed until the patient inhales.

It opens easily at the start of inspiration and automatically closes at the end of inspiration, without requiring the patient to exert effort during expiration.

During expiration, the valve redirects air through the vocal cords, mouth and nose → ↑ voice, ↑ olfaction and management of secretions.

Fact 690:

Can you use CPAP during **brainstem testing** if apnoeic oxygenation is a problem?

Yes

Fact 691:

What are the effects of theophylline and dipyridamole on the use of **adenosine**?

- *Theophylline*: ↓ effect of adenosine.
- *Dipyridamole*: ↑ effect of adenosine.

Fact 692:

What are the current recommendations for starting **highly active antiretroviral therapy (HAART)** in someone who is found to be HIV positive?

HAART should be initiated within seven days of a confirmed HIV diagnosis and detectable virology, regardless of CD4 count or clinical symptoms.

Early HAART initiation has been shown to ↓ severe AIDS and AIDS-associated illnesses.

Fact 693:

What happens to the awareness and wakefulness in **locked-in syndrome**?

Awareness and wakefulness are preserved.

Blinking and vertical eye movement are intact but there are no other voluntary movements (paralysis).

Occurs due to a bilateral pontine lesion transecting descending pathways, e.g. central pontine myelinosis or basilar artery thrombosis. Ascending and reticular activating system pathways are unaffected, the cortex is intact and an EEG will be normal.

Fact 694:

What is the value of **NT pro-BNP** testing for the diagnosis of heart failure in critical care?

- A normal NT pro-BNP in the untreated patient has an ↑ negative predictive value, so it is useful for ruling out heart failure.
- NT pro-BNP has a ↓ specificity in the critical care population therefore a high level is not diagnostic for heart failure.

Fact 695:

When can a **paradoxical CO_2 embolism** occur during laparoscopic surgery?

If there is intracardiac communication, e.g. a patent foramen ovale (PFO)

- During laparoscopic surgery, CO_2 creates a surgical field (pneumoperitoneum).
- It can enter abdominal vessels and reach the right heart.
- If there is a PFO, CO_2 may shift to the left heart and can potentially embolise to the systemic circulation.
- CO_2 embolisation is short-lived due to its high water solubility, leading to rapid absorption into the blood.

Fact 696:

How does the **Sickledex** test work?

- It is a qualitative screening test to detect HbS.
- When the reagent is added, it forms a cloudy, turbid suspension if HbS is present.
- This is present in either Sickle Cell Disease (S/S) or Sickle Cell Trait (A/S). It does not differentiate between these two, it simply detects the presence of HbS.
- If there is turbidity, then Hb electrophoresis is performed to determine the nature of the haemoglobinopathy.

Fact 697:

In which condition do you get a **sudden painless loss of vision** and severe retinal haemorrhages on fundoscopy?

Central retinal vein occlusion

Venous occlusion → ↑ venous pressure within the eyes → optic nerve swelling and venous haemorrhage

If only a segment of the retinal is affected, it is called branch retinal vein occlusion (BRVO).

- *Causes*: Glaucoma, polycythaemia, diabetes and hypertension
- *Complications*: Macular oedema and rubeosis iridis (neovascular glaucoma)
- *Treatment*: Prompt referral to ophthalmologist for possible laser photocoagulation therapy

Fact 698:

If someone is tested positive for both **HIV** and tuberculosis, which one would you treat first and why?

Anti-tuberculosis treatment should be started before anti-retrovirals. Starting anti-retrovirals first would ↑ the risk of immune reconstitution inflammatory syndrome (IRIS).

Fact 699:

What happens to the **haematocrit** in pregnancy?

↓ Haematocrit because there is a dilutional anaemia:

- ↑ Plasma volume by 50%
- ↑ RBC mass by 30%

Fact 700:

Why are younger children at a higher risk of **airway obstruction** when lying flat, like on a spinal board?

Relatively large occiput

The very short cricothyroid membrane also makes needle/surgical cricothyroidotomy difficult.

Fact 701:

What are some of the risk factors for developing **spontaneous bacterial peritonitis (SBP)**?

- Prior episode
- GI bleeding
- Ascitic protein < 1.0 g/dL
- Child-Pugh score

Fact 702:

What is the classical triad of **fat embolism syndrome (FES)**?

1	Hypoxaemia	Dyspnoea, tachypnoea, hypoxaemia, ARDS
2	Neurological features	Confusion, lethargy, agitation, coma, Purtscher's retinopathy, seizures, focal deficit
3	Petechiae	Petechial rash in non-dependent regions (conjunctivae, head, neck, axillae, thorax)

The classic triad may not always be present, and presentations can range from subclinical to multi-organ dysfunction and death.

It is a clinical diagnosis typically 12–72 hours after an identifiable insult, often related to fat release into the circulation (e.g. fractures in high yellow marrow areas like femoral or pelvic bones). Various scoring systems can assist in diagnosis.

Other features include:

- Pyrexia
- *Eyes*: Fluffy retinal exudates
- *CVS*: ↑ HR, RV dysfunction, biventricular failure, shock
- *Renal*: Oliguria, lipiduria, proteinuria, haematuria, hypocalcaemia
- Coagulation abnormalities which mimic DIC

Fact 703:

What does a **sentinel loop** signify on abdominal imaging, and what may cause this to occur in the upper abdomen and right lower quadrant?

A sentinel loop is a short segment of adynamic ileus close to an intra-abdominal inflammatory process. It can be seen both on AXR or CT:

- Upper abdomen: Pancreatitis
- Right lower quadrant: Appendicitis

Fact 704:

What are some of the indications for using **Digibind** in digoxin toxicity?

- Bradyarrhythmias not responsive to atropine
- VT/VF/Cardiac arrest
- Acute digoxin ingestion > 10 mg in adults
- Serum concentration > 15 nmol/mL
- Potassium > 5–6 mmol/L – this is a major concern as it increases the risk of AV block due to changes in the ionic gradient.

Digibind is given as an infusion over 30 minutes, and it typically starts to take effect within about 90 minutes. Following administration, there should be a reduction in all signs and symptoms of toxicity, including improvements in ECG changes.

Fact 705:

What is the most likely diagnosis if a young lady with a known history of **Graves' disease** presents with the following features:

- Agitation, abdominal pain, mild jaundice and diarrhoea.
- She is in fast atrial fibrillation with bibasal crackles and peripheral oedema.
- Her temperature is 39°C.
- LFTs are mildly deranged.
- WCC and CRP are normal.
- Pregnancy test is positive.

Thyroid storm – this is an extreme form of thyrotoxicosis where there is ↓ TSH and ↑ T3/T4.

Thyroid storm can be triggered in those with a background of hyperthyroidism who have been exposed to stressors, e.g. surgery, infection, trauma, myocardial infarction or pregnancy. This results in additional release of thyroid hormones to cause a hypermetabolic state:

- *CNS*: Agitation, delirium or psychosis
- *CVS*: High-output failure, atrial arrhythmias, hypertension (or hypotension)
- *Liver dysfunction*: Due to heart failure or the effect of excess thyroid hormones on the liver
- *GIT*: Nausea, vomiting, diarrhoea and abdominal pain

Fact 706:

How would you manage **abdominal compartment syndrome** in a post-laparotomy patient with ileus?

↑ Abdominal wall compliance

- ↑ sedation/analgesia/paralysis
- Reverse Trendelenburg positioning

↓ Intraluminal contents:

- ↓/stop enteral feeding
- Consider prokinetics
- Consider decompression with Ryle's/ rectal tube

Optimise regional perfusion:

- Avoid excess IV fluids as this can ↑ IAP
- Consider fluid removal (diuresis/RRT)
- Use noradrenaline to ↑ MAP (aim APP > 60 mmHg)

If this fails, consider surgical review for a decompressive laparotomy.

Fact 707:

What is the difference between a **persistent** and **permanent vegetative state**?

- *Persistent*: Vegetative stage for > 1 month
- *Permanent*: Vegetative stage for > 12 months

The prognosis is worse with a metabolic cause than with a traumatic cause.

Fact 708:

What is the pathophysiology of **thrombotic thrombocytopaenic purpura (TTP)**?

Failure of von Willebrand factor (vWF) breakdown

- vWF is a plasma glycoprotein that is produced in the endothelium as ultra-large multimers. It binds to factor 8 and has a role in activating platelets. It is inactivated when cleaved by ADAMTS13.
- TTP is caused by a deficiency or ↓ activity of ADAMTS13, where vWF multimers are not broken down. This may be genetic or acquired (autoantibody, e.g. malignancy, HIV, pregnancy or drugs).
- The resulting large vWF multimers trigger uncontrolled platelet activation.
- Microclots consume platelets (thrombocytopaenia), occlude small blood vessels and cause distal ischaemia.
- As red blood cells pass through narrowed vessels and the fibrin/ platelet mesh, they are haemolysed (microangiopathic haemolytic anaemia – MAHA).

The classic pentad of TTP is MAHA, thrombocytopenia, renal failure, neurological signs and fever.

Fact 709:

What steps are involved in conducting a **spontaneous breathing trial (SBT)**?

- The patient is allowed to breathe spontaneously. If attached to a ventilator, 'minimal ventilator settings' are used (e.g. PS 5–7 and PEEP 1–5).
- The trial should last 30–120 minutes.
- Objective measures are made of patient comfort and respiratory function.

Fact 710:

Why is nitrite dipstick testing an insensitive indicator of the presence of **bacteriuria**?

Nitrite is formed from the bacterial reduction of urinary nitrates. You need >10,000 bacteria per mL to turn a nitrite dipstick positive. Although 90% of common urinary pathogens are nitrite-forming, 10% have minimal or no nitrite-producing capacity.

Infection with non-nitrate-reducing organisms will result in a negative nitrite test. Therefore, a negative nitrite test does not rule out a UTI, but a positive one may strongly suggest infection.

Fact 711:

What are the leading causes of **maternal death** in the UK, not including COVID-19?

- The most common direct cause is thrombosis and thromboembolism.
- Cardiac disease is the leading indirect cause.
- Mental health-related causes, including suicide, and sepsis are the next most common contributors, representing both direct and indirect causes.

Fact 712:

How can **nerve conduction studies** help to distinguish between demyelinating and axonal lesions?

	Axonal	Demyelinating
	e.g. Critical illness polyneuropathy	e.g. Guillain–Barré syndrome
Amplitudes	**Decreased**	Normal
Distal latency	Normal	**Prolonged**
Conduction velocity	Normal	**Slow**

Fact 713:

What are four significant consequences of **thiamine (vitamin B1) deficiency**?

Dry beriberi	Wet beriberi
• Wasting and partial paralysis resulting from damaged peripheral nerves • Sensory ataxia	• High output cardiac failure • Peripheral oedema
Wernicke's encephalopathy	**Korsakoff's syndrome**
• Ataxia • Ophthalmoplegia • Confusion	Severe memory impairment (damage to areas like the thalamus and mamillary bodies)

Fact 714:

What are five elements of the care bundle to reduce **catheter-related bloodstream infection (CRBSI)** in the Matching Michigan programme?

1. Hand hygiene
2. Strict asepsis with full barrier precautions
3. Use of 2% chlorhexidine in 70% alcohol for skin preparation
4. Avoidance of the femoral route
5. Daily review, with removal of catheters as soon as they are no longer needed

Fact 715:

Through which receptors do **cyclizine**, **metoclopramide** and **ondansetron** mediate their antiemetic effects?

Cyclizine	Histamine receptors	H_1 receptors
	Acetylcholine receptors	Muscarinic receptors
Metoclo-pramide	Dopamine receptors	D_2 receptors
	Serotonin receptors	5-HT_4 receptors
Ondan-setron	Serotonin receptors	5-HT_3 receptors

Fact 716:

What are some risks of performing CPR in an **LVAD recipient**?

- Cannula dislodgement
- Anastomotic rupture

Chest compressions may not be effective. Current evidence is limited. It should be considered if attempts to restart or troubleshoot the LVAD fail.

Fact 717:

What pharmacological treatment for secondary prevention should be offered following an **acute coronary syndrome (ACS)**?

1. ACE inhibitor indefinitely. If intolerant, an angiotensin II receptor blocker (ARB) should be offered instead.
2. Beta-blocker indefinitely for ↓ LVEF. In those without ↓ LVEF, the beta-blocker may be discontinued after 12 months. Calcium channel antagonists (verapamil/diltiazem) are given when beta-blockers are contraindicated, provided there is no pulmonary congestion and the LVEF is normal.
3. Dual antiplatelet therapy, unless anticoagulation is indicated for another reason. Aspirin should be continued indefinitely. The second antiplatelet is continued for 12 months unless contraindicated.
4. Statin: High-dose indefinitely unless contraindicated.

Fact 718:

Why is **phenylephrine** useful in managing septic shock in someone with severe aortic stenosis?

Phenylephrine is a pure α_1-agonist and can be run peripherally.

Its two useful effects in this clinical context are as follows:

- ↑ DBP → ↑ coronary perfusion
- Reflex ↓ HR → helps diastolic filling

Fact 719:

What is **distal intestinal obstruction syndrome (DIOS)** in cystic fibrosis (CF)?

DIOS is the result of the accumulation of viscid faecal material within the bowel in CF. The intestine may be completely blocked (complete DIOS) or only partially blocked (incomplete DIOS). Once diagnosed, the goal is to relieve obstruction and prevent the need for surgery.

Mild cases are treated with good hydration, avoiding constipating drugs (e.g. opiates) and using laxatives, enemas and prokinetics. In more severe cases, gastrograffin may be used orally or via NG.

Fact 720:

How does **transducer height** impact on the blood pressure obtained from an arterial line?

- The transducer must be at the level of the patient's right atrium.
- An error reading equivalent to 7.5 mmHg occurs for each 10 cm discrepancy in height
  - Transducer below heart level: Falsely ↑ BP
  - Transducer above heart level: Falsely ↓ BP

Fact 721:

What do the different parameters on a **TEG (thromboelastogram)** indicate?

Parameter	Details
R-time (reaction time) 4–8 minutes	• Time to the first significant clot (fibrin) formation (a 2 mm amplitude on the tracing) • This reflects the concentration of soluble clotting factors in the plasma
K-time (kinetic time) 1–4 minutes	• This is the time for the amplitude of the tracing to increase from 2 to 20 mm (a stronger clot) • It is a measure of clot kinetics • Fibrinogen, platelets and intrinsic clotting factors are implicated
α-angle 47–74°	• This is the angle between a tangent to the tracing at 2 mm amplitude and the horizontal midline • It measures the speed of solid clot formation (the rapidity of fibrinogen build-up and cross-linking) • ↓ Platelets and ↓ fibrinogen can ↓ the angle
The maximum amplitude (MA) 55–73 mm	• This is the greatest vertical width achieved by the tracing • It represents the ultimate strength of the fibrin clot, i.e. overall stability of the clot • Platelet number, function and fibrin interaction are implicated
LY30/60 <7.5%	• % lysis of clot 30/60 minutes after MA • Represents fibrinolysis • When the decrease over 60 minutes is >15% of MA, hyperfibrinolysis is suspected

Fact 722:

How do you reduce the incidence of **Transfusion Related Lung Injury (TRALI)**?

• Universal leucodepletion of units of blood
• Using pooled plasma donations to dilute any antibodies
• The exclusive use of male donors for all FFP and plasma for platelet pools, reducing the transfer of anti-HLA antibodies often found in multiparous women
• Selective screening and excluding donors likely to have anti-leucocyte antigen antibodies

Fact 723:

What are some of the common laboratory findings in **primary acute adrenal insufficiency**?

Sodium			Potassium	
Glucose				
pH		↓	Urea	↑
HCO$_3$			ESR	
Hb (normochromic normocytic)			TSH	
Calcium			Lymphocytes and Eosinophils	

Fact 724:

How do **liver function tests** assist in distinguishing between cholestatic and hepatocellular injuries?

Cholestatic	ALP > 2 × upper limit of normal
	ALT/ALP ratio < 2
Hepatocellular	ALT > 3 × upper limit of normal
	ALT/ALP ratio > 5

Fact 725:

How is the **pulmonary capillary wedge pressure (PCWP)** measured and what does it estimate?

- PCWP is measured by advancing a PA catheter into a small pulmonary artery branch. The balloon is then inflated to allow a static column of blood between the catheter tip and the left atrium.
- PCWP offers insight into left atrial filling pressure, serving as a surrogate for left ventricular end-diastolic pressure (LVEDP). LVEDP, in turn, is utilised as an approximation of left ventricular end-diastolic volume (LVEDV), which represents preload.
- The normal range is about 4–12 mmHg.
- ↑ PCWP may indicate severe left ventricular failure or severe mitral stenosis.
- PCWP is also useful in differentiating cardiogenic shock (PCWP > 15 mmHg) from non-cardiogenic shock (PCWP ≤ 15 mmHg).

Fact 726:

How does **NAC** work in treating a paracetamol overdose?

- Replenishes glutathione stores in the liver
- Acts as a direct reducing agent (sulphhydryl group) directly on NAPQI (N-acetyl-p-benzoquinone imine)

In therapeutic doses, paracetamol is metabolised into glucuronide and sulphate conjugates, which are then excreted in the urine. However, a small amount is converted into NAPQI, a hepatotoxic substance. Normally, NAPQI is detoxified through conjugation with glutathione in the liver.

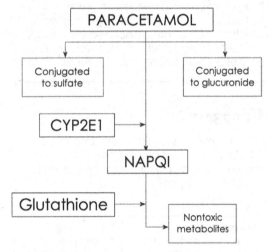

In a paracetamol overdose, glutathione stores are depleted. NAPQI cannot be detoxified, leading to hepatic (centrilobular necrosis) and renal toxicity. NAC replenishes glutathione stores, allowing for the detoxification of NAPQI. Additionally, NAC can directly detoxify NAPQI to some extent.

Fact 727:

How would you treat a young patient with **acute onset AF** without adverse signs?

Cardioversion is desirable and achievable (either chemically or electronically).

Fact 728:

What happens to the barometric pressure, PaO_2 and $PaCO_2$ with **altitude**?

↓ Barometric pressure
↓ PaO_2
↓ $PaCO_2$

Fact 729:

What is the impedance of wet skin compared to dry skin, and what is released into the urine following a **high-voltage electrical injury**?

The impedance of wet skin is 100 times less than dry skin. This allows much greater current to flow for a given voltage. High-voltage electrical injuries are associated with tissue/muscle damage and rhabdomyolysis. This causes myoglobinuria which ↑ the risk of AKI.

Fact 730:

In **pulse oximetry**, which wavelengths of light are absorbed by oxyhaemoglobin and deoxyhaemoglobin, and what is meant by the isobestic point?

660 nm (red light)	Absorbance of deoxyHb > oxyHb	The oximeter determines oxygen saturation by measuring absorbances at specific wavelengths and performing a calculation based on these measurements.
940 nm (infrared)	Absorbance of oxyHb > deoxyHb	
590 nm & 805 nm	Isosbestic points are wavelengths at which the absorption of light is equal for oxyHb and deoxyHb. This is not necessary to calculate oxygen saturation.	

Beer–Lambert's Law relates the concentration of a light-absorbing substance to its absorbance:

$$Absorbance = molar\ absorptivity \times path\ length \times concentration$$

Fact 731:

What is the common reason for patients undergoing **plasma exchange (PLEX)** to experience paraesthesia?

Citrate anticoagulation causes hypocalcaemia.

Fact 732:

What are the features of **post-cardiac arrest syndrome**?

- *Myocardial dysfunction*: Global stunning of the myocardium regardless of aetiology of arrest. This can result in a ↓ cardiac output and cardiogenic shock. Early echocardiography will show very poor function, but this generally improves. Early echocardiography should therefore be avoided unless there is suspicion of valve rupture or a LV aneurysm as a result of the initial insult.
- *Reperfusion syndrome*: All tissues suffer from global hypoperfusion which depends on the duration of downtime, the quality of CPR and peri-arrest hypotension/hypoxia. After ROSC, there is widespread systemic reperfusion. Reperfusion of ischaemic tissues release cytokines and hypoxic metabolites into the circulation. This causes vasoplegia and impaired oxygen utilisation in all tissues. Other effects include activation of coagulation and immunological pathways and adrenal suppression.
- *Hypoxic brain injury*: Hypoxemia results in the primary insult of brain cell apoptosis. Reperfusion disrupts cellular processes which results in a secondary insult through impaired cerebral autoregulation and cerebral oedema. Neuroprotective measures are crucial to avoid further brain insults due to, for example, sustained hypotension, pyrexia, seizures, hyperglycaemia and hyperoxia.

Fact 733:

When would you use antimicrobials in **acute pancreatitis (AP)**?

For infected pancreatic necrosis or for extra-pancreatic infections

Antimicrobials should be considered in AP if there is deterioration after 7–10 days. Procalcitonin can help to differentiate between SIRS and infection. Cultures should be considered, e.g. FNA of necrotic pancreatic tissue. Most evidence is for carbapenems as they penetrate pancreatic necrosis. Antifungals may also be needed.

Fact 734:

What is the mechanism by which hypoxia causes **hypoxic pulmonary vasoconstriction**?

Hypoxia causes:

- ↓ Production of ROS (redox second messengers) by mitochondria in pulmonary artery smooth muscle
- Inhibition of voltage-gated K^+ channels
- Depolarisation of smooth muscle cells
- Activation of L-type calcium channels
- ↑ Cytosolic calcium
- Hypoxic pulmonary vasoconstriction

Fact 735:

What are the typical blood tests that are suggestive of **iron deficiency anaemia**?

↓ MCV, MCH
↓ Ferritin, iron, transferrin saturation
↑ Total iron-binding capacity
↑ Red cell distribution width

Fact 736:

How should you manage someone with severe pre-eclampsia who develops **eclampsia** and has a normal post-seizure cardiotocography?

- 4 g bolus dose of magnesium over 5 minutes.
- Then an infusion at a rate of 1 g/hr for 24 hours.
- Any further seizures should be treated with a bolus dose of 2 g over 5 minutes.

Eclampsia is present when a seizure occurs as a result of pre-eclampsia. The fetus should be delivered once the patient is stabilised and after a course of steroids if appropriate. The mode of delivery is decided on a case-by-case basis. Magnesium may work by preventing cerebral vasospasm through blocking Ca^{2+} influx via NMDA-type glutamate receptors.

Fact 737:

What is the difference between **failure to pace** and **failure to capture** and what are some common causes post-cardiac surgery?

Failure to pace	Failure to capture
No attempt to pace when there should be	The attempt to pace is unsuccessful
There is absence of pacing spikes when the native rate is slower than the set rate	Pacing spikes are present but dissociated from ECG complexes
• **C**ross talk with dual chamber pacing: The atrial pacing spike is misinterpreted as native activity by the ventricular lead, causing it to inhibit ventricular pacing. • **O**ver sensing: Artefact is interpreted as native electrical activity, e.g. respiration, shivering • **L**ead disconnection or malfunction • **D**epletion of battery	• Displaced pacing wires • Alterations in resistance can occur due to electrolyte imbalances, drugs, recent defibrillation, ischaemia or inflammation/fibrosis at the lead tips
Settings on pacemaker are inappropriate	

Fact 738:

What findings on joint aspiration would indicate a possible diagnosis of **septic arthritis**?

- Turbid or purulent synovial fluid
- WCC > 50,000/mm³ (>90% neutrophils)

After confirming the diagnosis and giving antibiotics, joint washout should be performed to prevent damage. Other clues in diagnosis include:

- ↑ CRP: This is sensitive but may be raised for other reasons (therefore it is non-specific).
- Gram stain of joint fluid has a ↑ PPV but a ↓ NPV.
- Fever is common but has a sensitivity of about 57%, so its absence does not exclude the diagnosis.

Fact 739:

What are the features of the **diving reflex**?

Submergence → Trigeminal nerve (ophthalmic branch) → CNS → apnoea, bradycardia and vasoconstriction

- Apnoea prevents aspiration of water.
- Vasoconstriction redirects blood to brain and heart.
- Bradycardia ↓ cardiac oxygen consumption and balances vasoconstriction.

When apnoea stops → involuntary gasping → aspiration

Fact 740:

Which clinical features are suggestive of **ICU-acquired weakness (ICU-AW)**?

Aetiology	Exclusion of alternative causes of weakness not related to critical illness
Onset	Weakness after the onset of critical illness
Distribution	Symmetrical, widespread, flaccid muscle weakness with sparing of the cranial nerves
Duration	Noted > 2 occasions separated by > 24 hours
Effects	Dependence on mechanical ventilation or failure to mobilise

Fact 741:

How do you define **severe aortic stenosis** and why can patients develop syncope during exercise?

- Valve area: <1 cm²
- Mean gradient: >40 mmHg across valve

During exercise, the peripheral vascular system dilates to allow increased blood flow to reach the muscles and the cardiac output usually increases. In severe aortic stenosis, patients cannot increase their cardiac output sufficiently (low fixed cardiac output state), cerebral perfusion falls and this causes syncope.

Fact 742:

What type of analyser can confirm the presence of **carbon dioxide** in someone who was just intubated?

Infrared analyser – wavelength 4.28 μm for CO_2

This allows CO_2 to absorb IR in relation to its concentration. As the amount of CO_2 in the gas mix ↑, the amount of infrared light passing though the gas mix ↓ (Beer's law). The IR light passing through hits a sensor and the signal generated is analysed.

There are two types of capnograph:

- *Side stream*: There is a time delay but many gases/vapours can be analysed from one sample.
- *Main stream*: No time delay but ↑ dead space and ↑ bulkiness.

Fact 743:

Why is glyceryl trinitrate (GTN) preferred over labetalol to manage a hypertensive crisis in a **cocaine overdose**?

- Although labetalol has some α-blocking properties, it is primarily a beta-blocker.
- GTN would not cause coronary vasoconstriction or systemic hypertension which can theoretically can happen with a pure beta-blocker (unopposed α-stimulation).

Fact 744:

What are the principles of **airway pressure release ventilation (APRV)?**

- APRV is an open-lung mode of ventilation which uses an inverse ratio. It is used in potentially recruitable disease often when there has been a poor response to conventional ventilation.
- It uses long inspiratory times (e.g. T_{high} 5 seconds) and high mean airway pressures (e.g. $P_{high} \leq 30$ cmH$_2$O) to enhance oxygenation.
- Brief expiratory releases (e.g. T_{low} 0.5 seconds) at a lower pressure (e.g. P_{low} 0 cmH$_2$O) facilitate CO$_2$ clearance.
- These expiratory releases should be set so that the inspiratory cycle starts when expiratory flow is ≥75% peak expiratory flow. This is to avoid lung deflation and to maintain end-expiratory lung volume.
- The Vt (or release volume) with each release breath will depend upon the difference between the set P_{high} and P_{low}, the T_{low} and the compliance of the respiratory system.
- The patient is encouraged to breathe spontaneously over time-cycling alternation in pressure (NMB is therefore stopped and sedation is titrated to achieve this).

Fact 745:

Do **impregnated central lines** reduce the risk of blood stream infections?

Yes – catheters impregnated with antimicrobials (chlorhexidine/silver sulfadiazine) or antibiotics (minocycline/ rifampicin) are associated with a ↓ in catheter-related bacteraemia.

The CDC recommends taking this measure for patients with catheters anticipated to stay in for > 5 days if, despite implementing a comprehensive strategy to ↓ CLABSI (central line-associated bloodstream infection) rates, there has been no decrease in these rates.

Fact 746:

When should you consider a **pneumothorax** as the most likely pathology when using lung ultrasound?

- Absent lung sliding (barcode/ stratosphere on M-mode)
- Absent B-lines
- Absent lung pulse

If all of these are met, then look for a lung point where the two pleural layers re-join. If a lung point is found, then a pneumothorax is highly likely.

Fact 747:

What are some indications of **VA-ECMO** and **VV-ECMO?**

VA-ECMO	VV-ECMO
Circulatory failure, with or without concomitant respiratory failure	Any potentially reversible acute respiratory failure
• **C**ardiomyopathy as a bridge to VAD or decision • **H**ypertension (pulmonary) after pulmonary endarterectomy • **E**xtra-corporeal life support • **S**hock (cardiogenic) due to any cause • **T**ransplant (heart) when there is graft failure or a bridge to lung transplant • **S**urgery (cardiac) when weaning from bypass	• **H**aemorrhage (pulmonary) or massive haemoptysis • **E**xtra-corporeal support for lung rest, e.g. lung contusions, airway obstruction • **A**RDS • **T**ransplant (lung) when there is graft failure or a bridge to lung transplant • **S**tatus asthmaticus

Fact 748:

What finding during a TTE would make **catheter ablation** for atrial fibrillation contraindicated?

A left atrial thrombus

Fact 749:

What would a **flow-volume loop** show in tracheal stenosis?

Fixed upper airway obstruction – there is impedance to both inspiratory and expiratory airflow.

Fact 750:

What position should the head be placed for **airway management** in children?

Neutral because of large head, short neck, prominent occiput and relatively large tongue

---

Fact 751:

How do you calculate **oxygen delivery (DO_2)**?

DO_2: Amount of oxygen delivered per unit time

DO_2 = Cardiac output × oxygen content

Oxygen content (CaO_2)

= Oxygen bound to Hb + dissolved oxygen

= 1.34 × [Hb] × (SaO_2/100) + 0.003 × PaO_2

Fact 752:

What are the diagnostic criteria for **haemophagocytic lymphohistiocytosis (HLH)** using the HLH-2004 criteria?

The presence of at least five out of the eight total criteria:

- ↑ temperature (fever)
- ↑ ferritin > 500 ng/mL
- ↑ spleen (splenomegaly)
- ↑ TAGs (hypertriglyceridemia) +/– ↓ fibrinogen
- ↑ sIL2Ra ≥ 2,400 U/mL
- ↓ cell lines (≥2 cytopenias)
- ↓ or absent NK-cell activity
- Biopsy-proven haemophagocytosis

HLH is a hyperinflammatory state as a result of inappropriate and dysregulated activation of natural killer (NK) cells, CD8+ cytotoxic T-cells and macrophages that results in multi-organ failure and death.

It is either primary (the result of inherited genetic mutations which presents in childhood) or secondary (an inappropriate host response to infection, malignancy or autoimmune disease).

Fact 753:

What is the goal of urinary alkalinisation with sodium bicarbonate in **rhabdomyolysis**?

To ↑ solubility of brown granular casts by targeting urinary pH > 7

Myoglobin combines with Tamm–Horsfall protein within renal tubules, forming the distinctive 'muddy-brown' casts that can block urine flow within the tubules (particularly in acidic urine).

The use of urinary alkalinisation has been debated, as it has the potential to exacerbate hypocalcaemia and can result in calcium phosphate deposition in the kidney.

Fact 754:

What does the size of an **endotracheal tube (ETT)** refer to, why does the bevel face to the left, what is the purpose of Murphy's eye and what is the size of the proximal end connector that connects to the breathing system?

- Size of ETT: Internal diameter
- The bevel faces left to facilitate intubation
- Murphy's eye is an alternative port for gas flow should the bevel get blocked
- The proximal end connector that connects to the breathing system has a standard 15 mm outer diameter

Fact 755:

Why may someone with ascites fail a **spontaneous breathing trial**?

- Ascites occurs due to sodium and water retention (secondary hyperaldosteronism).
- Abdominal distension may splint the diaphragm and impair ventilation.
- Drainage may help facilitate extubation.

Fact 756:

How is the solubility of **midazolam** dependent on pH and how does it work?

- *pH < 3*: Open diazepine ring and is water soluble
- *Physiological pH*: As soon as it is injected and the pH increases, the ring closes and midazolam becomes readily lipid soluble (allowing it to cross the blood-brain barrier).

Acts on GABA-A → binds to a site distinct from the GABA binding site → potentiates GABA effects → ↑ chloride current → hyperpolarisation of cell membranes

Fact 757:

What is the priority in a haemodynamically unstable patient with **massive haemoptysis** with BP = 90/70, HR = 100 and SpO_2 = 85% on 15 L oxygen?

Secure airway and improve oxygenation to prevent asphyxiation, the leading cause of mortality.

Positioning the patient so that the affected lung is downward can help to prevent contamination of the unaffected lung. Prompt airway control allows bronchoscopy, diagnosis and treatment. If necessary, a DLT can be used for lung isolation.

Fact 758:

Which **toxicity** is indicated by the presence of high anion gap metabolic acidosis, high lactate, hypocalcaemia, a rising creatinine and oxalate crystals on urinalysis?

Ethylene glycol intoxication

Fact 759:

Can the fibrinogen be normal in **disseminated intravascular coagulation (DIC)**?

Yes – it may be normal in the early stages of DIC as it is an acute phase protein.

Fact 760:

What temperature should the injectate be, and what effect does a small injectate volume have on deriving **cardiac output** with a pulmonary artery catheter?

- The injectate should be extremely cold; its accuracy decreases as it approaches body temperature.
- A small volume of injectate will overestimate CO; It will equilibrate rapidly and generate a small curve (CO is inversely proportional to area under the curve).

Fact 761:

What is the mechanism of action of **rFVIIa (recombinant activated factor VII)** when administered in high, supra-physiological doses in major haemorrhage as an off-label indication?

- Initiates direct thrombin generation on platelets.
- May have a role in rare cases of acute massive haemorrhage which fail to respond to blood component therapy and surgical management.
- It should not be given in patients with a history of VTE or thrombotic tendency.

Fact 762:

What are some considerations of using **suxamethonium** in critical care?

- *Renal/Liver failure*: While it is metabolised rapidly by plasma cholinesterases, in liver/renal failure there are ↓ pseudocholinesterase levels which leads to ↑ duration of effect.
- Muscle fasciculations and myalgia due to microfibrillar rupture may be undesirable, e.g. in rhabdomyolysis or trauma.
- *Myasthenia gravis*: Need ↑ doses as there is relative resistance to depolarisation.
- ↑ Duration of effect in those on aminoglycoside antibiotics or cholinesterase inhibitors.
- Risk of life-threatening hyperkalaemia due to the development of extra-junctional ACh receptors in:
  o Burns >24 hours
  o Spinal cord injury > 72 hours
  o Prolonged immobilisation
  o Myopathies, e.g. Duchenne muscular dystrophy
  o Guillain–Barré syndrome (GBS)
- Contraindicated in malignant hyperthermia
- Mindfulness of suxamethonium apnoea (deficiency of plasma cholinesterase) and anaphylaxis

Fact 763:

How do you monitor **anticoagulation** during ECMO?

- Anticoagulation is usually with heparin.
- ACT (Activated Clotting Time) is the chosen method for measuring the anticoagulation.
- The ACT target is 180–210 seconds.

Fact 764:

What are the initial management priorities of a **traumatic cardiac arrest (TCA)**?

Focus	• Focus on interventions which can rapidly manage reversible causes: Hypoxia, hypovolaemia, tension pneumothorax and cardiac tamponade • Using point of care cardiac ultrasound
Deprioritisation	• Deprioritising external chest compressions, defibrillation and vasopressors
Management priorities	• Stopping catastrophic external haemorrhage (e.g. tourniquet, haemostatic dressings) • Ensuring adequate oxygenation and ventilation • Performing bilateral thoracostomies • Minimising internal haemorrhage (e.g. pelvic binder) • Rapid blood transfusion as per major haemorrhage protocols

Fact 765:

What is the most common reason for GI bleeding in patients who have a **continuous-flow left ventricular assist device (CF-LVAD)** and why does this occur?

AV malformations located in the upper GI tract

Bleeding is multifactorial and related to:

- The physiology of the LVAD itself:
  - ↓ Pulsatile flow → local hypoxia in GI mucosa → vessel dysplasia
  - ↓ Pulsatile flow → ↓ platelets and breakdown of vWF
- Use of anticoagulants
- Patient comorbidities

Octreotide can be effective in preventing recurrent GI bleeding that does not respond to standard treatment.

Fact 766:

What are some inherited conditions associated with an increased risk of cerebral aneurysms and **subarachnoid haemorrhages**?

- Autosomal dominant polycystic kidney disease
- Collagen vascular disease, e.g. Ehlers Danlos type 4
- Glucocorticoid-remediable aldosteronism
- Familial intracerebral aneurysms

Fact 767:

In drug overdose, when is **single-dose activated charcoal (SDAC)** and **multiple-dose activated charcoal (MSAC)** given?

SDAC	MSAC
If a potentially toxic dose of a drug was ingested within the last hour and the drug can be adsorbed by charcoal.	Ingestion of a life-threatening amount of a specific drug: • **P**henobarbital and Paraquat • **A**spirin • **C**arbamazepine • **T**heophylline • **Q**uinine • **D**apsone

Substances **NOT** adsorbed by charcoal include:

- Metals, e.g. iron, lithium
- Alcohol, glycols and esters
- Strong acids and alkalis
- Cyanide

Fact 768:

How does adrenaline cause a **type B lactic acidosis**?

Via β_2-receptors: Adrenaline induces glycolysis and pyruvate generation, which results in lactic acidosis

Fact 769:

What is a **catheter-related bloodstream infection (CRBSI)** and what is meant by differential time to positivity (DTP)?

CRBSI is a nosocomial bloodstream infection linked to the use of a vascular device. Following insertion, fibrin can coat the catheter and potentially can become colonised. Diagnosis is through quantitative culture of catheter tip or differences in growth between catheter and peripheral blood cultures. Treatment is to remove the vascular device and to give appropriate antibiotics.

To prevent unnecessary device removal, paired blood cultures are obtained from the device and a peripheral vein. A positive DTP indicates microbial growth from the device at least 2 hours earlier than the peripheral vein culture. However, this method's accuracy can vary and may lack sensitivity and specificity in some studies. In cases of suspected CRBI, prompt catheter removal is advisable, especially in unstable patients, without waiting for DTP results.

Fact 770:

Besides its efficacy, what advantage is there in initiating **itraconazole** for an Aspergillus infection?

Itraconazole has a steroid-sparing effect.

Fact 771:

What is the gold standard to measure **intracranial pressure (ICP)**?

A ventriculostomy, which involves using an EVD (external ventricular drain) with a pressure transducer. This is considered the gold standard because its accuracy, ease of calibration, capability for dynamic testing, and the ability to both drain CSF and administer drugs. The pressure is measured relative to atmospheric pressure, with the transducer positioned at the foramen of Munro. One of its biggest disadvantages is that it carries an ↑ risk of infection.

Fact 772:

What is the appropriate action if, while floating a **pulmonary artery catheter (PAC)**, the RV waveform doesn't transition to a PA waveform even after advancing it over 60 cm?

Deflate the balloon and carefully withdraw the catheter. This precaution is necessary avoid the catheter coiling or forming knots, and to ↓ the risk of damaging structures within the right ventricle.

Fact 773:

What are the diagnostic criteria for **chronic kidney disease (CKD)** if the eGFR is less than 60?

eGFR < 60 for > 3 months plus one of:

- **S**tructural abnormalities on imaging/histology
- **T**ubular disorders causing electrolyte abnormalities
- **A**CR ≥ 3 mg/mmol (≥30 mg/g)
- **S**ediment urinary abnormalities
- **H**istory of a renal transplant

The commonest causes of CKD that lead to ESRF in the UK include diabetes, hypertension and glomerular disease (e.g. IgA nephropathy, interstitial disease, idiopathic).

Fact 774:

What are the NICE criteria for performing an immediate CT-head in someone with a **head injury** who presents to ED?

- GCS < 13 when first assessed in ED
- GCS < 15 when assessed in ED 2 hours after injury
- Suspected open or depressed skull fracture
- Signs of base of skill fracture (haemotympanum, 'panda' eyes, CSF leakage from ears/nose, Battle's sign)
- Post-traumatic seizure
- Focal neurological deficit
- > 1 episode of vomiting

Fact 775:

Which metabolite of **ethylene glycol metabolism** can cause a spuriously elevated lactate?

Glycolic acid may cause a spuriously high lactate.

Fact 776:

How can you biochemically differentiate between an **NSTEMI** and **unstable angina**?

- *NSTEMI*: ↑ cardiac enzymes
- *Unstable angina*: Cardiac enzymes normal

Fact 777:

Why is **vecuronium** not usually recommended as a paralytic agent for rapid sequence induction?

Long onset of action

Recommended paralytics include suxamethonium or rocuronium.

Fact 778:

What is the mechanism of action of **furosemide** and what are some consequences of its use?

Furosemide is a loop diuretic

- It blocks the sodium–potassium–2 chloride (Na^+–K^+–2 Cl^-) cotransporter located in the thick ascending limb of the loop of Henle → osmotic diuresis and natriuresis
- Causes local vascular prostaglandin synthesis → venodilatation
- Other consequences:
  - ↓ Oxygen consumption in loop of Henle
  - ↓ Preload
  - Hypochloraemic metabolic alkalosis

Fact 779:

If you encounter an early trifurcation of three equal-sized openings resembling the **Mercedes Benz logo**, where is the bronchoscope's tip most likely positioned?

Right upper lobe – immediately divides into three equal segments – apical, posterior and anterior segments.

This is the only place in the upper bronchial tree where an equal trifurcation is commonly found.

Fact 780:

What is meant by **acute colonic pseudo-obstruction (Ogilvie syndrome)**?

Pseudo-obstruction is characterised by clinical features of a mechanical obstruction in the absence of a mechanical cause.

It is associated with conditions unrelated to direct abdominopelvic intervention, e.g. non-operative trauma, cardiac disease, infection, renal failure and orthopaedic surgery.

While the precise mechanism of acute pseudo-obstruction is unknown, autonomic dysfunction to the gut is the likely aetiology. The first-line of management is conservative. Neostigmine is indicated in patients who fail 24–48 hours of conservative therapy, or in those with severe bowel distension (>12 cm in diameter).

Fact 781:

Generally, which interventions would you give for abnormal **TEG values**?

TEG value	Intervention
↑ R-time	Fresh frozen plasma
↑ K-time	Cryoprecipitate
↓ α-angle	Cryoprecipitate +/– platelets
↓ MA	Platelets
↑ LY30	Tranexamic acid

Fact 782:

How does bladder function differ with a compressive lesion at the **conus medullaris** compared with a compressive lesion at the **cauda equina**?

Compressive lesion at the conus medullaris	Compressive lesion at the cauda equina
This is an UMN lesion, best thought of as bladder spasticity	This is a LMN lesion, best thought of as bladder flaccidity
A reflex neurogenic or 'automatic' bladder with overactivity, urgency and incomplete emptying	Overflow urinary incontinence due to a loss of bladder motor function so that the bladder passively fills

Fact 783:

How do you orally insert a **Sengstaken–Blakemore tube (SBT)** without an endoscope?

- Insert to approximately 55 cm (the gastro-oesophageal junction is ~40 cm from the incisors). Inflate the gastric balloon with 50 mL of air/saline/contrast and verify its position with a CXR. Once confirmed, fully inflate the gastric balloon with 250 mL of air/saline. Withdraw the tube until you encounter resistance. Traction is best achieved by taping it to the nose/face. Weighted traction using saline bags is no longer recommended as this can cause necrosis at the GOJ and angle of mouth. The gastric port should be aspirated to measure ongoing blood loss.
- If bleeding continues, the oesophageal balloon is inflated with air until a manometer reads 35–40 mmHg. The pressure is then ↓ to the lowest pressure required to prevent bleeding. Inflating the oesophageal balloon carries an ↑ risk of oesophageal necrosis and subsequent perforation.
- Oesophageal balloons should be deflated every few hours to assess for cessation of bleeding; gastric balloons are generally left inflated for 12–24 hours. The longer the balloons are left inflated and traction applied, the ↑ risk of necrosis. There is a 50% risk of re-bleeding following balloon deflation.

Fact 784:

What happens to **gas-filled cavities** with altitude and what are some clinical correlations of this?

Expansion of gas-filled cavities

Boyle's law explains this. At altitude, there is ↓ atmospheric pressure. An ideal gas' volume will therefore ↑. As the volume of a gas increases with altitude, care must be taken with gas in enclosed body cavities and in medical devices.

- Pneumothoraces may tension and must be drained.
- Endotracheal cuffs will expand and should be filled with saline.
- Gas within the gut lumen will expand and patients with GI obstruction should avoid altitude if possible or have an NGT placed.
- Pneumocephalus/ pneumoperitoneum/ pneumopericardium may also create pressure effects and should be drained or altitude avoided if possible.

Fact 785:

What is the role of allopurinol in the management of established **tumour lysis syndrome (TLS)**?

Allopurinol is a prophylactic agent used to prevent uric acid formation but does not affect breakdown of uric acid once TLS is established.

Fact 786:

What is **acute traumatic coagulopathy**?

- Occurs within minutes of trauma
- Modulated by tissue damage, inflammatory mediator release, ↑ levels of systemic anticoagulant factors and platelet dysfunction.
- INR > 1.2 is an accepted definition of trauma-induced coagulopathy.

Fact 787:

Which antibiotics are effective in the chemoprophylaxis of **invasive meningococcal disease (IMD)**?

Rifampicin, ciprofloxacin or ceftriaxone

Neisseria meningitidis is a Gram-negative diplococcus which causes IMD and is a notifiable disease. Close contacts should receive chemoprophylaxis regardless of their vaccination status. Chemoprophylaxis is also indicated for those who have been in direct contact with secretions from the patient's respiratory tract during medical procedures before or less than 24 hours after antimicrobial therapy was initiated (infection spreads with droplets).

Fact 788:

Which agents can you use to treat **status epilepticus**?

Status epilepticus is defined as ≥ 5 minutes of continuous clinical and/or electrographic seizure activity OR recurrent seizure activity without recovery in-between seizures.

First-line therapies	Benzodiazepines	Midazolam (IV/IM)
		Lorazepam (IV/IM)
		Diazepam (IV/PR)
Second-line therapies	Phenytoin (IV)	
	Valproate (IV)	
	Levetiracetam (IV)	
Third-line therapies	Propofol (IV)	
	Phenobarbital (IV)	
	Thiopentone (IV)	

Fact 789:

How do **linezolid** and **vancomycin** work in the treatment of Methicillin-resistant *Staphylococcus aureus* (MRSA)?

- *Linezolid*: Oxazolidinone antibiotic that inhibits bacterial protein synthesis.
- *Vancomycin*: Glycopeptide antibiotic that works by inhibiting bacterial cell wall synthesis.

Fact 790:

How would you treat **hyperchloraemic metabolic acidosis** with a normal lactate in a patient who has undergone neobladder formation after a radical cystectomy?

IV 1.26% sodium bicarbonate

This is a normal anion gap metabolic acidosis. The strong ion difference (SID) ↓ either because of an ↑ in chloride relative to strong cations or ↓ cations with chloride retention:

SID = (strong cations) − (strong anions)

$$SID = (Na^+ + K^+ + Ca^{2+} + Mg^{2+}) - (Cl^- + SO_4^{2-})$$

Abbreviated SID = $(Na^+) - (Cl^-)$

Normal SID is 42 mEq/L

- ↓ SID = acidosis
- ↑ SID = alkalosis

In this case, the ↓ SID and acidosis occurs because of intestinal/renal losses of K^+, Ca^{2+} and Mg^{2+}.

Sodium bicarbonate will ↑ sodium in relation to chloride to treat the acidosis.

The same principle applies in an externally draining pancreatic fistula.

Fact 791:

How may **ARDS** differ from **cardiogenic pulmonary oedema (CPO)** on lung ultrasound?

	ARDS	CPO
Bilateral B-lines	Yes	Yes
Homogenous B-lines	No	Yes
Subpleural irregularities	Yes	No
Reduced B-line in response to diuresis	No	Yes
Pleural sliding	Diminished	Greatly diminished
Pleural effusion	Evidence of septation	Free flowing effusion
Dynamic effect of recruitment	Litlle change with recruitment	↑ Size and aeration with recruitment

Fact 792:

What is the multimodal approach to manage pain in traumatic **rib fractures**?

- Paracetamol, NSAID and opioids
- Regional: Thoracic epidural, paravertebral, erector spinae plane, serratus anterior plane (for anterior rib fractures)
- Rib fixation: For flail requiring mechanical ventilation

Fact 793:

In which pairing of **respiratory rate** and **tidal volume** can a greater amount of CO_2 be removed when one component is increased while the other is decreased?

↓ RR + ↑ TV will eliminate more CO_2 than ↑ RR + ↓ TV.

Fact 794:

What is the most common causative organism of **infective endocarditis**?

Staphylococci have overtaken streptococci as the most common cause.

Fact 795:

Why are **continuous-flow LVADs** (second and third generation) preferred over pulsatile ones (first generation)?

↑ Survival, ↓ stroke and ↓ device failure (and therefore reoperation) compared with pulsatile devices

Fact 796:

What is the difference between **zero-order kinetics** and **first-order kinetics** of drug elimination?

Zero-order kinetics (Few drugs are eliminated in this way, e.g. ethylene glycol, phenytoin, salicylates)	First-order kinetics (most drugs are eliminated in this way)
A constant <u>amount</u> of a drug is eliminated per unit time	A constant <u>fraction</u> of a drug is eliminated per unit time
Elimination mechanisms are saturable	Elimination mechanisms are NOT saturable
Zero-order kinetics undergo constant elimination regardless of the plasma concentration

For example, 2.5 mg of a drug may be eliminated per hour. This rate of elimination is constant and is independent of the total drug concentration in the plasma. | The rate of elimination is proportional to the amount of drug in the body. The higher the concentration, the greater the amount of drug eliminated per unit time.

For example, a drug with a concentration of 100 and half-life of 1 hour will reduce to 50 in the first hour, 25 in the second hour and 12.5 in the third hour etc. |

Fact 797:

How does LiDCO differ from PiCCO in the measurement of **cardiac output**?

	PiCCO	LiDCO
Technique	Pulse contour analysis	Pulse power analysis
SV determination	Uses the arterial waveform contour to determine SV, recognising the dicrotic notch	Tracks changes in SV based on the power of the arterial waveform, without the need to identify specific parts
Assumption	Assumes that the area under the systolic portion of the arterial pressure trace is proportional to SV	Assumes that fluctuations of arterial pressure around the mean are proportional to SV
Method	Transpulmonary thermodilution and requires a central line	Transpulmonary lithium dilution and does not require a central line (calibration is affected by atracurium)
Arterial line requirement	Requires a special thermistor-tipped femoral line	Uses an existing arterial line
Volume responsiveness indicators	Both provide 'dynamic' indicators of volume responsiveness: Stroke volume variation (SVV), pulse pressure variation (PPV), systolic pressure variation (SPV)	
Volumetric markers of preload	• Global end-diastolic volume • Intrathoracic blood volume • Extravascular lung water (measures pulmonary oedema)	
Reliability with arrhythmias	Both are not reliable in the presence of arrhythmias	

Fact 798:

How do you interpret these **nerve conduction studies**:

* Normal conduction velocities
* Normal SNAP amplitude
* ↓ CMAP amplitude
* 5% CMAP amplitude reduction on repetitive nerve stimulation with no incremental response to muscle exercise

These findings are indicative of critical illness myopathy (CIM)

Additional points to consider regarding nerve stimulation:

* Repetitive nerve stimulation involves 10 supramaximal stimuli at 2–3 Hz. A reduction in CMAP amplitude of >10% from the first to the fourth response could suggest ↓ NMJ transmission, as seen in conditions like myasthenia.
* In pre-synaptic NMJ disorders, such as Lambert–Eaton syndrome and botulism, a ↓ CMAP amplitude is typical. In these disorders, after 10 seconds of muscle exercise or fast repetitive stimulation (20–50 Hz), there can be an increase in CMAP amplitude of more than 100%.

Fact 799:

Assuming that there is no change in heart rate, afterload and myocardial contractility, what determines an increase in **left ventricular preload**?

↑ End-diastolic volume

Fact 800:

How is a **straight blade/laryngoscope** used for intubating neonates and infants?

* Children typically have a relatively large, floppy U-shaped epiglottis.
* During paediatric intubation, a straight laryngoscope (such as the Wisconsin, Magill or Miller) is placed behind the epiglottis holding it in position.
* The operator then lifts up the epiglottis to view the cords.

Fact 801:

What are some of the absolute contraindications to liver transplantation in **acute liver failure**?

Cholangiocarcinoma, especially later-stages
AIDS
Malignancy (metastatic, uncurable, extrahepatic)
Pulmonary and cardiac disease (advanced disease)

Fact 802:

What are the different types of probes used for **ultrasound** in intensive care?

Probe	Approximate frequency range (MHz)	Resolution	Common uses in ICU
Linear	5–15	Highest spatial resolution for superficial structures	Vascular access, pleural sliding
Curvi-linear	2–5	Large footprint with good penetration	Thoracic and abdominal US
Phased array	1–5	Small footprint, poor superficial resolution, large field of view at depth	Cardiac, IVC, sometimes used for lung

Fact 803:

What is the current evidence for using **IV Vitamin C** in the management of adults with sepsis or septic shock?

Currently not recommended

Fact 804:

When is PCI the preferred coronary reperfusion strategy for **acute STEMI** patients?

- Presentation within 12 hours of symptom onset and
- Primary PCI can be delivered within 120 minutes of potential fibrinolysis administration

Fact 805:

What are the responsibilities and governing legislation of a **coroner**, and what is the objective of a coroner's inquest?

- A coroner, who is a judicial office holder appointed by the Crown, is usually a highly experienced and qualified lawyer, or a doctor if appointed before 2013.
- Their role is governed by the Coroners and Justice Act 2009.
- The main objective of a coroner's inquest is to determine four critical details about a death: the identity of the deceased, as well as the where, when, and how of their passing.

Fact 806:

Which treatments have been shown to reduce mortality in **tuberculous meningitis**?

Anti-tuberculosis treatment and corticosteroids

Fact 807:

How is **ethylene glycol** metabolised, what are its metabolites and what happens to the osmolal gap?

Metabolised by alcohol dehydrogenase

Ethylene glycol → glycolaldehyde → glycolic acid → glyoxylic acid → oxalic acid

Ethylene glycol is commonly found in antifreeze, detergents and metal polish. Intoxication produces a HAGMA with hyperosmolality.

Osmolal gap = measured osmolality – calculated osmolality (normal is <10 mOsm/L). In ethylene glycol toxicity, the osmolal gap is increased (>10 mOsm/kg).

Fact 808:

Why do you give **albumin** when performing large-volume paracentesis of ascites in alcohol-related liver disease?

To ↓ the risk of cardiovascular decompensation that can occur due to fluid shifts post-drainage.

Volume expansion with 8 g albumin should be given per litre of ascites removed. This is roughly equivalent to 100 mL of 20% albumin per 3 L ascites.

Fact 809:

How would you manage a sustained ICP spike in a patient with **isolated traumatic brain injury (TBI)**?

*   Optimise sedation and paralyse to ↓ $CMRO_2$
*   Treat seizures (early post-traumatic seizures are not associated with adverse outcomes)
*   Osmotherapy with either:
    *   NaCl 5% (hypertonic) saline 1–2 mL/kg. Can be repeated every 4–6 hours provided serum osmolality < 320 mOsm/kg and Na^+ < 155 mmol/L
    *   Mannitol 0.25–1 g/kg of 20% solution. Can be repeated provided serum osmolality < 320 mOsm/kg and normovolaemic.
*   Moderate hyperventilation to $PaCO_2$ 4.0–4.5 kPa to ↓ cerebral blood volume and ICP. This is a temporising measure and once ICP is controlled, adjust ventilation back to achieve $PaCO_2$ to 4.5–5.0 kPa.
*   If an EVD is present, CSF can be drained off.
*   Repeat imaging to exclude a surgically treatable lesion.
*   Thiopentone-induced burst suppression is used in refractory cases (guided by EEG or BIS).

Fact 810:

How can tracheal anatomy guide orientation during **bronchoscopy**?

*   *Anteriorly*: C-shaped cartilaginous tracheal rings
*   *Posteriorly*: Trachealis muscle

Fact 811:

What are some examples of intravenous **GP2b/3a inhibitors** that can be given during primary PCI?

Tirofiban, **E**ptifibatide, **A**bciximab

Activation of the GP 2b/3a receptor by fibrinogen stimulates the final common pathway in platelet aggregation. By blocking this, these agents function as powerful antiplatelet agents.

Fact 812:

Which patient groups are most affected by **traumatic brain injury (TBI)**?

There is a bimodal distribution

*   *Young adults*: Road traffic collisions
*   *Elderly adults*: Falls

Fact 813:

What are the underlying pathophysiological mechanisms for the three different types of **renal tubular acidosis (RTA)**?

Type 1	Type 2	Type 4
Distal RTA	**Proximal RTA**	**Hyperkalae-mic RTA**
Defect in the α intercalated cells in the distal tubule to secrete H^+ ions into the urine	Defect in proximal convoluted tubule to reabsorb bicarbonate into the blood	↓ Aldosterone production OR aldosterone resistance

Fact 814:

How does the target and cycle differ between **volume-controlled ventilation (VCV) and pressure-controlled ventilation (PCV)**?

Target: How flow is delivered during inspiration

Cycle: When inspiration ends

VCV = **flow**-targeted, **volume**-cycled

PCV = **pressure**-targeted, **time**-cycled

Fact 815:

What are some **adverse effects** of giving protamine to reverse unfractionated heparin (UFH)?

Pulmonary hypertension, CVS collapse, bronchospasm

Given at a dose of 1 mg for every 100 units of UFH. It has a partial effect against LMWH. It should be given slowly via a large-bore PVC and not when on cardiopulmonary bypass. Excessive doses have anticoagulant properties (rebound anticoagulation).

Fact 816:

Why opt for **remifentanil** to re-sedate an intubated patient with a history of alcohol excess, TBI and renal/liver impairment, who, when off sedation, exhibits tachycardia, hypotension and an ICP of 18 mmHg?

Remifentanil is metabolised by non-specific plasma and tissue esterases, preventing accumulation.

Fact 817:

What is the general effect of **triazole antifungals** on the cP450 system?

Inhibitors of cytochrome P450 isozymes

Fact 818:

How does **sacubitril-valsartan** work in the management of HFrEF?

- In HFrEF, activation of the RAAS contributes to detrimental effects such as vasoconstriction and cardiac remodelling. Conversely, the natriuretic peptide system, which is degraded by the enzyme neprilysin, provides beneficial effects like vasodilation and BP reduction.
- Sacubitril, a neprilysin inhibitor, works by preventing the breakdown of natriuretic peptides, thus enhancing their favourable cardiovascular effects. However, inhibiting neprilysin also increases levels of angiotensin II, as neprilysin is involved in its degradation. To counteract this rise in angiotensin II levels, sacubitril is combined with valsartan, an ARB.
- This combination allows for both augmentation of the protective effects of natriuretic peptides and mitigation of the potentially harmful effects of increased angiotensin II in the management of HFrEF.

Fact 819:

What did the **DECRA** and **RESCUEicp** trials show?

- DECRA (NEJM, 2011): In diffuse TBI, early decompressive craniectomy reduces ICP, duration of mechanical ventilation and ICU length of stay compared with standard care. However, it increased the risk of unfavourable neurological outcomes.
- RESCUEicp (NEJM, 2016): In TBI patients with persistently elevated ICP, decompressive craniectomy lowered mortality, but was linked to higher rates of poor neurological outcomes in survivors.

Fact 820:

What is the goal of **full targeted medical nutrition therapy** according to ESPEN (European Society for Clinical Nutrition and Metabolism)?

To deliver 70–100% of resting energy expenditure (REE)

If oral intake is not feasible, commence low-rate enteral nutrition, gradually escalating it over 48 hours.

Fact 821:

In a three-bottle **chest drainage system**, what is the role of each bottle?

- First bottle: Trap/collection bottle
- Second bottle: Underwater seal
- Third bottle: Manometer or pressure-regulating bottle which allows suction to be attached

Modern drains incorporate three separate bottles into one unit.

Fact 822:

Typically over which vertebral bodies is the **carina** typically visible on a chest X-ray?

T5–7

Fact 823:

How can you classify a **haemopoetic stem cell transplant**?

Source of stem cell	• Autologous: Patient's own cells (rare risk of GvHD) • Allogenic: From donor (higher risk of GvHD if unmatched)
Matching of donating cells	• Matched • Unmatched
Site of cell	• Peripheral • Bone marrow • Cord blood
Intensity of pre-transplant chemotherapy regime	• Myeloablative: Total destruction of patient's native bone marrow • Reduced intensity conditioning: Partially destroying the patient's native bone marrow, followed by tumour cell destruction by donor cells

Fact 824:

Approximately how many cases of **subarachnoid haemorrhage** does a CT scan miss?

10% of cases

A lumbar puncture should be performed if suspected

Fact 825:

When comparing dabigatran, apixaban, rivaroxaban and edoxaban, which **DOAC** has the highest renal elimination?

Dabigatran has the highest renal elimination (80%).

Edoxaban (50%), rivaroxaban (35%), apixaban (27%)

Fact 826:

How does **ganciclovir** work to treat CMV infections?

Inhibits viral DNA synthesis

It is a nucleoside analogue of guanosine that competitively inhibits viral DNA polymerase from incorporating dGTP.

Quantitative PCR is useful for monitoring disease.

Fact 827:

What are the long-term benefits of oxygen therapy for **chronic cor pulmonale**?

To prevent RV failure and to improve both life expectancy and quality of life.

Fact 828:

What is meant by changing the **gain** on an ultrasound?

Adjusting the gain modifies the amplification of reflected ultrasound waves, much like adjusting brightness.

Increasing the gain amplifies the returning signals, analogous to increasing the volume on a radio.

The gain should be fine-tuned to ensure that the interaction between sound and tissue produces optimal images of the specific structure being examined; too low makes it dark, too high causes excessive brightness, known as a 'snowstorm'.

Fact 829:

Which antiplatelets are recommended post-PCI in someone with a **STEMI**?

- Aspirin for life – this irreversibly inhibits COX and blocks the production of thromboxane.
- Prasugrel or Ticagrelor for 12 months – these are thienopyridines. They are more potent and effective at inhibiting the P2Y12 receptor and producing a more reliable clinical effect on platelet aggregation than clopidogrel.

Fact 830:

What is the **alveolar O_2 concentration** in someone whose $PaCO_2$ is 10 kPa on room air?

The alveolar gas equation: $P_AO_2 = PiO_2 - PaCO_2/R$

- PiO_2 = partial pressure of inspired oxygen = can be calculated by subtracting the partial pressure exerted by water vapour at body temperature:
  o $PiO_2 = 0.21 \times (100 \text{ kPa} - 6.3 \text{ kPa}) = 19.8$ kPa
- $PaCO_2 = 10$ kPa
- R = respiratory quotient = amount of CO_2 produced divided by the amount of O_2 consumed. With a normal diet = (200 mL/minute)/(250 mL/minute) = 0.8

Therefore:

$PAO_2 = PiO_2 - PaCO_2/R$

$PAO_2 = 19.8 - 10/0.8$

$PAO_2 = 19.8 - 12.5 = \textbf{7.3 kPa}$

Fact 831:

What type of acid base abnormality is associated with **cardiogenic shock**?

A mixed acidosis – both metabolic and respiratory acidosis

Fact 832:

Which artery is implicated if a patient has **crushing chest pain** and the following ECG changes in V_{1-3}:

- ST-segment depression of 3 mm
- Positive T waves
- Positive R waves

Posterior descending artery

- 85% of people: Arises from RCA
- 15% of people: Arises from circumflex artery

This is a posterior STEMI; if posterior leads were applied, it would a mirror image: ST elevation and Q waves in V_{1-3}.

Fact 833:

How do C-lines differ from B-lines on lung ultrasound in someone with **SARS-CoV-2**?

C-lines have the appearance of B-lines but they do not obliterate A-lines

In COVID-19 vertical lines often originate from sub-pleural consolidations and not from the pleural line itself. These lines, although similar to B-lines, are not strictly B-lines as they do not originate from the pleura and do not erase A-lines.

Fact 834:

What are the three major components of the **APACHE IV scoring system**?

1. *Acute physiology score (APS)*: Based on the worst physiological measurements recorded during the first 24 hours of ICU admission
2. *Age points*: Assigns points based on age. Older age is associated with an ↑ risk of mortality.
3. *Chronic health points*: Assigns points based on the number and severity of chronic health conditions, e.g. cancer and/or organ failure

Among these three, the APS typically has the greatest impact on the final APACHE IV score.

Fact 835:

How do you treat **haemophagocytic lymphohistiocytosis (HLH)**?

1. Supportive care
2. Identification and treatment of trigger, e.g. PJP
3. Attenuation of cytokine storm (specific HLH therapy):
   a. Corticosteroids, e.g. hydrocortisone or pulsed methylprednisolone
   b. Anakinra: A recombinant IL-1 antagonist
   c. IVIg
   d. Cytotoxics: Etopside

Fact 836:

What were the findings of the International Subarachnoid Aneurysm Trial (ISAT) regarding **endovascular coiling** in subarachnoid haemorrhages?

Compared to clipping, coiling was associated with:

- ↓ Death or severe neurological deficit at one year
- Sustained survival benefit at seven years
- ↓ Incidence of post-procedure epilepsy and cognitive decline
- ↑ Rebleeding in the first year post-treatment

Fact 837:

How would you confirm a diagnosis of **Pneumocystis jirovecii** in a ventilated patient with a solid organ transplant on anti-rejection therapy?

Samples from induced sputum or bronchoalveolar lavage

Pneumocystis jirovecii is often undetectable in sputum and requires specialised techniques like induced sputum with hypertonic saline or bronchoscopy with alveolar lavage. These samples are then stained using methods like silver stain, periodic acid-Schiff, or immunofluorescence for detection.

Fact 838:

What is the role of the **malate–aspartate** and **glycerol–phosphate shuttles**?

- The malate–aspartate and glycerol–phosphate shuttles transfer NADH produced in the cytosol during glycolysis into the mitochondria, where it can be used in the electron transport chain to produce ATP. They provide an indirect way to transport electrons across the mitochondrial membrane, since NADH itself cannot cross the membrane.
- The malate–aspartate shuttle is predominantly found in tissues with high energy demands, such as the liver, kidneys and heart, allowing efficient ATP production.
- The glycerol–phosphate shuttle, which is less efficient in terms of ATP production, is more common in tissues with lower energy demands, such as skeletal muscles and the brain.

Fact 839:

What is the difference between single, double and triple **blinding**?

- *Single blinding*: Only the subjects are blinded.
- *Double blinding*: The clinician/ researcher is also blinded.
- *Triple blinding*: The individual or group analysing the data are also blinded

Fact 840:

What is meant by **damping** in the context of invasive arterial blood pressure (IABP) monitoring?

Damping is the tendency of an object to resist oscillating.

- The IABP measuring system relies on transmitting oscillations from the artery to the transducer.
- Damping reduces the amplitude of these oscillations.
- Optimal damping means the system can respond quickly to input changes without excessive oscillations.
- This is measured by the damping factor (D):
  - Undamped, D = 0
  - Critically damped, D = 1
  - Optimally damped, D = 0.64 (captures pressure changes accurately without adding additional noise or oscillations)

	Over-damping	Under-damping
Effect on BP	↓ SBP & ↑ DBP	↑ SBP & ↓ DBP
Effect on MAP	No change in MAP	
Possible causes	Clots, air bubbles, kinking, excess tubing compliance	Long, non-compliant tubing

Fact 841:

What are some causes of a raised **osmolal gap** >10 mOsm/kg?

- Alcohols, e.g. ethanol, methanol, ethylene glycol
- Sugars, e.g. mannitol, sorbitol
- Lipids, e.g. hypertriglyceridaemia
- Proteins, e.g. Waldenstrom macroglobulinaemia, glycine (TURP syndrome)

Fact 842:

Is there a difference between small- and large-bore chest drains for managing a **spontaneous pneumothorax**?

No – small-bore drains are equally effective with fewer complications and less pain.

Fact 843:

Which ion channels does **amiodarone** affect?

- K^+ channels – Class 3 effect (primary effect)
- Na^+ channels – Class 1 effect
- Ca^{2+} channels – Class 4 effect

It also has β-blocker-like effects (Class 2 effect) but this is independent of ion channels.

Fact 844:

What happens to the serum sodium in **trans-urethral resection of prostate (TURP) syndrome**?

↓ Sodium (hyponatraemia)

TURP syndrome results from the intra-operative absorption of hypotonic 1.5% glycine-based irrigation fluid through open prostatic venous sinuses. This fluid does not contain electrolytes to ensure it is non-conductive to diathermy current.

Risk factors for TURP syndrome include irrigation fluid pressure, operative time, extent of resection (↑ surface area for absorption) and smoking.

Clinical features include:

- Volume overload
- Acute hyponatraemia, e.g. agitation, seizures, coma
- *Glycine toxicity*: Glycine is an inhibitory neurotransmitter. It contributes to volume overload and hyponatraemia and is also associated with cardiotoxicity, AKI (hyperoxaluria) and transient blindness.

Immediate management includes stopping surgery, providing multi-organ support and correcting hyponatraemia, e.g. with hypertonic saline.

Fact 845:

Typically, how much does the **platelet count** increase by with the transfusion of one unit of platelets?

If a platelet transfusion is indicated, one unit will typically raise the count by approximately $20–30 \times 10^9$/L

Fact 846:

What are some examples of drugs that can be used for **AF with pre-excitation** in a stable patient?

PIFA: Procainamide, **I**butilide, **F**lecainide, **A**miodarone

Using AV nodal blocking drugs (e.g. adenosine, beta-blockers, digoxin, or CCBs) may ↑ conduction via the accessory pathway, potentially leading to VT or VF.

Haemodynamic instability requires synchronised DCCV.

Fact 847:

Why may someone with an **LVAD** be at an increased risk of fungal infection?

Chronic immune activation → immunosuppression → ↑ risk of fungal infection

---

Fact 848:

What strategies can be employed to enhance the effectiveness of **renal replacement therapy (RRT)** in cases where acidosis persists despite its initiation?

- ↑ Blood flow
- ↑ Effluent dose
- ↓ Pre-dilution
- ↓ Interruptions
- Improve vascular access

Fact 849:

What are the possible causes of a **profound motor block** in a patient with an epidural?

- Received a large local anaesthetic bolus
- Catheter migration into the subarachnoid or extradural space
- Epidural abscess
- Epidural hematoma

Emergency management includes stopping the epidural infusion, re-evaluating and considering an urgent spinal MRI.

Fact 850:

What is the difference between **sensitivity** and **capture threshold** of a pacing box?

- Sensitivity is the minimum voltage (in mV) for sensing native electrical activity. A lower number means greater sensitivity. The 'pacing threshold' is the sensitivity at which the sense indicator flashes during each endogenous depolarisation when tested. Sensitivity is typically set at 30–50% of the measured pacing threshold (or at 2 mV if no underlying native rhythm is present).
- The capture threshold is the minimum output required to stimulate an action potential in the myocardium, confirmed with a QRS complex following each pacing spike. Output is usually set at 2–3 x the measured capture threshold.

Fact 851:

What receptors do **vasopressin** act on and what are the physiological effects?

- V_1: Vasoconstriction everywhere other than pulmonary circulation
- V_2: H_2O absorption in distal convoluted tubule and collecting duct of the kidney
- V_3: ACTH release from anterior pituitary

Fact 852:

How do you calculate **sensitivity, specificity, positive predictive value (PPV)** and **negative predictive value (NPV)** using a two-by-two contingency table?

		Disease		Predictive value
		+	**−**	
TEST	**+**	True Positive (TP)	False Positive (FP)	**PPV** $\frac{TP}{TP + FP}$
	-	False Negative (FN)	True Negative (TN)	**NPV** $\frac{TN}{FN + TN}$
Sensitivity & specificity		**Sensitivity** $\frac{TP}{TP + FN}$	**Specificity** $\frac{TN}{FP + TN}$	

Fact 853:

What are some antibiotics and cardiovascular drugs that may exacerbate **myasthenia gravis**?

Antibiotics	Cardiovascular
• **F**luoroquinolones • **L**incosamides • **A**minoglycosides • **T**etracyclines • **C**olistin • **A**mpicillin • **M**acrolides • **P**olymyxins	• Calcium channel blockers • Beta-blockers • Procainamide • Quinidine • Magnesium • Statins

Fact 854:

What intervention should you consider in someone with an **acute sudural haematoma** who develops a pulmonary embolism one day following evacuation?

An IVC filter given the risk of a potentially lethal recurrent PE

Anticoagulation is risky with an acute haematoma and thrombolysis is contraindicated.

An IVC filter can be permanent or temporary.

Fact 855:

How do you define **contrast-induced acute kidney injury (CI-AKI)**, and what are some of the risk factors?

- ↑ Serum creatinine > 0.5 mg/dL or >25% from baseline within 48 hours after iodinated contrast media (CM)
- Aetiology:
  - o Vasoconstrictive effect of CM on large and small renal arteries → renal medullary ischaemia.
  - o Direct cytotoxic effect on the vascular endothelium and renal tubular cells → cell injury and death from reactive oxygen species.
  - o CM viscosity may play a role in pathogenesis.
- Risk factors:

Patient-related	Nonpatient-related
• Inpatient risk > outpatient risk • CKD with or without DM • Age > 75 • Albuminuria • Abnormal volume states, e.g. heart failure, hypovolaemia • Haemodynamic instability	• Contrast osmolality • Total contrast dose and sequential CM dosing • Concomitant exposure to nephrotoxic agents • Requirement for an intra-aortic balloon pump • It is unclear if IA has a greater risk than IV

Fact 856:

What are some of the major complications of **ECMO**?

- Complications of vascular access
- Major or significant bleeding, e.g. intracranial haemorrhage, major vessel rupture
- Circuit clots or systemic thromboembolism, e.g. strokes
- Specific to VA-ECMO:
  - o Limb ischaemia
  - o LV distension and pulmonary haemorrhage
  - o Cardiac chamber thrombosis

Fact 857:

What is the **deep sulcus sign** on a CXR suggestive of?

Pneumothorax

The costophrenic angle is abnormally deepened.

Fact 858:

How does an excess of immunoglobulins in **multiple myeloma** affect serum sodium levels?

It can lead to pseudohyponatremia.

Fact 859:

What are the pathophysiological changes and diagnostic criteria for **hepatorenal syndrome causing acute kidney injury (HRS-AKI)** (formerly type 1 HRS)?

The pathophysiology is multifactorial:

- Pro-inflammatory cytokines contribute to splanchnic vasodilatation, portal hypertension and ↓ SVR
- ↓ SVR leads to ↓ BP
- This results in an ↑ cardiac output and activation of the RAAS, ADH and sympathetic nervous system, resulting in renal vasoconstriction, Na^+ & H_2O retention, ascites and hyponatremia
- ↑ Renal vasoconstriction → ↓ GFR → ATN

The criteria for diagnosis:

- Cirrhosis + ascites; acute-on-chronic liver failure
- **D**rugs: No current/recent nephrotoxic drugs
- **R**enal disease: No macroscopic signs of parenchymal renal disease, e.g. no proteinuria, no microscopic haematuria, no abnormal renal US
- **A**KI: ↑ creatinine ≥ 0.3 mg/dL in 48 hours or ≥ 50% from baseline or urine output ≤ 0.5 mL/kg/hr for ≥ 6 hours
- **M**inimal/no response to two consecutive days of diuretic withdrawal and plasma volume expansion (HAS 1 g/kg/day up to a max 100 g/day)
- **A**bsence of shock

Fact 860:

What are the requirements, indications and goals of a **resuscitative thoracotomy** in a traumatic cardiac arrest?

Requirements	• ETT • Shock or cardiac arrest in the presence of a suspected correctable intrathoracic lesion or a specific diagnosis (e.g. cardiac tamponade, penetrating cardiac injury or aortic injury) • Evidence of ongoing thoracic haemorrhage
Accepted Indications	• Penetrating injury + arrest + previous signs of life • Blunt injury + arrest + previous signs of life
Goals	• Alleviate cardiac tamponade • Conduct open cardiac massage • Interrupt aortic blood flow to enhance perfusion to the heart and brain • Control life-threatening thoracic bleeding • Control broncho-venous air embolism

This should be started within 10 minutes of the cardiac arrest, if indicated. Outcomes are better in penetrating injuries than in blunt injuries.

Fact 861:

What are some likely reasons for unconsciousness in a patient with an **extensive burn**?

• Hypoxia, e.g. inhalation injury, carbon monoxide poisoning, cyanide poisoning
• Shock (hypotension)
• Alcohol and drug intoxication
• Head injury, e.g. TBI

Fact 862:

What are the effects of **hypothermia** on the renal, endocrine, gastrointestinal, haematological and immune systems?

System	Effect/s
Renal	• Renal vasoconstriction, ADH resistance and ↓ reabsorption of solutes → 'cold diuresis' • Metabolic acidosis • ↑ K^+, ↑ Mg^{2+}
Endocrine	• ↓ Pancreatic insulin secretion → ↑ glucose
Gastrointestinal	• ↓ GI motility • ↓ Hepatic blood flow and drug metabolism • ↓ Glucose/fat metabolism
Haematological	• ↑ Clotting time, ↑ viscosity and thrombocytopaenia → ↑ bleeding risk
Immune	• ↓ WCC and function → impaired immunity → ↑ risk of infection

Fact 863:

What happens to the serum calcium in **ethylene glycol poisoning**?

↓ Levels due to precipitation with oxalate

Fact 864:

What are the advantages of **high-flow nasal oxygen (HFNO)**?

• Provides warmed humidified oxygen.
• Delivers a precise FiO_2 of up to 1.0 at high-flow rates of e.g. 60 L/min, matching or surpassing peak inspiratory flow.
• Anatomical reservoir of O_2 in nasopharynx and oropharynx → CO_2 washout → ↓ dead space and ↓ work of breathing.
• Provides some CPAP/PEEP when the mouth is closed.
• ↑ Mucociliary clearance.

Fact 865:

How much pleural fluid is typically needed for a **pleural effusion** to show on a CXR?

>150–200 mL

Fact 866:

What is the most common opportunistic infection of the central nervous system in patients with **acquired immune deficiency syndrome (AIDS)**?

Toxoplasmosis

Fact 867:

What are the two phases of **amniotic fluid embolism (AFE)**?

AFE is an immune, not embolic, condition. It is a clinical diagnosis. Foetal antigens in amniotic fluid trigger an anaphylactoid reaction, leading to symptoms like hypotension, hypoxia, seizures and coagulopathy without another clear cause. It can happen during labour, soon after delivery or during dilation and evacuation.

- *Phase 1*: Amniotic fluid and foetal cells entering the maternal circulation trigger biochemical mediator release, causing pulmonary artery vasospasm and acute pulmonary hypertension. ↑ RV pressures and RV dysfunction lead to hypoxemia, hypotension and related myocardial and microvascular damage.
- *Phase 2*: LV failure and pulmonary oedema develop. Biochemical mediators trigger DIC leading to massive haemorrhage and uterine atony.

The key factors in the management are early recognition, prompt resuscitation and delivery of the fetus.

Fact 868:

How does carbon monoxide (CO) poisoning cause **rhabdomyolysis**?

CO poisoning → muscle tissue hypoxia → muscle cell damage → release of toxic muscle contents

---

Fact 869:

What effect do neuromuscular blocking drugs have on **somatosensory evoked potentials (SSEPs)**?

No effect since the study focuses on the sensory, not motor, pathway

---

Fact 870:

What are some causes of **expiratory limb obstruction** in a ventilator circuit?

- *Tubing*: Kinked tubing, incorrect tubing diameter, e.g. using neonatal tubing for a larger child
- Expiratory filter blockage, e.g. secretions, blood
- Expiratory valve malfunction
- Water condensation

Fact 871:

What type of statistical test would you use to analyse blood pressure data in a **randomised controlled trial**?

Parametric tests

BP is a form of quantitative data characterised by a normal distribution.

Fact 872:

Why are organ transplant recipients who receive calcineurin inhibitors at risk of developing **posterior reversible encephalopathy syndrome (PRES)**?

- PRES is associated with an abrupt ↑ in BP. It is a syndrome of headaches, confusion, seizures and visual disturbance. It is characterised by vasogenic oedema predominantly in the parietal and occipital lobes. These show up as diffuse hyperintense lesions in the white matter on T2-weighted MRI.
- Calcineurin inhibitors like ciclosporin and tacrolimus can cause hypertension as a side effect. This is thought to be mediated by activation of the renal NaCl Co-transporter (NCC).
- Rapid control of the hypertension should reverse the features of PRES.

Fact 873:

What are the preconditions for **brainstem testing**?

- Irreversible brain damage of known aetiology
- Unconscious, apnoeic and mechanically ventilated
- The condition should not result from factors that can be fully or partially reversed, e.g. CVS and respiratory instability, metabolic and endocrine disturbances, hypothermia, sedative medications or potentially treatable causes of apnoea, e.g. neuromuscular disorders or muscle relaxants.

If depressant drugs have been used, five half-lives should have passed before testing. If there is any doubt, specific drug levels should be measured.

Fact 874:

Why is **Entonox** not used for analgesia in cases of pneumothorax, intestinal obstruction and during myringoplasty?

Entonox is 50% nitrous oxide and 50% oxygen.

It can diffuse into gas-filled cavities. It can therefore exacerbate a pneumothorax, make intestinal pain worse and make inner ear surgery difficult.

It is useful in childbirth and in orthopaedic manipulation as a patient-controlled analgesic via a demand valve.

Fact 875:

How would you treat new onset **tonic-clonic epilepsy** in someone of child-bearing age?

- Start lamotrigine
- Supplement with folic acid as anticonvulsants may disrupt intestinal folic acid absorption

Although sodium valproate is first line for generalised tonic clonic seizures, it can cause neural tube defects. Folic acid deficiency also poses a risk for neural tube defects.

Fact 876:

What conditions is **ribavirin** used to treat?

This is an antiviral used to treat RSV infection, hepatitis C and some viral haemorrhagic fevers.

Fact 877:

Which nerve is affected in **winging of the scapula**?

Long thoracic nerve (nerve root C5–7)

Fact 878:

What types of shock can occur in **amniotic fluid embolism**?

- *Obstructive*: Pulmonary artery vasoconstriction on exposure to immunologically active substances
- *Cardiogenic*: LV dysfunction
- *Distributive*: Part of SIRS with capillary leak
- *Haemorrhagic*: Because of the development of DIC

Fact 879:

What are some causes of **stridor** in children?

Congenital abnormalities		Non-congenital	
Nasal	- Choanal atresia - Septum deformities	Acute	- Foreign body - Airway burns - Bacterial tracheitis - Epiglottitis - Anaphylaxis - Croup
Cranio-facial	- Pierre Robin syndrome - Apert syndrome	Sub-acute	- Peritonsillar abscess - Retropharyngeal abscess
Laryngeal	- Laryngomalacia - Subglottic/tracheal stenosis - Vocal cord paralysis - Tracheomalacia	Chronic	- Vocal cord dysfunction - Laryngeal spasm - Neoplasms - Multiple system atrophy

Fact 880:

In the context of solid organ transplants, when is the recipient at the greatest risk of **CMV infection**?

- *Donor*: CMV positive
- *Recipient*: CMV negative

Fact 881:

Are there any variations in conducting **chest compressions** on a pregnant patient in the third trimester?

The hand placement might require adjustment to a higher position on the sternum.

Fact 882:

What is the approximate volume required within the pericardium to manifest **Beck's triad**?

- Acute: About 100 mL (e.g. trauma, aortic dissection).
- Chronic: About 1,500 mL (e.g. uraemia, pericarditis, autoimmune diseases, malignancies, radiation-related issues).

Fact 883:

What could be the potential reasons if, immediately after **endotracheal intubation**, there is limited chest movement and elevated airway pressures?

- **P**neumothorax
- **O**bstruction from secretions
- **K**inked endotracheal tube
- **E**ndobronchial intubation
- **D**ynamic hyperinflation due to bronchospasm
- **D**istension of stomach

Fact 884:

What is the purpose of temporarily storing the shock energy of a **defibrillator** in a capacitor, and why are inductors integrated into the system?

Batteries can store energy but cannot release it quickly enough for effective defibrillation. Capacitors are capable of rapidly discharging energy when charged to high voltages, making them suitable for this purpose.

For successful defibrillation, it's essential to maintain a sustained current over a few milliseconds. However, the current and charge from a capacitor discharge exponentially and quickly diminish. Inductors are added to the system to prolong the duration of the current, ensuring effective defibrillation.

Fact 885:

What are the features of **autonomic dysreflexia (AD)**?

AD is a complication of spinal cord injury at or above T6. It leads to uncontrolled sympathetic responses to noxious stimuli below the injury level. This occurs because there are functioning sensory afferent sympathetic fibres below the injury level but a loss of descending inhibitory fibres.

- Noxious stimulus below lesion → uninhibited sympathetic response → diffuse vasoconstriction in many arterial networks. This leads to systemic hypertension and ↑ risk of a hypertensive crisis, despite maximal parasympathetic vasodilatory efforts above the level of the injury.
- ↑ BP → stimulation of baroreceptors → ↑ vagal tone to heart → ↓ HR (bradycardia)
- Skin changes are observed as follows:
  - o *Below lesion*: Pale and dry skin due to vasoconstriction
  - o *Above lesion*: Flushed skin, diaphoresis and piloerection due to vasodilation

Treatment involves addressing noxious stimuli below the lesion (e.g. urinary retention, faecal impaction, pressure sores) and using rapidly acting antihypertensive medications like GTN, nifedipine, hydralazine or labetalol for hypertension. Bradycardia can be managed with atropine or glycopyrrolate.

Fact 886:

What are some contraindications to **proning** for ARDS?

- Spinal instability
- Pregnancy
- Pelvic fracture
- Severe haemodynamic instability
- ↑ Intracranial pressure
- ↑ Intra-abdominal pressure

Fact 887:

Is giving **hydrocortisone** time-critical in anaphylaxis?

Nope

Fact 888:

What is the primary reason for mortality following a substantial **inhalation injury**?

Respiratory failure

This arises from a combination of factors, including the inhalation of particulate matter leading to airway and pulmonary damage, and subsequent inflammatory responses that can result in ARDS.

Fact 889:

How do you classify strokes using the **Bamford classification**?

Total anterior circulation stroke	Lacunar syndrome	Posterior circulation syndrome
All three of these: • Unilateral weakness (and/or sensory loss) of the face, arm and leg • Homonymous hemianopia • Higher cerebral dysfunction (dysphasia, visuospatial disorder)	One of these: • Pure sensory stroke • Pure motor stroke • Sensori-motor stroke • Ataxic hemiparesis	Any one of these: • Cerebellar dysfunction • Isolated homonymous hemianopia or cortical blindness • Brainstem signs
Partial anterior circulation stroke: Two of the above		

Fact 890:

How does a **transthoracic echocardiogram** assist in assessing a high-risk or massive pulmonary embolism (PE) in unstable patients?

- Eliminates the risk of moving an unstable patient for a CTPA scan.
- Aids in diagnosis, e.g. RV dilation, pulmonary hypertension, direct visualisation of thrombus, McConnell's sign
- Rules out other causes of cardiovascular instability, e.g. valvulopathy, left ventricular dysfunction or pericardial tamponade.

Fact 891:

What thyroid function tests differentiate between **primary hypothyroidism** and **sick euthyroid syndrome**?

Primary hyperthyroidism	Sick euthyroid
↓ T3 ↓ T4 ↑ TSH	↓ T3 ↓ or normal T4 ↓ or normal TSH

In sick euthyroid, thyroid replacement is not necessary because increased T3 tissue receptor synthesis maintains clinical euthyroidism even when there is biochemical evidence suggesting otherwise.

Fact 892:

What are examples of **Gram-positive** bacteria?

Gram-positive bacteria have an inner cell membrane and an outer thick peptidoglycan layer. This allows the bacteria to take up the purple-coloured Gram stain.

Cocci				Bacilli
Staphylococcus			**Strep**	**'ABCDL'**
Co-agulase +ve	Coagulase –ve		See table below	Actinomyces Bacillus Clostridia Dipheria (Corynebacterium) Listeria
Aureus	Novo-biocin sensitive	Novo-biocin resistant		
	Epidermidis	Saprophyticus		

Streptococcus					
Partial haemolysis (α haemolytic)		Complete haemolysis (β haemolytic)		No haemolysis (γ)	
Unencapsulated	Encapsulated	Group A	Group B	Enterococci	
Viridans, e.g. S. mutans, S. mitis	S. pneumonia	S. pyogenes	S. agalactiae	S. faecium, S. faecalis	S. bovis

Fact 893:

What is the definition of **proteinuria** in nephrotic syndrome?

≥3 g in 24 hours

Nephrotic syndrome is the triad of proteinuria, oedema and hypoalbuminemia.

Fact 894:

What is the typical fluid infusion rate to keep an A-line patent?

2–4 mL/hr pressurised NaCl 0.9%/heparinised saline

Fact 895:

In managing **infected pancreatic necrosis**, what additional interventions should be considered beyond antibiotic therapy?

- Fine needle aspiration for culture
- Percutaneous drainage
- Surgical necrosectomy

Fact 896:

How do you confirm **NGT placement**?

- If an aspirate is obtained, test the aspirate on a pH indicator. If the aspirate pH is <5.5, the NG tube can be used.
- If no aspirate can be obtained, or the pH is >5.5, then perform a CXR:
  - The CXR should include the upper oesophagus and extend to below the diaphragm.
  - The NG tube should bisect the carina, and must not follow the course of either of the main bronchi.
  - The NG tube should remain in the midline down to the level of the diaphragm.
  - The tip of the NG tube should be clearly visible and below the left hemidiaphragm.
  - The tip of the NG tube should be approximately 10 cm beyond the GOJ (i.e. within the stomach).

Fact 897:

What is meant by the **precision** of a test?

The ability to produce consistent and reproducible measurements when the test is repeated.

Fact 898:

What are the main causes of a **pulmonary-renal syndrome** in someone with diffuse alveolar haemorrhage and glomerulonephritis-induced acute kidney injury?

ANCA-associated vasculitis	Anti-GBM disease
Granulomatosis with polyangiitis	Also known as Goodpasture's disease
Microscopic polyangiitis	
Eosinophilic granulomatosis with polyangiitis	

Fact 899:

What are the most prevalent types of protein, lipid and carbohydrate in **total parenteral nutrition (TPN)**?

- *Protein*: Amino acids
- *Lipid*: Triglycerides
- *Carbohydrate*: Glucose

Fact 900:

Why is **ethylene oxide** used for industrial sterilisation?

It is a highly penetrative gas capable of killing bacteria, spores and viruses.

It is used for the industrial sterilisation of heat-sensitive equipment, e.g. plastics, sutures and single-use equipment.

Fact 901:

Besides managing intracranial pressure, what other neuroprotective strategies help mitigate secondary brain injury in individuals with **traumatic brain injury**?

Maintain adequate oxygen delivery	• Adequate MAP to achieve CPP $\geq$ 60 mmHg to optimise perfusion and $\downarrow$ ischaemia to the penumbra • PaO_2 >10 kPa • $PaCO_2$ 4.5–5.0 kPa • Deep sedation/paralysis to avoid coughing and vomiting
Optimise cerebral venous drainage	• 30-degree head up • Avoid tight endotracheal tube ties • Avoid excessive PEEP
Minimise cerebral oedema	• Na^+ 145–150 mmol/L
Minimise $CMRO_2$	• Avoid hyperthermia • Prevent seizures • Normoglycaemia

Fact 902:

What are the effects of mechanical ventilation on the **right ventricle**?

$\uparrow$ Intrathoracic pressure $\rightarrow$ $\downarrow$ venous return (preload) and $\uparrow$ right ventricular afterload

Fact 903:

How do **V/Q mismatch** values differ between the lung base and apex in a healthy individual, and what distinguishes a shunt from dead space?

V/Q at bases	V/Q at apex	Overall V/Q of the lung
0.6	3	~1 (almost all blood returning to the left heart is oxygenated)

- **Shunt**: V/Q ratio of 0 (perfusion without ventilation), e.g. intra-pulmonary shunts (e.g. dense consolidation) or intra-cardiac shunts (e.g. septal defects).
- **Dead space**: V/Q ratio of infinity (ventilation without perfusion), e.g. a massive pulmonary embolism.

Fact 904:

What are some causes of **right raised hemi-diaphragm**?

- Right phrenic nerve palsy
- Lung conditions causing volume loss, e.g. lobar collapse, lobectomy, pneumonectomy and pulmonary hypoplasia
- Abdominal pathology, e.g. tumour, subphrenic abscess, bowel distention and ascites

Fact 905:

How is **lactate** normally cleared?

- Around 1–2% is excreted unchanged in the urine.
- 98–99% is oxidised by lactate dehydrogenase into pyruvate, which then follows one of two paths:
  - Pyruvate enters the mitochondria and is converted into acetyl-CoA, which is further metabolised in the citric acid cycle (Krebs cycle) for energy production.
  - Alternatively, pyruvate can be converted into oxaloacetate and, eventually, into glucose through gluconeogenesis, which is a part of the Cori cycle.

This process of lactate clearance, particularly the conversion to glucose, primarily occurs in the liver and, to a lesser extent, in the kidneys.

Fact 906:

What are the anatomical borders of the **'triangle of safety'** for intercostal drain insertion?

- *Anterior*: Lateral border of pectoralis major
- *Posterior*: Lateral border of latissimus dorsi
- *Inferior*: Horizontal line from nipple (or fifth ICS)
- *Superior*: Base of axilla

Fact 907:

What is the relationship between **dexmedetomidine** and **atipamezole**?

- Dexmedetomidine induces sedation as an α_2-agonist.
- Atipamezole is a highly selective α_2-antagonist, which is used to reverse this sedative effect.

Fact 908:

What is **acute epiglottitis** (supraglottitis) and why is it more common in adults than children?

- Epiglottitis is cellulitis of the epiglottis and its adjacent supraglottic structures (e.g. aryepiglottic folds, arytenoid cartilages, vallecula).
- It's more common in adults due to widespread immunisation against *Haemophilus influenzae* B in children.
- Bacterial pathogens are implicated include *Haemophilus parainfluenzae*, *Streptococcus pneumoniae* and *Streptococcus pyogenes*.
- Definitive diagnosis involves direct visualisation of the epiglottis via laryngoscopy or flexible nasoendoscopy.
- Empiric antibiotic treatment with third-generation cephalosporins (ceftriaxone, cefotaxime) and vancomycin is recommended.

Fact 909:

What are some causes of a **prolonged QT** on an ECG?

Congenital	• Romano–Ward syndrome (autosomal dominant) • Jervell–Lange–Neilson (autosomal recessive, associated with congenital deafness)
Pathologies	• Myocardial ischaemia • Subarachnoid haemorrhage • Hypothermia
Electrolyte abnormalities	• Hypokalaemia • Hypomagnaesaemia • Hypocalcaemia
Antiarrhythmics	• Amiodarone • Sotolol • Quinidine
Antimicrobials	• Quinolones, e.g. levofloxacin, moxifloxacin, • Macrolides, e.g. erythromycin, clarithromycin • Antimalarials, e.g. quinine • Antiprotozoal, e.g. pentamidine • Azole antifungals, e.g. fluconazole, ketoconazole
Antiemetics	• Ondansetron
Antacids	• Cisapride
Psychiatric drugs	• TCAs (tricyclic antidepressants) • SSRIs (selective serotonin reuptake inhibitors) • Phenothiazines • Butyrophenones (e.g. haloperidol)

Fact 910:

How is the **WETFLAG acronym** employed when managing children aged 1–10 years?

			Example of a 2-year-old
W	Weight (kg)	(Age + 4) × 2	(2 + 4) × 2 = 12 kg
E	Energy	4 J/kg	12 × 4 = 48 J
T	Tube (uncuffed ETT)	Age/4 + 4	2/4 + 4 = 4.5 uncuffed tube
Fl	Fluid (bolus) of crystalloid	Trauma — 10 mL/kg	10 mL × 12 kg = 120 mL bolus
		Non-trauma — 20 mL/kg	20 mL × 12 kg = 240 mL bolus
A	Adrenaline	10 mcg/kg = 0.1 mL/kg of 1 in 10,000 solution	10 µg × 12 kg = 120 µg 1:10,000 = 1.2 mL
G	Glucose	2 mL/kg 10% dextrose	2 mL × 12 kg = 24 mL 10% dextrose

Fact 911:

Which **state of matter** has volume but no definite shape?

Liquids

Solids have a definite volume and shape. Gases have no finite shape or volume.

Fact 912:

How do you estimate **blood volume** and **systolic blood pressure** in a four-year-old boy?

Blood volume	Systolic blood pressure
80 mL/kg up to 2 years 70 mL/kg thereafter	(Age × 2) + 80
Est weight = 2(4+4) = 16 kg Therefore 70 × 16 = 1,200 mL	(4 × 2) + 80 = 88 mmHg

Fact 913:

What is the difference between **tachyphylaxis** and **densensitation**?

- Tachyphylaxis is a rapid ↓ in the response to a drug over a short period, typically minutes to hours. This often results from the acute depletion of neurotransmitters. An example is ephedrine, which can quickly deplete noradrenaline stores.
- Tolerance or desensitisation is a gradual ↓ in activity of a drug over a period of days or week, e.g. opioids/dobutamine (down-regulation of receptors), barbiturates (liver enzyme induction) and nitrates (depletion of sulphydryl groups in smooth muscle).

Fact 914:

What should you be mindful of when using standard **non-depolarising neuromuscular blocking drugs** in ICU?

Benzylisoquinolines	
Atracurium	Associated with bronchospasm due to histamine release
Cis-atracurium	Most haemodynamically stable but expensive
Aminosteroids	
Rocuronium	• Highest risk of anaphylaxis • Prolonged duration of action in hepatic and renal impairment • Reversed by sugammadex

Fact 915:

What is the mechanism behind **invasive arterial blood pressure (IABP)** measuring?

- The A-line connects to pressurised fluid in rigid tubing.
- Intra-arterial pulsations travel to the pressure transducer, which includes a sensitive diaphragm and strain gauge in a Wheatstone bridge setup.
- Pulsations deform the diaphragm, altering strain gauge resistance.
- An electronic device detects these resistance changes.
- Fourier analysis processes the data to create the blood pressure waveform.

Fact 916:

What makes a barium swallow unsuitable for diagnosing **Boerhaave syndrome**?

Extravasation can worsen mediastinal inflammation with subsequent fibrosis.

VATS with fundic reinforcement is the gold standard of treatment.

Fact 917:

Which blood product would you give next to someone with massive **haematemesis** who has already received a major transfusion and these are his urgent post-transfusion blood tests:

- ↑ PT 15.5 seconds (12–15)
- ↑ APTT 35.5 seconds (25–35)
- ↓ Fibrinogen 0.3 g/L (1.5–4)
- ↓ Hb 105 g/L (130–180)
- ↓ WCC 3.4 × 10⁹/L (4–11)
- ↓ Platelets 115 × 10⁹/L (150–400)

Cryoprecipitate – contains large amounts of fibrinogen.

A fibrinogen level < 0.5 g/L is strongly associated with microvascular bleeding. A fibrinogen level > 1.5 g/L should be the target in major haemorrhage.

Fact 918:

How can the reticulocyte count help differentiate anaemia caused by a **parvovirus infection** from a haemolytic crisis in someone with sickle cell disease?

- The reticulocyte count is ↓ in a parvovirus infection.
- The reticulocyte count is ↑ in a haemolytic crisis.

Parvovirus ↓ erythropoiesis which leads to an aplastic crisis.

Fact 919:

How do **Erb's palsy** and **Klumpke's palsy**, both potential birth-related brachial plexus injuries, differ from each other?

	Erb's PALSY	Klumpke's palsy
Part of plexus	Upper plexus (C5–C7)	Lower plexus (C8–T1)
Mechanism of injury	Shoulder dystocia during birth	Excessive arm traction during birth
Some clinical features	Sensory loss down lateral arm 'Waiter's tip' position: • Shoulder adducted • Elbow extended • Arm internally rotated • Forearm pronated	• Sensory loss in medial forearm and hand • Complete claw-hand • Wasting of small muscles in hand • Horner's syndrome may co-exist

---

Fact 920:

How do generic scores compare to specific liver scores in predicting outcomes in **liver failure**?

It depends on various factors:

1. *Liver disease severity*: Specific liver scores like MELD and Child-Pugh may be more accurate in advanced liver failure and decompensated cirrhosis due to their focus on liver-specific abnormalities.
2. *Multi-organ dysfunction*: In critically ill liver failure patients with multiple organ involvement, generic scores such as APACHE and SOFA may offer a more comprehensive evaluation of overall illness severity and mortality risk.
3. *Liver failure cause*: The underlying cause of liver failure can influence score effectiveness. Scores like MELD, tailored to certain liver conditions like chronic liver disease and cirrhosis, may perform better in these scenarios.

No single scoring system is universally superior in predicting liver failure outcomes. Clinicians typically combine scoring systems and clinical judgment to assess liver disease severity and to guide management.

Fact 921:

What is a **quality-adjusted life-year (QALY)**?

A QALY quantifies the health impact of a medical intervention or prevention program using the formula:

QALY = Years of life × utility value

The utility value ranges from 1 (perfect health) to 0 (death):

- If someone enjoys perfect health for one year, they gain 1 QALY. (1 year of life × 1 utility value = 1 QALY)
- If someone experiences perfect health for half a year, they gain 0.5 QALYs. (0.5 years of life × 1 utility value = 0.5 QALYs)

QALYs facilitate the calculation of cost–utility ratios for interventions, enable comparisons between different interventions and aid in resource allocation decisions.

Fact 922:

Why may **coronary artery bypass grafting (CABG)** mimic sepsis?

CABG triggers a systemic inflammatory response. Both on-pump and off-pump CABG techniques can elicit this response.

Fact 923:

Would administering IV radiological contrast be appropriate for someone at risk of **acute kidney injury**?

Yes – the diagnostic benefits of using contrast for accurate pathology visualisation often outweighs the risk

The notion of contrast-induced nephropathy, characterised by a reduction in kidney function following contrast use, lacks robust evidence which links it to significant adverse outcomes.

A 2023 multi-site study reported no significant relationship between the use of contrast and sustained AKI at hospital discharge, or the necessity for dialysis within 180 days in those with pre-existing AKI (PMID: 36715705).

Consensus recommendations support its use in stable renal disease and in patients with pre-existing AKI. In severe AKI, think about the potential need for RRT.

Fact 924:

Which organism is associated with **infective endocarditis** in the context of colorectal cancer?

Streptococcus gallolyticus (also known as *Streptococcus bovis*)

Fact 925:

What are some features of **severe pre-eclampsia**?

Severe pre-eclampsia is defined by the presence of any of the following:

A	Pulmonary oedema
B	
C	SBP ≥ 160 mmHg or DBP ≥ 110 mmHg
D	Papilloedema, clonus, severe headache, visual disturbance
E	Significant tissue oedema
F	Renal failure
G	ALT or AST > 70 IU/L, right upper quadrant/ epigastric tenderness, vomiting, HELLP syndrome
H	Platelets <100 × 10^9 /L

Fact 926:

Applying the **Stewart approach**, what would be sodium/chloride base excess (BE) effect if the serum Na$^+$ is 140 mmol/L and serum Cl$^-$ is 117 mmol/L?

Sodium/chloride BE effect:

= ([Na$^+$] – [Cl$^-$]) – 40

= (140 – 117) – 40 = –17

When the sodium/chloride base excess is in the negative range, it is referred to as hyperchloremic acidosis.

Fact 927:

What are the two subtypes of **hepatorenal syndrome-non-AKI (HRS-NAKI)** (formerly type 2 HRS)?

HRS-NAKI	
HRS acute kidney disease	**HRS chronic kidney disease**
Cirrhosis + ascites	
No other cause of kidney disease	
eGFR < 60 for < 3 months	eGFR < 60 for ≥ 3 months

Fact 928:

What is the mechanism of action of **quetiapine**?

Therapeutic effects:

- 5-HT_{2A} antagonism in the frontal cortex
- D_2 antagonism in the mesolimbic pathway
- 5-HT_{1A} partial agonism

Side effects:

- α_1 *antagonism*: ↓ BP
- H_1 *antagonist*: Sedative effects and weight gain

Fact 929:

When does a **delayed haemolytic transfusion reaction (DHTR)** occur?

> 24 hours after a transfusion

An unexplained fever and ↓ Hb typically develops 5–10 days after the transfusion.

A DHTR occurs in those previously sensitised to non-ABO antigens through past transfusions. Upon re-exposure with a new transfusion, an anamnestic response causes a rapid antibody titre increase, resulting in a positive Direct Antiglobulin Test (Direct Coombs' test) and fragile ballooned spherocytes on blood film. Additional features include:

- ↑ Unconjugated bilirubin (dark urine)
- ↑ LDH ↑ reticulocytes
- ↓ Haptoglobin

Fact 930:

What happens to the ventilation and perfusion in the **lateral decubitus position** in a healthy spontaneously breathing patient?

The lung on the dependent side will exhibit ↑ ventilation and perfusion compared to the nondependent lung.

Fact 931:

What are the features and pathophysiology of **propofol infusion syndrome (PRIS)**?

Acute refractory ↓ HR + 1 or more of the following:

- **M**etabolic acidosis (base deficit > 10 mmol/L)
- **E**nlarged/fatty liver
- **R**habdomyolysis (↑ CK, ↑ K^+, AKI) or myoglobinuria
- **L**ipaemic plasma (↑ triglycerides)

Pathophysiology:

- Impaired mitochondrial fatty acid metabolism → ↓ fatty acid utilisation → ↑ accumulation → arrhythmias
- Direct mitochondrial respiratory chain inhibition → ↓ oxygen utilisation → anaerobic respiration → ↑ lactate
- Direct myocardial depressant → cardiac dysfunction

Risk factors ('SCAMPI'):

- **S**tarvation (↓ carbohydrate intake) releases FFAs
- **C**atecholamine or glucocorticoid administration
- Young **A**ge (↓ glycogen storage)
- Subclinical **M**itochondrial disease
- **P**ropofol Dose > 4 mL/kg/hr for > 48 hours
- Critical **I**llness

Fact 932:

For meningitis with a risk of **Listeria monocytogenes**, which antibiotic complements cefotaxime and dexamethasone treatment?

Ampicillin

Fact 933:

How would you define **Wolff–Parkinson–White syndrome**?

The presence of an accessory pathway capable of causing symptomatic tachyarrhythmias due to pre-excitation

Fact 934:

What is the most frequent complication following an **inferior myocardial infarction**, and what is the underlying reason?

Cardiac dysrhythmias, e.g. complete heart block

This occurs because an infarction in this area can lead to ischaemic compromise of the SA and AV nodes in most individuals. The right coronary artery is often implicated in this situation.

Fact 935:

What are common pathological causes of **hyperphosphatemia**?

- *Renal disease*: ↓ excretion
- *Hypoparathyroidism*: ↓ excretion

Fact 936:

What intervention involving glucose control has been shown to reduce the incidence of **ICU-AW**?

Tight glycaemic control with intensive insulin therapy

This however goes against the NICE-sugar protocol and is therefore not practiced.

Fact 937:

What is a **U-wave** on an ECG and in which conditions is it most commonly seen?

A small (0.5 mm) positive deflection immediately following the T-wave. Most commonly seen in bradycardia and severe hypokalaemia.

Fact 938:

How would you manage a 10-year-old boy with a background of autism and pica, who exhibits ataxia, microcytic hypochromic anaemia and **multiple radiopaque spots** on his abdominal X-ray?

Whole bowel irrigation – this is lead poisoning.

The child ingested lead from non-food items, possibly paint chips. Early symptoms are non-specific, and blood tests may reveal anaemia and basophilic stippling. The recommended treatment is gastrointestinal decontamination to prevent further lead absorption.

Fact 939:

Why is **dexamethasone** started empirically along with ceftriaxone in a 16-year-old presenting with fever, headache, neck pain and photophobia?

- Associated with a ↓ hearing loss, neurologic complications and mortality in *S. pneumoniae* meningitis. This is the most common cause of bacterial meningitis in adults in the developed world.
- Adjunctive dexamethasone should be given just before or concurrently with the initial antibiotic dose. It should only be continued if the CSF Gram stain and/or the CSF/blood cultures reveal *S. pneumoniae*.

Fact 940:

What are some complications of **hyperoxia**?

A	• Tracheobronchitis • Mucosal damage
B	• Alveolar toxicity → ARDS • Absorption atelectasis • ↓ Respiratory drive • Pulmonary vasodilation: CO_2 narcosis can develop in patients dependent on a hypoxic drive, e.g. COPD
C	• Vasoconstriction → Hypertension • Bradycardia (reflex) • ↓ Cardiac output
D	**CNS**	• ↓ Cerebral blood flow • Amnesia • Seizures
	Ophthalmic	• Myopia (reversible) • Cataract formation • Retrolental fibroplasia (children)

Fact 941:

How do **calcium channel blockers (CCBs)** influence the impact of non-depolarising muscle relaxants?

CCBs → ↓ calcium release from nerve terminals → prolonged effect of non-depolarising muscle relaxants

Fact 942:

What is the definition of **multidrug-resistant tuberculosis (MDR-TB)**?

Strains of *Mycobacterium tuberculosis* that are resistant to at least isoniazid and rifampicin.

Fact 943:

What are some scenarios where **high-flow nasal oxygen (HFNO)** is a favoured indication?

• When NIV is unsuitable, e.g. oesophageal surgery
• In situations where intubation is not appropriate, e.g. palliative symptom relief
• To facilitate intubation, e.g. pre-oxygenation, apnoeic oxygenation
• To prevent T1RF after cardiac surgery
• For oxygenation during procedures with sedation that require mouth access, e.g. bronchoscopy, TOE, endoscopy

Some potential areas of clinical application where there is evolving evidence include:

• Acute hypoxemic respiratory failure
• Post-surgical respiratory failure
• Acute heart failure/pulmonary oedema
• Hypercapnic respiratory failure, e.g. COPD
• Pre- and post-extubation oxygenation
• Obstructive sleep apnoea

Fact 944:

What is the **half-life** ($t_{1/2}$) of the following drug:

Time following injection (hours)	Plasma concentration (mcg/mL)
2	400
6	100
10	25
14	6.25

Extrapolating further values:

Time following injection	Plasma concentration
0	800
2	400
4	200
6	100
8	50
10	25
12	12.5
14	6.25

$T_{1/2}$ is the time it takes for the initial plasma concentration to fall by 50%. Therefore, $t_{1/2}$ = **2 hours**

Fact 945:

Which bacteria are most commonly responsible for causing **meningitis** in different age groups?

<3 months	3 months–2 years	2–50 years	>50 years
Listeria monocytogenes	Neisseria meningitides (meningococcus)		
	Streptococcus pneumoniae (pneumococcus)		
Escherichia coli			
Group B streptococcus			*L. monocytogenes*
	Haemophilus influenza		

Fact 946:

What are the most likely reasons for a **raised lactate** following trauma?

- *Type A lactic acidosis*: Occurs in hypoperfusion states with excessive anaerobic metabolism
- *Type B*: Results from the inability of organs, such as the liver, to metabolise lactate

Lactate has consistently demonstrated prognostic value in trauma patients. There is minimal distinction between venous and arterial lactate levels.

Fact 947:

In cases of persistent ST elevation following **thrombolysis** for a STEMI, is it advisable to administer a second dose of thrombolysis?

No – repeat fibrinolysis is contraindicated.

Rescue PCI is indicated instead.

Fact 948:

Why might initiating **erythromycin** for pneumonia increase the bleeding risk in someone on warfarin for atrial fibrillation?

Erythromycin → CYP3A4 inhibition → ↓ hepatic metabolism of warfarin → ↑ prothrombin time/INR

Fact 949:

Which assay is suitable for monitoring the anticoagulant effects of **low molecular weight heparin** in an individual with a burn injury?

Anti-factor Xa assay

Fact 950:

At what points in relation to the A-line trace and ECG should the inflation and deflation of an **intra-aortic balloon pump (IABP)** occur?

	Inflation	Deflation
Cardiac cycle	In diastole	At the beginning of systole, before the aortic valve opens, in the isovolumetric contraction phase
A-line	Dicrotic notch	Just before the upstroke on the A-line trace
ECG	Middle of the T wave on the ECG	R wave on the ECG
Effects	↑ Coronary perfusion because of ↑ diastolic pressure and ↓ LV wall tension	↑ CO through ↓ afterload (and therefore ↓ cardiac work, ↓ oxygen demand and ↓ LV-EDP)

Fact 951:

What tubing characteristics prevent **overdamping** in the system transmitting pulsatile fluid from an arterial catheter to the transducer system?

The tubing should be stiff (non-compliant), short in length and wide in diameter.

Fact 952:

How is **cystatin C** helpful in assessing renal clearance?

Cystatin C is a small protease inhibitor unaffected by muscle mass, making it valuable for renal clearance calculations in situations of extreme body weight and in paediatrics. In AKI, cystatin C levels ↑.

Other biomarkers, like TIMP-2 for tubular stress, and NGAL and KIM-1 for tubular damage, are not yet in clinical use.

Fact 953:

How do you treat **propofol infusion syndrome (PRIS)**?

- Stop propofol and use another sedative
- RRT to treat acidosis, remove propofol and other toxic metabolites
- Cardiorespiratory support, e.g. chronotropic agents, VA-ECMO
- Carbohydrate loading and minimising lipid intake

Fact 954:

Which drugs and electrolyte imbalances can enhance the effects of **non-depolarising neuromuscular blockers**?

Drugs	Electrolyte disturbances
• Local anaesthetics • Inhalational anaesthetics, e.g. halothane • Lithium • Antibiotics, e.g. aminoglycosides, tetracycline • Ca²⁺-channel blockers, e.g. verapamil	• ↓ K⁺ • ↓ Ca²⁺ • ↑ Mg²⁺

Fact 955:

How does **rasburicase** work to reduce the risk of acute kidney injury in tumour lysis syndrome (TLS)?

In TLS, ↑ cell turnover → ↑ purine metabolism → ↑ uric acid → crystals deposit in renal tubules/ducts → AKI

Rasburicase catalyses the oxidation of uric acid (which has low solubility) to the more water soluble allantoin.

↓ Uric acid means ↓ crystal deposition in the kidney.

Fact 956:

What is **procalcitonin (PCT)**?

- **Origin and clearance**: PCT is a prohormone of calcitonin produced by thyroid C-cells. The liver and kidneys play roles in its clearance.
- **Production in sepsis**: In sepsis, it arises from extra-thyroid tissue (e.g. neuroendocrine cells in the lung and intestine) in response to pro-inflammatory stimuli such as bacterial endotoxin and inflammatory cytokines.
- **Specificity for sepsis**: PCT is more specific for bacterial sepsis than CRP, peaking within 6 hours and having a half-life of about 24–36 hours. It aids in distinguishing bacterial from non-bacterial inflammation.
- **Use in antibiotic stewardship**: While PCT peaks quickly, it is not recommended for starting antibiotics but helps guide antibiotic duration as levels ↓ when bacterial infection is appropriately treated.
- **Limitations**:
  o PCT is less useful in assessing viral/fungal infections as its levels are not typically elevated in these conditions.
  o PCT can be elevated in non-infective conditions, e.g. burns, trauma, major surgery, ESRF and paraneoplastic production, e.g. medullary thyroid carcinoma or SCLC.

Fact 957:

What are some mechanisms by which bacteria develop **antibiotic resistance**?

Mechanism	Description	Example
Modification	Modifying structure of antibiotic	Adding acetyl groups to aminoglycosides
Degradation	Enzymatic degradation of antibiotics	β-lactamases
Efflux	Removal of antibiotic from the cell using energy from ATP hydrolysis	Pseudomonas has a pump for many antibiotics
Target modification	Alteration of antibiotic binding targets	Peptidoglycan remodelling on the cell wall by MRSA
Sequestration	Proteins bind to antibiotics to stop them from binding to their targets	Bleomycin-binding proteins

Resistance relies on mutation and genetic transfer mechanism such as:

- *Transformation*: Bacteria take up free DNA and incorporate it into its own genome.
- *Transduction*: Transfer of genetic material from one bacterium to another by a bacteriophage (virus).
- *Conjugation*: Direct transfer of DNA circles (plasmids) between two bacterial cells that are in physical contact.
- *Transposition*: Movement of genetic elements, known as transposons or 'jumping genes', within a genome.

Fact 958:

What are the clinical features associated with various types of **cerebral herniation syndromes**?

Type of herniation	Clinical features	Examples of causes
Lateral transtentorial (uncal)	Ipsilateral CN3 palsy, contralateral hemiplegia/ posturing (Kernohan notch phenomenon)	Temporal lobe mass lesion where the medial temporal lobe moves under the tentorium cerebelli
Central transtentorial	Coma with progression from bilateral decorticate to decerebrate posturing and loss of brainstem reflexes	Diffuse cerebral oedema or hydrocephalus causes downward displacement of the diencephalon
Subfalcine	Coma with asymmetric motor posturing (contralateral > ipsilateral)	Frontal or parietal mass lesions cause cingulate gyrus to move under the falx cerebri
Cerebellar (upward or downward)	Sudden progression to coma (limited space in the posterior fossa) with bilateral motor posturing in someone with cerebellar signs	Cerebellar mass lesion forcing the cerebellar tonsils through the foramen magnum

Fact 959:

What are some possible clinical indications for an **intra-aortic balloon pump (IABP)**?

- Cardiogenic **S**hock
- **W**eaning from cardiopulmonary bypass
- Refractory unstable **A**ngina or ventricular arrhythmias
- Acute **M**yocardial infarction, including acute mitral regurgitation and/or VSD development post infarction
- **P**ost-operative support in cardiac surgery
- **S**tructural heart disease, e.g. cardiomyopathy, LVF

Fact 960:

What are the key intra-operative management goals in someone with **mitral regurgitation (MR)**?

In MR, a proportion of blood ejected by the LV flows back into the LA. Overtime, this leads to LA dilation and pulmonary hypertension (P-HTN).

Intra-operative management goals include:

- Avoid hypoxia, hypercarbia, acidosis and excessive inspiratory pressures which can worsen P-HTN
- ↑ LV stroke volume by maintaining or ↑ preload
- Balance this with ↑ HR → ↓ time for regurgitation
- ↓ Regurgitant fraction by ↓ afterload, e.g. vasodilatation to ↑ forward flow

Fact 961:

What is the treatment approach for **acute pancreatitis** induced by elevated triglyceride levels?

Insulin – this ↓ triglyceride levels by activating lipoprotein lipase which metabolises chylomicrons. If this does not work, then plasmapheresis is an alternative.

Fact 962:

What makes **dexmedetomidine** a suitable choice for managing hyperactive delirium in someone with ileus, a QTc > 450 ms, and who is receiving pressure support ventilation via a tracheostomy?

Can be administered intravenously, does not have respiratory-depressant effects and is less prone to causing QTc prolongation when compared to other agents.

Medications like haloperidol prolong the QTc interval, benzodiazepines can exacerbate delirium, atypical antipsychotics lack IV formulations and propofol has respiratory suppressant effects.

Delirium is an independent predictor of ↑ mortality at six months and ↑ LOS.

Fact 963:

What are some ways of reducing the risk of **electrical injury** in ICU?

- *Mains isolating transformer*: Isolates the power supply from the ground, preventing current flow through a person in contact with faulty equipment.
- *Earth leakage circuit breaker*: Shuts off the electrical supply upon detecting stray currents.
- *Common earth connection*: Links all earthing points in a patient care area, minimising the risk of microshock.
- *Use of Class II equipment*: Provides double insulation, ensuring that even with one fault, no part of the casing accessible to the patient carries a live current.

Fact 964:

How do you manage suspected **hepatorenal syndrome**?

- Volume repletion using 20% human albumin solution at 20–40 grams per day
- Vasoconstriction with terlipressin (0.5–2 mg every 4–6 hours) to redirect blood flow to vital organs via splanchnic vasoconstriction
- Treating concurrent infections, e.g. SBP
- Providing supportive care
- Considering liver transplantation for eligible cases

Fact 965:

How can you classify **scoring systems**?

Class	Description	Examples
Physiological (illness severity)	Uses physiological variables, assuming that greater derangement indicates both a sicker patient group and a poorer prognosis	• APACHE II–IV • SAPS (Simplified Acute Physiology Score) • MODS (Multiple Organ Dysfunction Score) • P-POSSUM (Physiological and Operative Severity Score for the enUmeration of Mortality and morbidity)
Ongoing assessment	Uses data over a longer period of time rather than at a single point to allow assessment of response to an intervention	• SOFA (Sequential Organ Failure Assessment) score • NEWS (National Early Warning Score)
Disease Specific	Organ specific	• MELD in liver disease • CURB-65 in community acquired pneumonia • Well's Score in PE
Interventions	The more interventions a patient requires, the higher the score and the sicker they are perceived to be	• TISS (Therapeutic Intervention Scoring System): measures the amount and complexity of nursing interventions required for each ICU patient
Anatomical	Uses anatomical regions	• ISS (Injury Severity Score)

Fact 966:

What is the **Standardised Mortality Ratio (SMR)**?

SMR = Observed mortality rate/Expected mortality rate

- Score > 1 worse than expected
- Score < 1 better than expected

Expected deaths are typically predicted by applying a scoring system to the patient population, e.g. APACHE II.

While this ratio is employed to assess service quality, it possesses numerous limitations.

Fact 967:

How is **sepsis** defined?

- *Definition*: Life-threatening organ dysfunction caused by a dysregulated host response to infection.
- *Clinically*: Acute increase of SOFA score ≥ 2 points.

Fact 968:

What dermatomal level is **xiphisternum** and **umbilicus**?

- Xiphisternum: T6
- Umbilicus: T10

Fact 969:

In which adult medical conditions can **hyperoxia** lead to worsened outcomes?

- **S**troke (acute)
- **M**yocardial infarction (acute)
- **A**rrest: Post-cardiac arrest syndrome
- **L**ung diseases with hypoxic drive
- **L**ung injury (acute)
- **S**evere head injury

Fact 970:

Why is a **bronchospastic** ETCO$_2$ trace shaped like this?

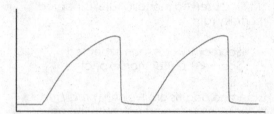

- In bronchospasm, alveolar units with poor ventilation ($\downarrow$ V/Q) empty later in expiration than those with high ventilation ($\uparrow$ V/Q)
- These late-emptying units accumulate more CO$_2$ from the blood
- The ETCO$_2$ is therefore a reflection of alveoli with the longest time constants (time constant = compliance $\times$ resistance)

Fact 971:

What is the **cerebral perfusion pressure (CPP)** and how is it relevant in head injury?

CPP = MAP – ICP

Under normal conditions, ICP ranges from 0 to 10 mmHg, primarily regulated by autoregulation of cerebral blood flow (CBF). In a head injury, this autoregulation is disrupted, and CBF becomes directly linked to CPP. The desired CPP target is in the range of 60–70 mmHg.

Before ICP monitoring is established, the target MAP is 80–90 (assuming ICP is at 20 mmHg) to ensure an adequate CPP. Once ICP monitoring is established, then treatment is targeted at maintaining CPP 60–70 mmHg.

Fact 972:

What type of performance device is a **Hudson mask**?

Variable performance device – delivers a variable FiO$_2$

FiO$_2$ is influenced by the oxygen flow rate and peak inspiratory flow rate. When a patient's inspiratory effort exceeds the supplied oxygen flow rate, which can occur due variations in tidal volume, inhalation speed and respiratory rate, air will be entrained at a variable ratio throughout the respiratory cycle.

Fact 973:

How do the **hepatic extraction ratios** of warfarin and phenytoin compare to those of morphine and propranolol?

- *Low hepatic extraction ratio*: Warfarin & phenytoin
- *High hepatic extraction ratio*: Morphine & propranolol

Fact 974:

Which drugs can provide symptomatic relief for **acute pericarditis**?

NSAIDs, corticosteroids and colchicine

Fact 975:

What does trial data state about the use of **intra-aortic balloon pump (IABP)**?

In the IABP Shock II (2012) trial, there was no difference in mortality between patients who had acute myocardial infarction complicated by cardiogenic shock and were randomly assigned to either IABP or conservative management (medical therapy).

Fact 976:

Why is the **expired fraction of oxygen (FeO$_2$)** a useful marker of preoxygenation in an RSI?

FeO$_2$ > 90% is sufficient to ensure de-nitrogenation of the FRC, which is the determining factor of oxygen desaturation during apnoea.

Fact 977:

How should circulatory failure in **sepsis** and **septic shock** be managed?

- *IV fluids*: Give 30 mL/kg of balanced crystalloid within 3 hours and consider albumin if large volumes of crystalloid are given.
- *Vasoactive agents*: Initiate noradrenaline as the first-line agent, targeting a MAP ≥ 65 mmHg. If MAP remains inadequate with noradrenaline at 0.25–0.5 µg/kg/min, consider adding vasopressin.
- *Corticosteroids*: If there is an ongoing requirement for vasopressors, introduce IV corticosteroids.
- In cases of cardiac dysfunction despite adequate volume and blood pressure, consider an inotropic agent, e.g. dobutamine or switching to adrenaline.

Fact 978:

Which graft is preferred for a **coronary artery bypass graft (CABG)** for left coronary lesions?

Left internal mammary artery graft

↓ Future intervention, ↓ morbid events, ↑ graft patency

Fact 979:

Can **propofol infusion syndrome (PRIS)** be prevented with early nutrition?

Yes

In the presence of carbohydrate, lipid metabolism slows.

Fact 980:

How does **intraparenchymal ICP monitoring** compare to subdural, subarachnoid or extradural systems in terms of accuracy?

Intraparenchymal monitoring is the most accurate compared to the other methods.

Fact 981:

What are the indications for **one-lung ventilation (OLV)**?

- Prevent contamination of the other lung (e.g. haemorrhage or bronchiectasis)
- Regulate ventilation distribution (e.g. bronchopleural fistula, traumatic bronchus rupture or large bullae)
- Facilitate surgical access (in select cases) (e.g. thoracic aortic aneurysm, pneumonectomy, oesophagectomy)

OLV is typically accomplished using a double-lumen tube (DLT), the insertion of an endobronchial blocker, or intentional endobronchial intubation. DLTs are larger than standard ETTs, with a 13 mm external diameter and smaller lumens, each measuring 5 mm.

Fact 982:

What does a **Clinical Pulmonary Infection Score (CPIS)** > 6 suggest?

The presence of pulmonary infection/VAP

CPIS is a diagnostic scoring based on six variables.

Each element is scored 0–3, with 3 indicating most severe derangement: (1) Temperature, (2) leucocytosis, (3) P/F ratio, (4) CXR infiltrates, (5) volume & character of secretions and (6) results of microbiological analysis.

Fact 983:

When may a **tracheo-oesophageal fistula** develop?

Commonly seen with injury to the posterior tracheal wall during tracheostomy. Excessive secretion production and recurrent aspiration may suggest this complication.

Fact 984:

How does **protamine** work to reverse heparin?

Protamine (positively charged) reverses heparin (negatively charged) by forming an inactive complex that is cleared by the reticuloendothelial system.

Fact 985:

Why doesn't **amiodarone** require adjustment in renal failure?

Amiodarone is excreted almost completely in bile

It is metabolised by CYP34A to N-desethylamiodarone and has a half-life of about 25 days.

Fact 986:

If a drug has a **half-life** of 4 hours, what proportion of it will be eliminated 20 hours after ingestion?

20 hours = 5 half-lives

50% + 25% + 12.5% + 6.25% + 3.125% = 97%

Therefore 97% of the drug will be eliminated.

Fact 987:

What are requirements for admission to **HDU**?

- Support for a single organ (excluding mechanical ventilation), e.g. renal support or vasopressors
- Maintained with a nurse-to-patient ratio of 1:2

Fact 988:

What is the observed association between ECMO use and the occurrence of **venous thromboembolism (VTE)**?

- Studies have identified a relationship between ECMO use and the incidence of VTE.
- It's important to exercise caution when interpreting this association due to the descriptive nature of these studies and variations in data.

Fact 989:

What are some causes of **distributive shock**?

- Sepsis
- Anaphylaxis
- Neurogenic shock
- Acute adrenal insufficiency (absence of hormones which normally maintain vascular tone)

Fact 990:

Which neuraminidase inhibitors can you use to treat **influenza A** in someone with respiratory failure?

- Oseltamivir first line
- Zanamivir second line

Influenza viruses are single-strand RNA viruses, classified into types A, B and C. Influenza A is more virulent and common, while influenza B is milder but can cause outbreaks. Influenza C leads to mild or asymptomatic illness. Types A and B have subtypes based on haemagglutinin and neuraminidase antigens. Transmission occurs through respiratory secretions via droplets, aerosols, or direct contact, with an incubation period of 1–3 days.

Fact 991:

What is the cause of a **high anion gap metabolic acidosis (HAGMA)** in an elderly patient with low BMI receiving flucloxacillin and paracetamol for cellulitis?

Pyroglutamic acidosis – a rare cause of HAGMA

Pyroglutamic acid (or 5-oxoprolinemia) is typically metabolised by 5-oxoprolinase. In cases of glutathione depletion, there is ↑ activity of γ-glutamyl cyclotransferase, leading to ↑ pyroglutamic acid.

Risk factors for pyroglutamic acidosis include:

- Glutathione depletion (e.g. malnutrition, pregnancy, sepsis or paracetamol use)
- Inhibition of 5-oxoprolinase (e.g. flucloxacillin)

Treatment involves addressing contributing factors (e.g. stopping paracetamol and flucloxacillin) and administering NAC/methionine to restore glutathione levels.

Fact 992:

What meant by the **'p-value'**?

The probability of observing results as extreme as, or more extreme than, the ones observed, assuming the null hypothesis is true.

Fact 993:

Where does the majority of blood drain in a **persistent left-sided SVC (PLSVC)**, and what are the risks of using a central line inserted into it?

PLSVCs drain blood either into:

- *The coronary sinus (in the right atrium)*: There is a risk of arrhythmias with central line use.
- *The left atrium*: There is a risk of systemic air embolism with central line use.

PLSVCs are typically smaller than right-sided SVCs, making them less tolerant of high-flow rates, such as during haemofiltration.

Diagnosis frequently happens by chance, often when a chest X-ray taken after the insertion of a central line shows the line positioned on the left side of the chest.

Fact 994:

Is clonus typically observed in **neuroleptic malignant syndrome (NMS)**?

Nope

It is more commonly associated with serotonin syndrome.

Fact 995:

What is the mechanism of toxicity in **calcium channel blocker (CCB) overdose**?

The three classes of CCBs affect L-type channels in cardiac myocytes, vascular smooth muscle and beta islet cells:

Dihydropyri-dines	Non- dihydropyridines	
	Phenylalky-lamines	Benzothiaz-epines
Nifedipine Amlodipine Nicardipine Nimodipine	Verapamil	Diltiazem

Toxic effects include:

Cardiac	• Verapamil and diltiazem suppress cardiac contractility, SAN automaticity and AVN conduction. • Dihydropyridines have a milder impact on pacemaker cells and myocardial contractility.
Vascular smooth muscle	• Verapamil and dihydropyridines induce significant vasodilation, leading to systemic hypotension. • Diltiazem causes less vasodilation.
Metabolic	• Hypo-insulinaemia and insulin resistance • The adaptive response of the myocardium, which normally shifts from using free fatty acids to carbohydrates as its main energy source, is compromised. This is caused by impaired glucose uptake and disrupted calcium-dependent mitochondrial activity that is essential for glucose breakdown.

Fact 996:

How should you address low haemoglobin and low ferritin in someone who receives erythropoietin treatment for anaemia associated with **chronic kidney disease**?

Intravenous iron

Erythropoietin may not be effective when ferritin levels are low. If haemoglobin remains low despite adequate iron, consider increasing the dose of erythropoietin.

Fact 997:

Which **electrolyte** should be the initial priority for replacement if someone has:

- Confusion, lethargy and tingling in the extremities
- A self-terminating seizure
- Muscle weakness accompanied by positive Chvostek's and Trousseau's signs
- An ECG displaying ST depression, T-wave flattening, U-waves and a QTc of 500 ms

IV magnesium

Symptomatic manifestations of hypocalcaemia, hypokalaemia and hypomagnesaemia warrant prioritising Mg^{2+} replacement as the initial treatment approach.

Fact 998:

How does the level of **spinal cord injury** affect respiratory function?

Level of injury	Effect	Need for ventilation
Above C3	Diaphragmatic paralysis	Immediate and long-term. Early tracheostomy is encouraged. A surgical tracheostomy is preferred with an unstable C-spine.
C3–C5	Partial phrenic nerve denervation causes diaphragmatic weakness/ paralysis	80% of patients will require ventilation within 48 hours
Above T8	Weakness of intercostal and abdominal muscles	Impaired sputum clearance may require brief ventilation
Below T8	Weakness of abdominal muscles	Brief ventilation may be needed due to a weak cough and impaired sputum clearance

Note that cord ischaemia spreads bidirectionally from the injury site within the first 72 hours, potentially causing an ascending neurological level and clinical deterioration. Early on, there may be flaccid areflexia and hypotonia below the lesion level before upper motor neuron signs appear. Over the initial weeks, muscle spasticity ↑, leading to ↑ thoracic wall tone and ↓ chest wall compliance. Autonomic dysfunction can result in ↑ secretions and bronchospasm.

Fact 999:

What are the major potential complications of **sickle cell disease**?

Thrombotic	Bony pains, abdominal crises, chest crises, neurological signs or priapism
Aseptic necrosis	Humeral or femoral heads
Aplastic crises	Triggered by parvovirus B19 infection
Haemolytic anaemia	↑ Risk with dehydration, infection, hypoxaemia and cold temperatures
Sequestration crises	Occurs in children with rapid enlargement of the liver and spleen
Hyposplenism	Due to auto-infarction in childhood
Renal failure	Due to renal medullary infarction or glomerular disease
Osteomyelitis	Typically caused by unusual organisms, e.g. Salmonella

Fact 1000:

How may reduced albumin levels impact the unbound drug concentration in someone with a **burn injury**?

↓ Albumin → less drug–protein binding → ↑ proportion of unbound drug

Fact 1001:

Which agents are used to control **hypertension** in pre-eclampsia?

Depends on pre-existing treatment, side effects and risk. Examples include labetalol, nifedipine, hydralazine and methyldopa with a target BP ≤ 135/85 mmHg. Epidural analgesia may also be considered as an adjunct.

Note that thiazides, ACE inhibitors and ARBs are associated with ↑ risk of congenital abnormalities.

Fact 1002:

What is the difference between variable performance and fixed performance **oxygen delivery devices**?

Variable performance (patient dependent)	Fixed performance (patient independent)
Delivered FiO_2 is variable and depends on patient factors, device used and oxygen flow rate	Delivers a specific FiO_2
• Nasal cannula • Hudson mask • Non-rebreathe mask	• Venturi

Fact 1003:

What is a ventilator-associated event (VAE)?

A VAE is characterised by a decline in respiratory status following a stable or improving ventilator period, along with signs of infection or inflammation and laboratory evidence of respiratory infection. They are classified as:

Ventilator-associated condition (VAC)	
After two days of stability or improvement, there is now worsening oxygenation. Patients should have at least one of the following: • ↑ FiO_2 ≥ 0.2 for ≥ 2 days • ↑ PEEP ≥ 3 for ≥ 2 days	
Infection-related ventilator-associated condition (IVAC)	
VAC + abnormal temperature or WCC + new antimicrobial requirement	
Possible/ Probable VAP	
IVAC + purulent secretions and/or positive culture	
Possible VAP	**Probable VAP**
Gram stain evident of purulent pulmonary secretions	Gram stain evident of purulent pulmonary secretions
OR	AND
Positive pathogenic pulmonary culture	Positive pathogenic pulmonary culture

Fact 1004:

What are the options to **anticoagulate** a RRT circuit?

In RRT, blood interaction with the filter circuit triggers platelet activation and the coagulation cascade. Anticoagulation is recommended to prevent filter clotting, preserve filter membrane permeability and extend filter lifespan.

First-line: citrate	Regional anticoagulation ↓ bleeding risk but is contraindicated in severe liver disease or shock due to the risk of citrate accumulation/ toxicity.
Second-line: Heparin	• UFH is titratable, easily monitored and can be reversed. • LWMH is not titratable with no definitive reversible agent. • Citrate and heparin show no mortality difference in comparison.
Others	• Patients with HIT: Direct thrombin inhibitors (lepirudin, argatroban, bivalirudin) or anti-thrombin-dependent factor Xa inhibitors (danaparoid, fondaparinux) can be used. Argatroban is recommended by KDIGO in HIT unless there is severe liver disease. • Epoprostenol acts as a platelet inhibitor but is not recommended by KDIGO due to limited efficacy when used alone, potential hypotension and ↓ filter longevity.

Fact 1005:

What occurs if you discontinue the infusion of a drug with a short and stable **context-sensitive half-time (CSHT)**?

It will wear off very quickly and predictably after stopping the infusion. An example of this is remifentanil.

CSHT is the time it takes for an infused drug's plasma concentration to drop by 50% upon discontinuation. Drugs like fentanyl with a more prolonged CSHT will take much longer to wear off and are less predictable.

Fact 1006:

What happens to the **arterial waveform** in response to shock states?

	MAP	DBP	Pulse pressure	Pulse pressure variation	Dicrotic notch
Vasodilation	↓	↓	↑	-	Shifts downwards
Hypovolaemia	↓	↑	↓	↑	-
Impaired ventricular function	↓	↑	↓	-	-

Fact 1007:

What are some of the physiological responses to **altitude**?

Respiratory system	Cardiovascular system
• Acute: ↑ minute ventilation as peripheral chemoreceptors respond to hypoxia • Chronic: ↑ tidal volume due to thoracic remodelling	• Acute: ↑ HR and ↑ BP due to ↑ sympathetic activity • Chronic: Hypoxia stimulates haemopoiesis, raising haematocrit levels, and eventually, HR and SV normalise.
Neurological system	**Renal system**
• ↓ Cognitive function • ↑ Risk of delirium	• ↑ Diuresis → haemoconcentration → ↑ haematocrit • ↓ Serum bicarbonate (due to hypocapnia)

Fact 1008:

Why is **lorazepam** better than diazepam in treating status epilepticus?

- *Half-life*: Lorazepam is less lipid-soluble than diazepam with a distribution half-life of 2–3 hours versus 15 minutes for diazepam
- *Receptor effects*: Lorazepam binds GABAergic receptors more tightly resulting in a longer duration of action.

Fact 1009:

When present, what is the significance of the fourth and fifth positions of a **pacemaker** code?

- *Fourth position*: The ability of the pacemaker to alter the rate based on physiological demand. R if rate modulation is present, O if not.
- *Fifth position*: Denotes if the pacemaker is pacing at more than one site in the atrium (A), ventricle (V) or both (D). If not present, O is used.

Fact 1010:

How does hydroxyurea work in the management of **sickle cell disease (SCD)**?

Stimulates the production of foetal haemoglobin (HbF), which carries oxygen more effectively and is less likely to polymerise (sickle) compared to HbS.

Fact 1011:

Which three elements are required for a **fire** to start?

Heat, Oxygen and Fuel

Fact 1012:

What is the mechanism of action of the drug used to treat **Scarlet Fever**?

Penicillin is used as it targets *Streptococcus pyogenes*. It binds to transpeptidase to block the cross-linking of peptidoglycan cell walls, ultimately resulting in bacterial cell lysis.

Fact 1013:

Who is at risk of developing **portal hypertensive gastropathy (PHG)**?

Those with portal hypertension

The gastric mucosa in PHG shows congested capillaries, appears red and oedematous, often in the proximal stomach, and can develop a mosaic pattern. In severe PHG, the mucosa becomes fragile and prone to bleeding upon contact.

Fact 1014:

What effect does brown-red nail polish have on **pulse oximeters**?

It leads to the underestimation of oxygen saturations.

Fact 1015:

What potential risks should you consider when selecting medication for intubating someone with a **traumatic brain injury**?

Risk	Consideration
Exaggerated reflex sympathetic response to laryngoscopy	Consider using fentanyl or remifentanil
Hypotension due to induction agents	Consider dose reduction if using propofol or thiopentone
Exacerbation of raised intracranial pressure	• Give analgesia, keep head in neutral position, avoid neck constraints and consider osmotherapy. • Although ketamine is no longer contraindicated in ↑ICP, it may ↑ BP

Fact 1016:

What is the significance of performing a transthoracic echocardiogram (TTE) in cases of **pericarditis**?

To determine the presence of a pericardial effusion and to evaluate for concomitant myocarditis.

Fact 1017:

What is the primary explanation for an elderly patient having an elevated baseline **pulse pressure**?

↓ Aortic compliance

Fact 1018:

What is the most common **CMV disease** in HIV?

CMV retinitis

Fact 1019:

When are tunnelled lines appropriate for administering **total parenteral nutrition (TPN)**?

If TPN is required for >30 days, e.g. bowel failure

Long-term TPN is changed to cyclical administration as it is more physiological.

Short-term TPN (e.g. bowel rest following surgery or inefficiency of enteral intake) needs dedicated port/access, e.g. PICC line or CVC with dedicated port

---

Fact 1020:

How does **serotonin syndrome (SS)** differ clinically from **neuroleptic malignant syndrome (NMS)**?

	SS	NMS
Agent	Serotoninergic drug	Dopamine antagonist (or withdrawal of dopamine agonist)
Onset	Abrupt (within 24 hours)	Gradual (days to weeks)
Course	Rapidly resolving (within 24 hours)	Prolonged (days to weeks)
CNS & ANS	Altered mental status and autonomic instability	
Neuro-muscular	Myoclonus & tremor	Lead-pipe rigidity
Reflexes	↑	↓
Pupils	Mydriasis	Normal

Fact 1021:

Which phase of the cardiac action potential is responsible for the tall, tented T-waves seen in **hyperkalaemia**?

Phase 3 – the T-wave corresponds to repolarisation, which is due to efflux of potassium.

Fact 1022:

How should **acute decompensated cardiac failure** be managed in someone with distress, diaphoresis and tachypnoea?

1. Supplementary oxygen. Excess oxygen administration can cause vasoconstriction, ↑ afterload and worsen heart failure.
2. IV loop diuretics (e.g. furosemide) for diuresis, ↓ preload and venodilatation. Resistant cases may require adding a thiazide diuretic or initiation of RRT.
3. Opiates (e.g. diamorphine) provide anxiolysis, ↓ catecholamine levels and have a venodilator effect.
4. Vasodilators (e.g. glyceryl trinitrate, SNP) ↓ afterload and ↓ preload. Overall helps to ↑ stroke volume. Should not be given if SBP < 90 mmHg.
5. CPAP if refractory hypoxia for ↑ alveolar recruitment, ↑ oxygenation, ↓ work of breathing and ↑ cardiac output.
6. Cardiogenic shock may require inotropes, vasopressors +/– circulatory assist devices +/– revascularisation:
   a. Inodilators, e.g. milrinone, enoximone
   b. Inotropes, e.g. levosimendan, dobutamine
   c. Inopressors, e.g. noradrenaline, adrenaline
   d. Mechanical support, e.g. IABP, VAD, VA-ECMO

Once symptomatic relief has been achieved, management can shift its focus to addressing the underlying cause, such as ischaemia, arrhythmias, tamponade, emboli, aortic disease or cardiomyopathy.

Fact 1023:

What is the dose of **intralipid** in treating a ventricular fibrillation arrest in someone with an epidural catheter?

- Initial 1.5 mL/kg bolus.
- Infusion of 15 mL/kg/hr.
- Further boluses of 1.5 mL/kg at 5-minute intervals if the patient remains in cardiac arrest (maximum 3).
- Double the infusion rate after 5 minutes if the patient remains in cardiac arrest.
- Maximum cumulative dose of 12 mL/kg.

Fact 1024:

What are the storage temperatures and shelf-life durations for common **blood products**?

	Storage temperature	Approximate shelf-life
Platelets	Room temperature 20–24°C and therefore ↑ risk of bacterial contamination	5 days
Red blood cells	2–6°C	35 days
Fresh frozen plasma	−30°C to maintain factor 5 and 8 activity	1–2 years. Has to be used within 24 hours of thawing.

Fact 1025:

What does the following **volume/time** graphic on a mechanical ventilator suggest?

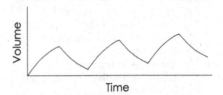

Dynamic hyperinflation – although a constant TV is being delivered, the waveform does not return to baseline and becomes progressively higher. This indicates that not all the gas entering the lungs with each breath is exhaled.

Managing this may require treating the underlying cause, e.g. bronchospasm, ↑ expiratory time and disconnection the circuit to allow trapped gas to escape.

Fact 1026:

How does a transducer function in an **invasive arterial blood pressure (IABP)** monitoring system?

A transducer transforms energy from one form to another.

In this instance, it converts kinetic energy into electrical energy, which is subsequently measured, analysed, processed and displayed.

Fact 1027:

What are the potential complications of **tracheostomy** insertion?

Immediate	• Problems with oxygenation (decruitment, bronchospasm, lung collapse, aspiration) • Bleeding • Damage to structures, e.g. oesophagus, thyroid, recurrent laryngeal nerve • Subcutaneous emphysema • Risk of death
Short-term	• Wound infection or problems with healing • Bleeding • Tracheo-innominate artery fistula • Accidental decannulation • Inadequate sputum clearance
Long-term	• Tracheal stenosis • Tracheomalacia • Changes in strength/pitch of voice • Scarring

Fact 1028:

At which point in the respiratory cycle is it most appropriate to remove a **chest drain**?

Expiration

This minimises the risk of air being drawn into the pleural space when the drain is removed.

Fact 1029:

How do you diagnose and treat **hyperosmolar hyperglycemic state (HHS)**?

Diagnosis includes all of the following:

• Dehydration
• Osmolality > 320 mOsm/L
• Glucose > 30 mmol/L
• Absence of significant ketosis

Management:

• Initial management is with NaCl 0.9% (+/– potassium) without insulin until the osmolality stops decreasing–then change to 0.45% saline.
• Insulin should only be started (FRII 0.05 units/kg/hr) at presentation if there is significant ketosis (urine > 2+ or blood > 1 mmol/L) OR if the blood glucose & osmolality are not falling in spite of adequate fluid resuscitation.

Fact 1030:

How does the overall mortality rate of **acute endocarditis** caused by S. aureus compare to that associated with intravenous drug use?

Acute endocarditis due to S. aureus is associated with a high mortality rate (30–40%), except when it is associated with intravenous drug use.

Fact 1031:

What are the basics of **ABO compatibility**?

ABO group	Red cell antigens	Antibodies in serum	Compatible red blood cells	Compatible plasma	
O	None	Anti-A Anti-B	O	AB	O A B
A	A	Anti-B			A
B	B	Anti-A			B
AB	A and B	None			A B AB

Some key points:

- AB: No antibodies, universal recipients for red cells.
- O: No antigens, universal donors for red cells.
- *Plasma compatibility*: Reverse of red cells (O is universal recipient, AB is universal donor).
- *Rh-negative females of childbearing age*: Should receive Rh-negative red cells and platelets to prevent developing anti-D antibodies. For other patients, Rh compatibility is preferred but not critical.

Fact 1032:

What are some differences between paediatric and adult **airways and breathing**?

Feature	Paediatric	Adult
Head	Large occiput	Smaller occiput
Breathing preference	Nose in infants	Mouth
Tongue	Large	Small
Epiglottis shape	Floppy, U-shaped	Firm, flatter
Epiglottis level	C3, 4	C5, 6
Larynx	Funnel-shaped, anterior	Column/cylindrical
Trachea	Narrow, short (bifurcates at T2)	Wide, long (bifurcates at T4)
Narrowest airway point	Subglottic region	Glottis
Soft tissues	More lax	More rigid
Airway resistance	Higher (smaller diameter)	Lower (larger diameter)
Minute ventilation (MV)	Higher (RR drives MV)	Lower
Lung compliance	Low in newborns, increases with age	About 200 mL/cmH$_2$O
Inspiratory reserve	Lower (closing volume > FRC until about 8 years)	Higher
Diaphragm use	About 95% for quiet breathing	About 40% for quiet breathing

Fact 1033:

In **high-frequency oscillatory ventilation (HFOV)**, which factors are responsible for oxygenation and CO_2 removal?

- HFOV achieves ventilation with ↓ TVs (1–3 mL/kg) at ↑ frequency (3–15 Hz). An electromagnetic piston on the inspiratory limb rapidly moves a flexible diaphragm, causing pressure oscillations (delta P) around the mean airway pressure.
- Settings include mean airway pressure (MAP), delta P, I:E ratio and frequency. TV cannot be directly set. $ETCO_2$ monitoring is not possible.
- Compared to conventional ventilation, there is ↓ peak airway pressure but ↑ mean airway pressure.
- Gas exchange occurs through various mechanisms, including bulk flow, pendelluft, cardiogenic mixing, and molecular diffusion.

To ↑ oxygenation	1.	↑ FiO_2
	2.	↑ Mean airway pressure (MAP)–↑ risk of barotrauma
To ↑ CO_2 removal	1.	↑ Delta P: This refers to the magnitude of mechanical diaphragm oscillation.
	2.	↓ Frequency to ↑ tidal volume: Note that the lower the frequency, the larger the changes in pressure per cycle and the greater the risk of lung injury. A typical starting frequency is 5 Hz (300 breaths/min) and is titrated to achieve adequate CO_2 clearance.
	3.	↑ % of inspiratory time

Fact 1034:

For individuals in the terminal stages of life, when might it be considered beneficial to retain the **pacemaker function** of a biventricular pacemaker with a defibrillator?

- In cases of pacemaker dependency (where disabling the pacemaker would lead to immediate death due to inadequate native rhythm)
- In severe heart failure, the pacemaker's cardiac resynchronisation function may be retained for symptom management while deactivating the defibrillator function.

Deactivating the ICD function should be done by a cardiac physiologist in non-emergencies or with a ring magnet in emergencies to prevent end-of-life shocks.

Fact 1035:

What are the usual initial doses of lorazepam, midazolam, and diazepam for the treatment of **generalised convulsive status epilepticus** in adults?

Lorazepam	IV	4 mg
Midazolam	Buccal	10 mg
Diazepam	IV/Rectal	10–20 mg

Fact 1036:

How does the dose of **IV dopamine** impact on its action?

Dose (µg/kg/min)	Receptor activated	Effect
Low dose (<2.5)	Dopaminergic receptors	• ↑ Renal blood flow and promotes diuresis • ↑ Mesenteric blood flow
Intermediate dose (2.5–10)	β-receptors (+ dopamine)	↑ HR, ↑ contractility, ↑ CO
High dose (>10)	α-receptors (+ β + dopamine)	↑ SVR and ↑ PVR

Although it cannot penetrate the blood–brain barrier, it can stimulate the chemoreceptor trigger zone externally, resulting in nausea and vomiting.

Fact 1037:

How does the **Well's score** help determine the clinical probability of a DVT or PE?

DVT		PE	
DVT likely	2 points or more	PE likely	More than 4 points
DVT unlikely	1 point or less	PE unlikely	4 points or less

Fact 1038:

What makes **citrate toxicity** more probable in cases of liver dysfunction or during shock states when it is used as regional anticoagulation in renal replacement therapy (RRT)?

- Citrate, administered pre-filter, chelates calcium.
- Subsequent hypocalcaemia impairs thrombin formation.
- A post-filter calcium infusion replaces chelated calcium which has been filtered into the effluent, while some citrate–calcium complexes return to the body. The liver and muscles metabolise citrate in these complexes to produce bicarbonate → mild metabolic alkalosis.
- In cases of liver dysfunction or muscle hypoperfusion (shock), there is ↓ citrate metabolism → ↑ risk of citrate toxicity
- Signs of citrate toxicity include:
  - HAGMA: Citrate is acidic
  - ↓ Ionised calcium, ↓ potassium, ↓ magnesium
  - ↑ Total:ionised calcium ratio > 2.5

Fact 1039:

Why is the **thoracic duct** susceptible to injury with a left subclavian central venous catheter (CVC) approach?

It enters left brachiocephalic vein at the junction of the subclavian and internal jugular vein.

Fact 1040:

What are some possible interpretations of a raised **pulmonary capillary wedge pressure (PCWP)** of 25 mmHg?

	Interpretation	Explanation
1	Hypervolaemia	Excess fluid volume leads to ↑ LVEDV and ↑ PCWP
2	Cardiac tamponade or constrictive pericarditis	↑ pressure around the heart leads to ↑ PCWP, even when LVEDV may be normal or decreased
3	Myocardial dysfunction	Poor heart muscle function, often due to ischaemia, results in diastolic dysfunction and ↑ PCWP, with normal or ↓ LVEDV

This is why using PCWP as a measure of fluid responsiveness may not be the most accurate.

Fact 1041:

In a double-blinded randomised controlled trial investigating whether a drug improves survival, what would the **null hypothesis** be?

Survival is not different between the groups

Fact 1042:

What is the most likely issue if someone with a **left-sided double-lumen tube (DLT)** intended to protect the right lung exhibits absent right-sided breath sounds, reduced tidal volumes and increased ventilatory pressures, but with a centrally aligned trachea on examination?

Displacement of the DLT

The left bronchial cuff has moved upward and out of the left main bronchus. It is now positioned at the carina, thereby obstructing the right main bronchus. Consequently, oxygen is only reaching the left (pathological) lung, and none is reaching the right (healthy) lung.

To address this issue, deflate both the bronchial and tracheal cuffs, advance the tube under direct guidance, and then reinflate the cuffs.

Fact 1043:

How do you calculate **MAP** from arterial pressure?

MAP = DBP + 1/3(pulse pressure)

Pulse pressure = SBP–DBP

Fact 1044:

Which antimicrobials are used for **selective decontamination of the digestive tract (SDD)**?

IV	Cefotaxime	For overgrowth of normal admission flora, e.g. *S. pneumonia, H. influenza, E. coli* and *S. aureus*. An antipseudomonal cephalosporin may be added for those at risk of Pseudomonas colonisation.
Oral paste and enteral suspension	Amphotericin B	To ↓ oral and intestinal colonisation of yeasts, e.g. Candida
	Polymixin E + Tobramycin	To ↓ oral and intestinal colonisation of aerobic Gram-negative rods
Enteral	Vancomycin	Added when MRSA is endemic

Fact 1045:

Why does **atracurium** affect lithium dilution in cardiac output studies?

- Drift of the measurement electrode occurs in the presence of atracurium.
- A prior bolus of atracurium is not a contraindication to using this to calculate cardiac output as long as it has been metabolised and is not in the circulation.

Fact 1046:

What is the difference between **absolute** and **relative** humidity?

ABSOLUTE HUMIDITY (g/m³)	RELATIVE HUMIDITY (%)
Defined as the mass of water vapour present in a unit volume of air, measured at a specific pressure and temperature. For example, air at room temperature (20°C) when fully saturated contains 17 g of water vapour per cubic metre (g/m³), whereas at body temperature (37°C), it contains 44 g/m³.	This is the ratio of the current partial pressure of water vapour in the air to the saturated vapour pressure of water at the same temperature, expressed as a percentage. Relative humidity has an inverse relationship with temperature. In a closed system, if the temperature increases, relative humidity decreases, and vice versa.

Fact 1047:

Which component of **brainstem testing** loses validity in cases of high spinal injury?

The apnoea test

In this setting, cessation of brainstem function can be established only by confirming the absence of other brainstem reflexes and by using ancillary investigations, e.g. blood flow in larger cerebral arteries, brain tissue perfusion and neurophysiology.

Fact 1048:

Which risk factors carry the highest risk for **gastrointestinal bleeding** in critical care?

- Mechanical ventilation without enteral nutrition
- Chronic liver disease
- Concerning coagulopathy
- ≥2 of the following:
  - AKI
  - Sepsis
  - Shock

Fact 1049:

What is the most likely cause of **hyponatremia** if someone with a seizure has these results:

- Low serum Na 113 mmol/L
- Low serum osmolality 270 mOsm/kg
- Low urine Na 10 mmol/L
- Low urine osmolality 60 mOsm/kg

Water intoxication

This is the diagnosis as all parameters are reduced.

In water intoxication, water intake exceeds that of water excretion.

Fact 1050:

What are the two prerequisites for a **micro-shock** to induce ventricular fibrillation?

1. A direct conduit for electrical current to reach the myocardium
2. A current source

A microshock is a low-level current (50 µA) that directly affects the myocardium. It can occur through central lines, intracardiac pacemakers with external leads and oesophageal probes. Type CF equipment, like ECG leads and pressure transducers designed for direct cardiac connection, offers the highest protection by utilising isolated circuits with a maximum leakage current of <10 µA.

Fact 1051:

What are the key management priorities for individuals with a **spinal cord injury**?

Ensuring adequate perfusion and preventing ischaemic or secondary injury:

- Spinal precautions, e.g. C-spine immobilisation, log roll
- Prevent secondary injury, e.g. avoid hypoxia, hypotension, hyperglycaemia and hyperthermia
- Timely transfer to specialist centre

Fact 1052:

How does a **heat and moisture exchanger (HME)** work?

- An HME collects moisture from exhaled gases through condensation, returning it to dry inhaled gases for humidification. It can achieve 60–70% relative humidity at 28°C.
- HMEs, with a typical pore size of 0.2 µm, can filter out particles, bacteria and viruses that are smaller than 0.1 µm in diameter.
- HMEs are made from glass fibre and use pleating to ↑ surface area → ↓ airflow resistance and ↑ efficiency.

Fact 1053:

Which **lateral position** is ideal for ventilating a person with right-sided pneumonia to optimise oxygenation?

Left lateral decubitus position (good lung down)

- Hypoxemia results from ↓ ventilation and relatively maintained perfusion in affected lung units
- 'Good lung down' can improve V/Q by increasing perfusion in the healthy lung, enhancing oxygenation, and reducing the shunt fraction. It also assists in recruiting alveoli in the non-dependent, diseased lung by increasing transpulmonary pressure.

Fact 1054:

Which drugs are used to raise gastric pH above 3.5 for **stress ulcer** prevention?

- *First line*: Proton pump inhibitors, e.g. omeprazole and lansoprazole, irreversibly bind and inhibit the hydrogen/potassium ATPase enzyme on parietal cells, which are responsible for producing gastric acid.
- *Second line*: Histamine-2 receptor blockers, e.g. famotidine and ranitidine, competitively inhibit histamine binding to gastric parietal cells.
- *Sucralfate*: Forms a physical barrier between gastric secretions and mucosal epithelial cells. Not widely used due to difficulty in administration.
- Antacids, e.g. magnesium hydroxide, are less commonly used because of the frequency of administration, gastrointestinal side effects and derangement in electrolyte levels that may result from treatment.
- *Enteral feeds*: Neutralise gastric acidity, promote mucosal blood flow and stimulate the release of protective substances like prostaglandins and mucus, potentially reducing stress ulcers and gastrointestinal bleeding.

Evidence regarding their impact on *C. difficile* infection, length of stay and duration of ventilation is less convincing.

Fact 1055:

What generally happens to the range of normal **vital signs** as a child gets older?

- ↓ HR, RR, urine output
- ↑ SBP
- SpO_2 stays the same

Age (years)	HR	RR	SBP	SpO_2	Urine output
<1	110–160	30–40	80–90	95–98	1–2
1–2	100–150	25–35	85–95	95–98	1–2
2–5	95–140	25–30	85–100	95–98	1–2
5–12	80–120	20–25	90–110	95–98	>1
>12	60–100	15–20	100–120	95–98	>0.5

Fact 1056:

What are the risk factors for developing **citrate toxicity** during renal replacement therapy with regional citrate anticoagulation?

↓ Citrate clearance	Exacerbating factors
• Hepatic dysfunction • Shocked states	• ↓ Calcium (hypocalcaemia) • ↓ Albumin (hypoalbuminaemia)

Fact 1057:

What are some examples of **Gram-negative** bacteria?

They have a thinner peptidoglycan layer surrounded by an outer cell membrane and appear pink on microscopy with Gram-staining:

Cocci	Bacilli (Anything other than 'ABCDL')	
	Coliforms	**Others**
Neisseria Moraxella	**S**almonella **E**SCHAPPM (see below) **E**. Coli **K**lebsiella	**P**seudomonas **A**cinetobacter **B**acteroides

- The ESCHAPPM group sometimes have β-lactamase activity: **E**nterobacter spp, **S**erratia spp, **C**itrobacter freundii, **H**afnia spp, **A**eromonas spp, **P**roteus spp, **P**rovidencia spp, **M**organella morganii
- Haemophilus and Bordetella are Gram-negative cocco-bacilli

Fact 1058:

What is the **Haldane effect**?

The ability of deoxygenated haemoglobin to carry more CO_2 than in the oxygenated state.

Fact 1059:

What are the three independent variables in **Stewart's acid–base hypothesis**?

- PCO_2
- Total weak acid concentration
- Strong ion difference (SID)

Fact 1060:

Which 'red flag' patient groups require diagnostic caution when performing **brainstem death testing**?

- Testing < 6 hours of the loss of the last brainstem reflex
- Testing < 24 hours of the loss of the last brainstem reflex, where aetiology primarily anoxic damage
- Therapeutic **D**ecompressive craniectomy.
- **R**ewarming for hypothermia (24-hour observation period following rewarming to normothermia is recommended).
- **A**etiology primarily located to the brainstem or posterior fossa.
- Prolonged **I**nfusions of fentanyl.
- Patients with **N**euromuscular disorders.
- **S**teroids for space-occupying lesions, e.g. abscesses.

Fact 1061:

What are some risk factors for **post-extubation stridor**?

Patient factors	• Female • Children • Short neck • Trauma history • Airway conditions (e.g. stenosis, tracheomalacia) • Small height-to-ETT ratio
INTUBATION FACTORS	• Airway manipulation • Traumatic intubation • Prolonged attempts • Oro-endotracheal intubation • Larger tube size
Post-intubation factors	• Intubation > 36 hours • Agitation during intubation • High cuff pressures • Recurrent intubations

---

Fact 1062:

Why can **diabetes insipidus (DI)** occur in pregnancy?

Three possible reasons:

- *Cranial DI*: ↓ Vasopressin (ADH) secretion from the posterior pituitary
- *Nephrogenic DI*: ↑ Renal tubule resistance to ADH
- *Placental breakdown*: The placenta produces vasopressinases (cysteine–aminopeptidases) that ↑ ADH metabolism

---

Fact 1063:

Why isn't **phenytoin** recommended for dosulepin overdose-related seizures or cardiac arrhythmias?

Dosulepin, a tricyclic antidepressant, shares sodium channel-blocking properties with phenytoin. Using phenytoin in a dosulepin overdose can ↑ the risk of cardiac arrhythmias and seizures.

Fact 1064:

What happens to the bleeding time, prothrombin time and APTT in **von Willebrand disease (vWD)**, **Haemophilia** and **Vitamin K deficiency**?

	Bleeding time	PT/INR	APTT
vWD	Prolonged as vWF is needed for platelet adhesion	Normal	Prolonged – vWF binds to factor 8
Haemophilia A	Normal – platelets not affected	Normal	**Prolonged**
Haemophilia B	Normal – platelets not affected	Normal	**Prolonged**
Vitamin K deficiency	Normal	**Prolonged**	**Prolonged**

Fact 1065:

What is meant by **discrimination, calibration** and **validity** when applied to mortality prediction models?

- *Discrimination*: Evaluates the model's ability to differentiate between survivors and non-survivors using the area under the receiver operating curve (AUROC). An AUROC > 0.7 is reasonable, and > 0.9 is excellent. For example, APACHE II has an AUROC of 0.85, and APACHE III has an AUROC of 0.90.
- *Calibration*: Measures how closely predicted values align with actual values. For instance, the Baux score, used to predict burns mortality, demonstrates robust discrimination but has poor calibration, leading to less precise predictions of actual mortality rates.
- *Validity (generalisability)*: Reflects the applicability of study findings to different settings. For instance, qSOFA is valid for screening outside of the ICU but has limited validity within the ICU.

Fact 1066:

What are some obstructive causes of **jaundice**?

Neoplastic	Autoimmune	Other
Pancreatic cancer	Primary sclerosing cholangitis	Common bile duct stone
Cholangio-carcinoma		Portal lym-phadenopathy

Fact 1067:

How does **dexmedetomidine** work?

Similar to clonidine but 8x higher affinity for the α_2-receptor. It is selective presynaptic α_2-agonist in:

- *Brain*: ↓ CNS excitation especially in the locus coeruleus → sedation and anxiolysis.
- *Spinal cord*: Activation of the α_{2c}-receptor subtype at the dorsal horn → augments endogenous opiate release and inhibits noradrenaline release in the propagation of pain signals → analgesia and opioid sparing effect.
- *CVS*:
  o Initial transient vasoconstriction in vascular smooth musculature (postsynaptic α_{2b})
  o Followed by a ↓ BP and ↓ HR (postsynaptic α_{2a} in the CNS) → ↓ peripheral sympathetic tone and augmentation of cardiac vagal activity

It is completely cleared by first pass hepatic metabolism.

Since it provides sedation without ↓ respiratory drive, it can be used as a sedative during weaning from mechanical ventilation, particularly in hyperactive delirium.
When compared to benzodiazepines, dexmedetomidine *may* be associated with ↓ duration and/or incidence of delirium.

Fact 1068:

Which adrenergic agents are typically employed to manage hypertension in individuals with a **phaeochromocytoma** when organ failure is not present?

Alpha blockade, e.g. oral phenoxybenzamine

The dose is sequentially increased until normotension is achieved or adverse effects become intolerable, e.g. nasal congestion or postural hypotension.

Beta blockade may safely be commenced once adequate alpha blockade is in place to control tachycardia or tachyarrhythmias.

Fact 1069:

What drug would you give to rapidly reverse the anticoagulant effects of **rivaroxaban** in someone with active major bleeding?

Andexanet alfa (AndexXa)

This is a recombinant form of human factor Xa which binds specifically to apixaban or rivaroxaban, thereby reversing their anticoagulant effects.

If this is not available, 4-factor PCC can be used (e.g. Kcentra, Beriplex, Octaplex).

Fact 1070:

How would you convert 5 mg of prednisolone to equivalent doses of **dexamethasone, hydrocortisone and methylprednisolone**?

- Dexamethasone 0.75 mg
- Methylprednisolone 4 mg
- Hydrocortisone 20 mg

Fact 1071:

What is the **systemic vascular resistance** if the MAP is 141mmHg, cardiac output is 4L/min and CVP is 1mmHg?

SVR = (MAP−CVP)/CO = (141−1)/4 = 35 mmHg.min.mL

Fact 1072:

What is **donated blood** routinely screened for in the UK?

- Hepatitis B virus
- Hepatitis C virus
- HIV
- HTLV
- Treponemal infection, e.g. Syphilis

Fact 1073:

What does the **'rule of four'** mean in chronic metabolic compensation for respiratory acidosis?

- For every 1.33 kPa ↑ in $PaCO_2$, there is a corresponding ↑ in HCO_3^- of 4 mmol/L.
- This compensation mechanism is observed in conditions such as COPD and increased dead space ventilation.

Fact 1074:

What are some examples of **serotonergic drugs**?

- Reuptake inhibitors: SSRIs (e.g. sertraline), SNRI (e.g. venlafaxine), TCAs, ondansetron
- Direct agonists, e.g. triptans
- Metabolism alteration, e.g. MAOi (e.g. phenelzine), linezolid, methylene blue
- Release enhancers, e.g. opioids, ecstasy, cocaine

Fact 1075:

What would you expect the state of a **weak acid** to be if it is at a pH below its pKA?

Weak acids will predominantly exist in their non-ionised form when the pH is below their pKa, because of the abundance of protons in the acidic environment, which prevents it from ionising.

Fact 1076:

What is the **Injury Severity Score (ISS)** in trauma?

An anatomical score to classify severity of trauma. The body is divided into six regions. Each region has the Abbreviated Injury Scale (AIS) applied to its injuries:

Body region		
1	Head	
	Neck	
2	Face	
3	Thorax	
4	Abdomen	
5	Upper extremity	
	Lower extremity	
6	External and other areas	

Score	Abbreviated Injury Scale (AIS)
1	Minor
2	Moderate
3	Serious
4	Severe
5	Critical
6	Unsurvivable

The three most injured regions' scores are then squared and added together to give the ISS (maximum of 75). An ISS score > 15 indicates major trauma. An AIS of 6 in any region automatically gives an ISS of 75 (unsurvivable).

The uncertainty surrounding the specific nature of traumatic injuries makes it impossible to calculate this score at the location of trauma.

Fact 1077:

How does **renal failure** affect the pharmacokinetic properties of drugs?

Absorption	• Uraemic gastroparesis and ↓ mesenteric blood flow can lead to ↓ drug absorption
Distribution	• Electrolyte and fluid balance changes in renal failure affect drug distribution. For example, water-soluble drugs like vancomycin have an ↑ Vd due to tissue oedema. • ↓ Plasma protein binding, as a result of accumulated metabolic products and changes in albumin levels, can increase the fraction of free (unbound) drug, leading to ↑ drug activity and potential toxicity. • ↓ Renal blood flow and ↓ tissue uptake further alters drug distribution.
Metabolism	• While most drug metabolism occurs in the liver, renal failure can indirectly affect this process. Accumulation of uraemic toxins may downregulate or impair liver drug-metabolising enzymes. • If a drug has significant renal elimination of its metabolites, there will be ↓ clearance. • ↓ Renal metabolism due to ↓ renal blood flow and/or ↓ renal enzymatic activity also leads to ↓ metabolic clearance.
Elimination	• ↓ GFR leads to ↓ clearance of drugs that are primarily eliminated by the kidneys, resulting in ↑ elimination half-life, ↑ accumulation and ↑ risk of toxicity. • Drugs may compete for specific renal clearance pathways, which can lead to further accumulation of one or both drugs when administered concurrently.

Fact 1078:

How soon after a blood transfusion has started does an **acute haemolytic transfusion reaction (AHTR)** occur and what usually causes this?

- An AHTR typically develops within 1 hour after the transfusion has started.
- It is usually caused by ABO incompatibility.
- Symptoms include fever, chills, haemoglobinuria, flank pain and discomfort at the infusion site.
- This may progress to acute renal failure and/or disseminated intravascular coagulation (DIC).
- The management includes immediate cessation of the transfusion and supportive care.

Fact 1079:

What are the most likely causes of a non-traumatic **subarachnoid haemorrhage (SAH)**?

- Rupture of aneurysm (85%), with the vast majority lying in the anterior Circle of Willis
- Arteriovenous malformation
- Cerebral venous sinus thrombosis
- Cerebral vasculitis
- Moyamoya disease

Fact 1080:

What are some conditions that result in **metabolic alkalosis** with concomitant hypokalemia?

Low/normal BP		High BP	
Genetic	Acquired	Genetic	Acquired
Bartter syndrome Gitelman syndrome Autosomal dominant hypocalcaemia with hypercalciuria	Diuretic use Vomiting	Liddle Syndrome HSD-11β inactivating mutation	Conn disease/ secreting adenoma of the adrenal glands/ bilateral hyperplasia Cushing disease/ tumour of the adrenals Chronic administration of corticosteroid Natural liquorice abuse

Fact 1081:

How does the bronchial limb of a **right-sided double-lumen tube (DLT)** differ from a left-sided DLT?

The right bronchus being shorter than the left bronchus necessitates the inclusion of a ventilation slot (hole) in right-sided tubes to aid in ventilating the right upper lobe.

Fact 1082:

What causes **Lyme disease** and what are its three stages?

Caused by *Borrelia burgdorferi* and transmitted by Ixodes spp. ticks:

Early infection
A rash, resembling a bull's eye target (erythema migrans), typically appears at the site of the bite and may spread. On the earlobe, a purple nodule called a borrelia lymphocytoma can develop.
Disseminated disease
• *Neurological*: Meningitis, cranial nerve palsies, peripheral neuritis, painful radiculopathy • Muscle weakness and spread of erythema migrans • *Cardiac*: Heart block and arrhythmias • *Joints*: Migratory arthralgia and mono-oligoarthritis
Late disease
Peripheral neuropathy develops months to years after the initial infection and does not respond well to antibiotics.

Fact 1083:

How do **isoniazid** and **rifampicin** affect the cytochrome P450 system?

- *Isoniazid*: P450 enzyme inhibitor
- *Rifampicin*: P450 enzyme inducer

Fact 1084:

What do the three peaks of the **ICP waveform** represent?

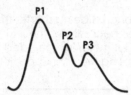

The ICP waveform is similar to the arterial waveform.

P1	**Percussion wave**	Represents arterial pulsation, which is transmitted via the choroid plexus. This is the highest of the three waveforms.
P2	**Tidal wave**	Represents intracranial compliance. As intracranial compliance ↓, the amplitude of P2 initially equals and then exceeds P1 (indicates intracranial hypertension).
P3	**Dicrotic wave**	Due to closure of the aortic valve.

Note that a reduction in CSF volume, such as that seen following CSF drainage, could result in a waveform with lower amplitude but no change in morphology.

Fact 1085:

How does molecular weight (MW) and molecular charge influence filtration at the **Bowman's capsule**?

- MW < 30,000 Da are freely filtered, e.g. electrolytes, glucose and amino acids.
- Proteins, e.g. albumin (MW 70,000 Da) are filtered in very small quantities.
- Negatively charged molecules are less likely to be filtered as the basement membrane and podocytes are negatively charged.

Fact 1086:

What is the commonest cause of **hyperthyroidism** in pregnancy?

Graves' disease

Fact 1087:

Does the use of post-extubation **non-invasive ventilation** in high-risk patients reduce the need for reintubation?

Yes it does.

Fact 1088:

Why is a **passive leg raise (PLR)** helpful in determining fluid responsiveness in a mechanically ventilated patient with known severe congestive cardiac failure?

- Lifting the legs by 45° induces a gravitational transfer of blood from the lower limbs
- It auto-transfuses about 300–500 mL of blood into the central circulation to mimic the haemodynamic effects of a fluid bolus (↑ preload)
- This test requires real-time monitoring of haemodynamic parameters, e.g. cardiac output and/or stroke volume
- A ≥ 10% increase in stroke volume or cardiac output suggests fluid responsiveness
- A key benefit of this approach is its reversibility, which avoids the risks of unwarranted fluid administration

Fact 1089:

When may the **PCWP** overestimate or underestimate LVEDP?

PCWP > LVEDP	PCWP < LVEDP
PCWP may give a higher-than-actual reading of the LVEDP in situations where there are external pressures influencing the measurement. These external pressures are not a reflection of LV function.	PCWP may give a lower reading that the actual LVEDP in scenarios where the internal pressure of the LV is elevated, but this increase is not captured by the PCWP-measuring catheter.
• Mitral stenosis • PEEP • Pulmonary hypertension	• Poorly compliant left ventricle • LVEDP > 25 mmHg

Fact 1090:

What are the common causes of a high and normal anion gap **metabolic acidosis**?

High anion gap	Normal anion gap
Ketones **U**raemia **S**alicylates **M**ethanol **E**thylene Glycol **L**actate	↑ Urinary bicarbonate loss, e.g. RTA type 2, acetazolamide
	↑ GI bicarbonate loss, e.g. diarrhoea, ileostomy, ureterosigmoidoscopy, pancreatic fistulae
	↓ Renal hydrogen secretion, e.g. RTA type 1
	Iatrogenic acids, e.g. TPN, NaCl 0.9%

Fact 1091:

What is the first **cardiac shunt** to close at birth?

Foramen ovale

The immediate closure occurs due to a reversed pressure gradient between the right atrium (RA) and left atrium (LA).

Fact 1092:

What are the key features of **severe malaria** in adults?

A	Pulmonary oedema	
B		
C	Shock	Compensated or decompensated
	Impaired consciousness	GCS < 11
D	Prostration	Significant weakness requiring assistance for sitting, standing, walking
	Multiple seizures	>2 episodes in 24 hours
	Hypoglycaemia	<2.2 mmol/L
F	Renal impairment	• Creatinine > 265 µmol/L • Urea > 20 mmol/L
	Metabolic acidosis	• Base deficient > 8 mEq/L • Bicarbonate <15 mmol/L or lactate >5 mmol/L
G	Jaundice	Bilirubin > 50 µmol/L + parasite count >100,000/µL
	Severe malarial anaemia	• Haemoglobin ≤ 70 g/L • Haematocrit ≤ 20%
H	Significant bleeding	• Bleeding from the nose, gums or venepuncture sites • Haematemesis and melaena
I	Hyperparasitaemia	P. falciparum parasitaemia > 10%

Fact 1093:

How would you manage a spontaneously breathing patient with a patent upper airway whose **tracheostomy** was displaced hours after insertion, resulting in a low SpO_2?

Verifying the patency of the tracheostomy is key. Attempts to bag ventilate via a displaced tracheostomy can cause catastrophic surgical emphysema.

- Call for expert help
- With capnography present, look, listen and feel for breathing
- If breathing, apply high-flow oxygen to both the tracheostomy site and the face
- Remove inner tube and pass a suction catheter down the tracheostomy tube. If this is unsuccessful, deflate the tracheostomy cuff and reassess breathing. If the patient does not improve, remove the tracheostomy.
- If not breathing or still has ↓ SpO_2 after removing the tracheostomy, attempt bag ventilation of the oral airway. The tracheostomy site may need to be covered to allow effective ventilation. Alternatively, a paediatric mask can be used for cautious mask ventilation of the tracheostomy stoma.
- If necessary, consider oral intubation. If this is difficult, the tracheostomy site may be intubated with airway assistance devices, e.g. a fibre-optic bronchoscope, using either an oral tube or a tracheostomy tube.

Fact 1094:

What is the pathology of **disseminated intravascular coagulation**?

Main pathological feature (thrombosis)	Consequence (Bleeding)
Uncontrolled, inappropriate, widespread activation of the haemostatic system	Extensive coagulation depletes platelets, uses up fibrinogen and clotting factors and triggers widespread systemic fibrinolysis,
This leads to fibrin deposition, platelet aggregation and microvascular occlusion	
Significant microvascular occlusion then leads to tissue hypoxia and organ dysfunction, e.g. ARDS, renal and hepatic failure	e.g. bleeding from previous surgical or vascular access sites and widespread bruising

Many diseases linked to DIC involve various procoagulant factors such as tissue factor, lipopolysaccharide, endotoxin or intracellular contents. Remember **'SORTS'**:

- **S**evere sepsis, e.g. Gram-negative bacteria or organisms that produce endotoxins
- **O**bstetric complications, e.g. placental abruption, eclampsia, amniotic fluid embolus
- **R**eactions to drugs
- **T**rauma especially in burns, multiple injuries or long-bone fractures
- **T**ransfusion reactions
- **T**ransplant rejection
- **S**olid tumours and haematological malignancies

Fact 1095:

What is the gold standard investigation to diagnose suspected **obstructive sleep apnoea (OSA)**?

Polysomnography (sleep study)

At the end of the investigation, the number of apnoea/hypopnoea episodes whilst asleep is quoted as the Apnoea/Hypopnoea Index (AHI). This grades the severity of OSA.

Patients can be screened for the likelihood of OSA using the Epworth (≥10 indicates excess sleepiness) and STOP-BANG (5–8 is high probability of moderate/severe OSA) scoring systems.

Fact 1096:

What is the **RASS** and **Ramsay** sedation scale?

- *RASS*: Scored from +4 (combative and violent) to −5 (unrousable). A score of 0 (alert and calm) is desired.
- *Ramsay*: Used in studies. It doesn't evaluate agitation but mainly assesses rousability. Scores range from 1 (anxious and restless) to 6 (unresponsive), with 3–4 considered optimal.

Fact 1097:

What are the three levels of **burn services** and when would you refer to each?

	Burn centres	Burn units	Burn facilities
Description	Highest inpatient care level for the most complex cases, with dedicated wards, immediate theatre access, and specialised critical care.	An intermediate level of inpatient care, featuring a dedicated ward capable of handling moderately complex injuries.	A basic level of inpatient care, suitable for non-complex injuries, often without a dedicated burn ward, potentially using a standard plastic surgical ward.
Referral criteria	TBSA > 25% + inhalation injury TBSA > 40% without inhalation injury	TBSA ≥10% Any burn ≥ 5% if non-blanching Circumferential burns Burns affecting specific areas (e.g. face, feet, hands, perineum, genitalia)	Any full-thickness burn TBSA > 2% but < 10% even in the presence of inhalation injury
	The referral thresholds dictate the appropriate burn service. Discuss chemical, electrical or non-significant burns that do not fall into these categories.		

Fact 1098:

How long will a full **CD oxygen cylinder** last when used with a transport ventilator, if the fresh gas flow is 4 L/min and the ventilator gas consumption is 1 L/min, given its internal capacity of 2 L at a pressure of 230 bar?

The volume of oxygen in the cylinder can be calculated by applying Boyle's law: $P_1 \times V_1 = P_2 \times V_2$

- P_1 is the pressure of a full cylinder (230 bar).
- V_1 is the volume of oxygen at that pressure (2 litres).
- P_2 is the final pressure (1 bar = atmospheric).
- V_2 is the volume of oxygen available.

$230 \times 2 = 1 \times V_2$

$V_2 = 460$ L

Total flow = 4 L/min + 1 L/min = 5 L/min

Therefore, the cylinder will last 460/5 minutes = **92 minutes**

Fact 1099:

What are the most common causes of **acute pancreatitis**?

Gallstones, alcohol and hypertriglyceridemia

Fact 1100:

What has most likely occurred if someone with **antiphospholipid syndrome (APS)** develops hyponatremia, hyperkalaemia and hypotension?

Loss of adrenal function – either due to venous thrombosis or haemorrhagic infarction

APS is an autoimmune condition causing hypercoagulability (arterial and venous thrombosis), pregnancy-related complications (e.g. recurrent miscarriage) and the presence of antiphospholipid antibodies. Catastrophic APS is a rare, rapidly progressing form of the disease with a high mortality rate of approximately 50% despite treatment. Management includes specialist care, heparin, IVIg/plasma exchange and immunomodulation.

Fact 1101:

What are some of the absolute contraindications to **solid organ donation**?

CJD
HIV – active
Infection – uncontrolled, donor sepsis
Cancer – metastatic, uncurable or transmittable

The number of transplants is limited by donors. Every day three people die due to lack of available organs.

Fact 1102:

What is the expected **bicarbonate (HCO$_3$-)** level if the PaCO$_2$ is 9.3 kPa and the normal HCO$_3$- range is 24–30 mmol/L and the normal CO$_2$ range is 4.7–6.0 kPa?

- Using Boston rules, in respiratory acidosis, a 1 kPa increase in PaCO$_2$ corresponds to a 0.75 mmol/L increase in HCO$_3$-.
- A PaCO$_2$ of 9.3 kPa is 3.3 higher than upper normal.
- This should increase the HCO$_3$- by 3.3 × 0.75 = 2.5
- If the normal HCO$_3$- range is 24–30 mmol/L
- Then the expected range is (24 + 2.5) to (30 + 2.5) mmol/L = **26.5–32.5 mmol/L**

Fact 1103:

What is the effect of **bronchospasm** on the phases of a capnography trace?

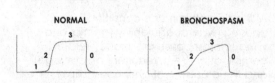

Bronchospasm causes a slow rise in phases 2 and 3 with a characteristic sloping waveform.

Fact 1104:

What are the **Ranson's criteria** and what score indicates severe acute pancreatitis?

Galaw and Chobbs

At admission	Non-gallstone pancreatitis	Gallstone pancreatitis
Glucose (mmol/L)	>11	>12.2
Age (years)	>55	>70
LDH (U/L)	>350	>400
AST (U/L)	>250	>250
WBCs (cells/mm³)	>16,000	>18,000
During initial 48 hours		
Calcium (mmol/L)	<2	<2
Haematocrit decrease (%)	>10	>10
Oxygen (PaO$_2$ kPa)	<8	<8
BUN increase (mmol/L)	>1.8	>0.7
Base deficit (mmol/L)	>4	>5
Sequestered fluid (litres)	>6	>4

A score of >3 at 48 hours indicates the presence of severe pancreatitis and carries a 15% mortality.

Fact 1105:

Why avoid fenestrated tubes initially for a **tracheostomy**?

- ↑ Risk of aspiration
- ↓ Efficiency of ventilation (leaks)
- ↑ Work of breathing

Fact 1106:

How would **excess heparin** and **prolonged storage** affect the readings of an ABG?

Condition	Effect on blood gas parameters	
Excess heparin	↓ $PaCO_2$ and ↓ PaO_2	
	↓ Calculated HCO_3-: ↓ $PaCO_2$ causes a proportionate ↓ in calculated HCO_3- (Henderson–Hasselbalch equation)	
	Minimal impact on pH: Despite its acidity, heparin doesn't significantly change blood pH due to the buffering effect of haemoglobin and other proteins.	
Prolonged storage	↓ PaO_2 due to cell metabolism	Metabolism by white cells causes a ↓ PaO_2
	Varying effects on PaO_2 due to air bubbles	Dissolved oxygen in the sample equilibrates with the pO_2 in the air bubble (21 kPa), e.g. a hypoxaemic patient may have a falsely ↑ PaO_2 and a hyperoxic patient may have a ↓ PaO_2.

Fact 1107:

What is the target time from symptom onset to endovascular thrombectomy in an **acute ischaemic stroke**?

Within 6 hours

Fact 1108:

What are two significant neurological complications of **acute aortic dissection**?

- Ischaemic stroke
- Acute paraplegia secondary to spinal cord hypoperfusion

Fact 1109:

Which part of the arterial waveform represents **stroke volume**?

Area under systolic portion up to the dicrotic notch

If this is multiplied by HR, then CO can be estimated.

Fact 1110:

Can you directly set the tidal volume in **high-frequency oscillatory ventilation (HFOV)**?

Nope

- TV is provided by oscillations of pressure around the mean airway pressure.
- This is directly related to the driving pressure and inversely related to the frequency.

Fact 1111:

How do you manage **beta-blocker** overdose?

- Single dose activated charcoal within 1 hour of ingestion.
- Treat symptomatic bradycardia with atropine. May need to consider the use of second-line drugs (adrenaline, dobutamine or isoprenaline) +/– cardiac pacing.
- Glucagon is the considered the antidote (bolus + infusion) but has not been proven to be superior over standard organ support.
- Other strategies include high dose insulin euglycemic therapy (HIET) and intralipid.
- Dialysis may be effective in water-solute beta-blocker toxicity, e.g. atenolol overdose.

Note that:

- Propranolol toxicity resembles TCA overdose, due to sodium channel blockade. In cases of seizures or QRS prolongation, consider sodium bicarbonate.
- Sotalol, a class III antiarrhythmic, blocks potassium channels and may lead to torsades de pointes. If this occurs, magnesium sulphate should be used.

Fact 1112:

How does the prevention and treatment of established **tumour lysis syndrome (TLS)** differ?

Prevention of TLS	Established TLS
Aggressive hydration with intravenous fluid	
Rasburicase: Recombinant urate oxidase	
Allopurinol is a xanthine oxidase inhibitor to prevent the formation of uric acid. Rasburicase is more effective than allopurinol in the prevention of TLS.	Correct electrolyte disturbances: • *Hyperkalaemia*: Insulin/dextrose, salbutamol, bicarbonate, potassium binders • *Hyperphosphataemia*: Phosphate binders • Calcium replacement only if symptomatic • Renal replacement therapy for refractory acute kidney injury and electrolyte abnormalities

Fact 1113:

How can **critical illness myopathy** be subdivided?

• Thick-filament (myosin) loss
• Cachectic myopathy
• Acute rhabdomyolysis
• Acute necrotising myopathy

Fact 1114:

How does serum lactate help assess liver transplantation eligibility in paracetamol toxicity according to the **modified King's College criteria**?

Consider liver transplantation if:

• Lactate > 3.5 mmol/L at 4 hours post-resuscitation OR
• Lactate > 3 mmol/L at 12 hours post-resuscitation or 24 hours after paracetamol ingestion

Fact 1115:

How do you treat **disseminated intravascular coagulation (DIC)**?

• Treat the underlying cause
• Therapeutic heparin for vascular thrombosis in the absence of bleeding.
• For severe bleeding or high-risk cases, consider blood products. For example, consider giving:
  o Platelets if counts <20 × 10⁹/L in high-risk patients
  o FFP in active haemorrhage or in high-risk patients before invasive procedures if PT or APTT is >150% of the normal range
  o Cryoprecipitate in active bleeding when fibrinogen is <1.5 g/L

Fact 1116:

How do you test for **legionella and mycoplasma** in someone with a high CURB-65 score of 4?

• *Mycoplasma*: PCR of respiratory tract samples
• *Legionella*: Urinary antigen

CURB-65 score predicts mortality:

• **C**onfusion (AMTS ≤ 8 or new disorientation)
• **U**rea > 7 mmol/L
• **R**R ≥ 30 breaths/min
• **B**P (DBP ≤ 60 or SBP < 90 mmHg)
• Age ≥ **65** years

0–1	Low severity	<3% mortality at 30 days	Consider treatment in the community
2	Moderate severity	3–15% mortality at 30 days	Treat as inpatient
3–5	High severity	>15% mortality at 30 days	Treat in HDU/ICU

Fact 1117:

What are the risks associated with **inadequate sedation** in mechanically ventilated patients?

- Agitation, delirium, potential for self-harm, and psychological distress
- ↑ Work of breathing, ↑ O_2 consumption, ventilator dyssynchrony
- ↑ Sympathetic activity may lead to CVS events

Fact 1118:

What is the minimum **CHA$_2$DS$_2$VASC** score that indicates the consideration of anticoagulation in atrial fibrillation?

- *Males*: 1 point
- *Females*: 2 points

	Condition	Points
C	**C**ongestive heart failure (or LV systolic dysfunction)	1
H	**H**ypertension (or on hypertension medication)	1
A$_2$	**A**ge ≥75 years	2
D	**D**iabetes mellitus	1
S$_2$	Prior **S**troke, TIA or thromboembolism	2
V	**V**ascular disease (e.g. peripheral artery disease, myocardial infarction, aortic plaque)	1
A	**A**ge 65–74 years	1
Sc	**S**ex **c**ategory (i.e. female)	1

Fact 1119:

Is it recommended to routinely administer seizure prophylaxis following a **subarachnoid haemorrhage**?

No

Routine seizure prophylaxis is associated with poor outcomes and is not recommended.

Fact 1120:

Which molecules are better cleared with **haemodialysis (HD)** when compared to **haemofiltration (HF)**?

- HD removes small molecules (<500 Da) through diffusion across a semipermeable membrane, e.g. urea, creatinine, electrolytes and lithium. Blood and dialysate move in opposing directions, creating a countercurrent system that ensures a continuous diffusion gradient for optimal solute removal.
- HF is effective at removing medium-sized (500–5,000 Da, e.g. vancomycin) and large (>5,000 Da, e.g. cytokines, complement) solutes through convection. It involves producing ultrafiltrate by passing fluid over a semipermeable membrane under pressure, causing solute removal via solvent drag. Increasing post-dilution over pre-dilution enhances solute removal.

Drug clearance varies with pharmacokinetics, the rate of endogenous clearance and the efficiency of RRT.

Fact 1121:

Which imaging technique is most effective for evaluating the degree of internal bleeding associated with a **pelvic fracture** in trauma cases?

A CT with contrast is a sensitive diagnostic method. It can provide information about intraperitoneal blood volume and ongoing bleeding during the arterial phase.

Fact 1122:

What causes **tuberculosis (TB)**, what increases the risk of TB infection in European adults, and how and when should respiratory samples be collected to confirm active respiratory TB?

Organism	Risk factors for TB infection in European adults	Confirming active respiratory TB
Mycobacterium tuberculosis Transmitted by inhalation of aerosolised sputum	• Close contact with a TB patient • Institutional living or working, e.g. hospitals, homeless shelters, prisons • Immigration from high TB prevalence areas • HIV infection • Immunosuppression • Illicit drug use	Three sputum samples are required, including at least one early morning sample, which can be either spontaneously produced or obtained through deep coughing.

Fact 1123:

Which type of echocardiogram is better in diagnosing an **aortic dissection**?

TOE is superior to TTE.

A negative TTE does not rule out dissection.

Fact 1124:

What are some respiratory system effects of using **cold and dry gas** for ventilation?

• Impaired ciliary function
• Mucosal dysfunction
• Accumulation of thick secretions and mucus plugging
• Keratinisation and ulceration of the airway

This leads to

• ↓ Compliance
• ↓ FRC
• ↑ Energy expenditure

This is why humidification is important. On a tracheostomy, a 'Swedish nose' serves this purpose.

Fact 1125:

What is the most likely diagnosis if a post-partum lady previously managed for **pre-eclampsia** presents with confusion, weakness, flushing and bradyarrhythmias?

Hypermagnesaemia

Conduction disturbances and flaccid paralysis reflect that the magnesium level is likely to be > 5 mmol/L.

Peripartum sepsis and intracerebral haemorrhage are also differential diagnoses.

Fact 1126:

What is a **tracheoinnominate fistulas (TIF)**?

A TIF is a connection that forms between the innominate artery and the trachea. The innominate artery traverses the trachea between the sixth and ninth cartilage rings. It typically arises due to localised ischaemia or infection. Initially, an ulcer develops, and over several weeks following tracheostomy insertion, it can progress to a full-blown fistula. A TIF is characterised by severe bleeding (haemoptysis) and has a high mortality.

Risk factors for development include:

• Tracheostomy below the third tracheal ring
• High innominate artery location
• Factors increasing the risk of ischaemia or infection:
  o **P**rolonged intubation
  o **O**ver-inflation of the tracheostomy cuff
  o **S**teroid and immunosuppressant use
  o **T**racheitis
  o **E**xtension of a skin infection at the stoma site to deeper tissue
  o **R**ecurrent hypotension leading to ischaemia
  o **N**eck radiation therapy

Fact 1127:

What is the algorithm for managing unanticipated **difficult intubations** in adults according to DAS (Difficult Airway Society)?

- *Plan A*: Initial tracheal intubation plan, with manoeuvres to improve the chances of successful intubation, e.g. positioning, equipment changes and reducing cricoid pressure. A maximum of three attempts; a fourth attempt by a more experienced colleague is permissible.
- *Plan B*: Maintenance of oxygenation using a supraglottic airway device (SAD). A maximum of three attempts using a second-generation SAD.
- *Plan C*: Maintenance of oxygenation with 2-person face-mask ventilation + adjuncts.
- Plan D: This is 'can't intubate, can't oxygenate' (CICO) situation, requiring a 'front-of-neck' approach (cricothyroidotomy with scalpel-bougie-tube technique); #10 blade scalpel and a cuffed 6.0 ETT.

Fact 1128:

What is the pathophysiology of **critical illness polyneuropathy (CIP)**?

Axonal degeneration

- ↓ CMAP and SNAP amplitude
- Normal conduction velocity

Fact 1129:

What do the labels on this **oesophageal Doppler waveform** represent?

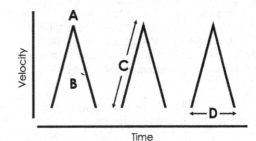

A	Peak velocity	Correlates with contractility
B	Stroke distance	Correlates with stroke volume
C	Mean acceleration	Correlates with contractility
D	Flow time	Inversely related to HR and afterload

Fact 1130:

How should you address **starvation ketosis** in a patient who is on a strict fasting regimen with no oral intake?

- A source of carbohydrate, e.g. IV Dextrose 5% (50–100 g/day of glucose is needed to prevent starvation ketosis) +/− IV insulin as required
- Vitamin supplementation, e.g. IV Pabrinex
- Maintenance fluids
- Monitoring and correction of electrolytes, e.g. K^+, PO_4^{3-}, Mg^{2+}

Fact 1131:

What's the likely diagnosis for a **post-CABG** patient on mechanical ventilation supported with milrinone and noradrenaline, exhibiting worsening tachycardia, a pulse pressure variation >20% on the arterial line, and the following cardiac output parameters: HR = 147, MAP = 65, CVP = 22, CI = 1.4, SVRI = 2,800, PAOP = 19, with a normal chest X-ray and minimal pericardial drain output?

$\downarrow$ CO + $\uparrow$ CVP + $\uparrow$ SVRI + reverse pulsus paradoxus = cardiac tamponade

- $\downarrow$ CO $\rightarrow$ $\uparrow$ HR and $\uparrow$ SVR to maintain MAP
- $\uparrow$ Intrapericardial pressure $\rightarrow$ $\downarrow$ RA compliance $\rightarrow$ $\uparrow$ CVP
- Reverse pulsus paradoxus ($\uparrow$ SBP during inspiration) is seen in IPPV, which is reflected as $\uparrow$ PPV.

In post-cardiac surgery, absent drain output doesn't exclude tamponade (clots in drains can hide blood loss and cause tamponade).

Fact 1132:

What is the relationship between body position and the likelihood of developing **ventilator-associated pneumonia (VAP)**?

- Semi-recumbent position $\rightarrow$ $\downarrow$ risk of VAP
- Supine position $\rightarrow$ $\uparrow$ risk of VAP

Fact 1133:

Is **activated charcoal** effective to treat an overdose of iron tablets?

No – iron does not bind to activated charcoal

- Tablets are radiopaque
- CXR/AXR can confirm ingestion
- Transition through the GI tract and bloodstream absorption can be delayed
- NPIS recommends whole bowel irrigation to $\downarrow$ absorption
- Desferrioxamine is recommended in severe toxicity, regardless of the iron level, e.g. metabolic acidosis, CVS instability, coma and hepatic dysfunction
- In other cases, consider desferrioxamine if the iron level reaches $\geq$ 90 µmol/L at 4–6 hours.
- While PPIs are not explicitly recommended in treatment guidelines, drugs that $\uparrow$ stomach pH $\downarrow$ absorption of iron.

Fact 1134:

How does **vasopressin** augment noradrenaline?

It works synergistically via different receptors to $\uparrow$ intracellular calcium and $\uparrow$ vascular tone.

Fact 1135:

What does the following oesophageal Doppler data suggest about a 70-year-old who is being mechanically ventilated for **pulmonary oedema** and is now hypotensive:

	Initial values	Post 250 mL crystalloid bolus
Flow time corrected (FTc)	270 ms	275 ms
Peak velocity	35 cm/s	32 cm/s
Stroke volume	40 mL	38 mL

- There is minimal response to a fluid challenge.
- This implies a state of fluid overload and being 'over the top' of the Starling curve.
- The ↓ FTc reflects an ↑ SVR.
- Peak velocity gives an indication of cardiac contractility (the normal range for this age group is 50–70 cm/s).

Fact 1136:

What is the anatomical basis for a **subdural haematoma**?

Bleeding between the dura and arachnoid mater is caused by the tearing of a bridging vein between the cerebral cortex and a draining venous sinus.

Fact 1137:

What are some of the different types of **bias** that can affect the validity of research and tests?

- *Lead-time*: When survival time seems better in the intervention group, but it's because of earlier disease detection, not the intervention itself.
- *Selection bias*: Participants chosen aren't representative of the broader population. Often occurs when participants self-select, e.g. respondents to a postal survey.
- *Attribution bias*: Arises when participants drop out of the study, and those who leave may have systematic differences compared to those who remain.
- *Recall bias*: Participants in retrospective studies remember things differently, potentially affecting the study's outcomes.
- *Observation bias (the Hawthorne effect)*: Participants' behaviour changes because they know they're being observed.

Fact 1138:

What is a **care bundle**?

A care bundle is a group of evidence-based interventions related to a condition that significantly improves patient outcome when used in combination, e.g. a VAP care bundle. Although different VAP bundles exist, an example of a bundle includes:

Daily sedation holds and assessment of readiness to extubate
Semi-recumbent position
Avoid unnecessary ventilator circuit changes
Gastric ulcer prophylaxis
Thromboprophylaxis
Oral hygiene
Subglottic suction tubes
Cuff pressure monitoring

The grade of evidence for each intervention should be high but some may be low/expert opinion. Adherence to all interventions is mandatory for success. Care bundles can function as an audit tool to assess delivery of interventions. Bundles should be constantly reappraised/updated.

Fact 1139:

Why may someone who takes **phenytoin** develop a raised mean corpuscular volume (MCV)?

Folate deficiency – this causes a macrocytic anaemia

Fact 1140:

What is the commonest gastrointestinal complication of **cocaine** use?

Bowel ischaemia secondary to vasoconstriction of the mesenteric circulation.

Fact 1141:

What impact does initial **ketamine** administration have on cerebral blood flow?

NMDA antagonism → ↑ release of excitatory neurotransmitters like glutamate → cerebral vasodilatation → ↑ **cerebral blood flow**

Fact 1142:

Why may someone with **cerebral tuberculosis (TB)** develop hydrocephalus?

A prominent pathological feature of cerebral TB is the formation of gelatinous exudates, which tend to affect the basal regions of the brain. These exudates have the potential to hinder the flow of CSF.

Fact 1143:

What is the **Vaughan Williams classification** of antiarrhythmic agents?

Class		Mechanism of action	Examples
I	Fast Na⁺ channel blockers	↓ Rate of rise of phase 0 of action potential	**Class Ia:** ↑ Action potential duration and refractory period (e.g. quinidine, procainamide)
			Class Ib: ↓ Action potential duration and refractory period (e.g. lignocaine, phenytoin)
			Class Ic: No effect on the action potential (e.g. flecainide, propafenone)
II	Beta-blockers	• ↓ AV conduction • ↑ Phase 4 duration • ↓ Contractility	Bisoprolol Metoprolol Esmolol
III	K⁺ channel blockers	• ↑ Phase 3 • ↑ Duration of action potential	Sotalol Amiodarone
IV	Ca²⁺ channel blockers	↓ SAN and AVN automaticity	Verapamil Diltiazem

---

Fact 1144:

What are some hepatic causes of **jaundice**?

	Neoplastic	Vascular	Infection
Cirrhosis & drugs	Hepatic metastasis	Heart failure (liver congestion) Hepatic ischaemia	Hepatitis (EBV, hepatitis viruses) Liver abscess Leptospirosis
Metabolic	**Autoimmune**	**Genetic**	**Pregnancy**
Primary and secondary non-alcoholic steatohepatitis	Primary biliary cirrhosis Autoimmune Hepatitis	Haemochromatosis A1AT deficiency Wilson disease Dubin–Johnson syndrome	Cholestasis of pregnancy (intrahepatic cholestasis) HELLP syndrome

Fact 1145:

How does **terbinafine** work as an antifungal?

- Inhibits squalene epoxidase
- This blocks the biosynthesis of ergosterol (a key component of fungal cell membranes) causing fungal cell membrane damage and cell death.

Fact 1146:

What are the three main mechanisms of **inhalation injury**?

Direct heat damage	Airway burns primarily affect the area above the vocal cords, leading to symptoms such as oedema, erythema and blistering. These symptoms can worsen in the days following the injury, and it is recommended to perform early intubation using an uncut endotracheal tube. Patients may experience breathlessness, hoarseness and stridor.
Irritation due to inhaled particulate matter	Inhaled soot contains toxic particles that get deposited in the airways and alveoli, leading to two distinct phenomena: 1. Activates an inflammatory cascade → ARDS 2. Mechanical obstruction → atelectasis and ↓ compliance
Biochemical dysfunction	• Hypoxic hypoxia: ↓ Ambient oxygen levels due to the fire and ↓ tissue oxygenation caused by carbon monoxide (CO) poisoning. • Cytotoxic hypoxia: Hydrogen cyanide has a high affinity for mitochondrial cytochrome oxidase which inhibits aerobic metabolism.

Facial burns are strongly associated with smoke inhalation. Inhalational injuries carry a higher mortality risk when compared to typical burn injuries.

Fact 1147:

What patient-specific data does an **oesophageal doppler monitor** utilise to estimate aortic cross-sectional area?

Age, height, weight

Fact 1148:

What are some patient-related risk factors for **delirium**?

- **A**ge > 65 and frailty
- **C**ognitive impairment
- **I**mmobility
- **D**rug/alcohol misuse
- **S**ensory impairment, e.g. visual/auditory

Occurs in up to 80% of ventilated patients: 10% hyperactive, 45% hypoactive and 45% mixed.

Fact 1149:

How does PEEP/CPAP help improve cardiac output in **acute left ventricular failure (LVF)**?

Acute LVF leads to pulmonary oedema. This reduces lung compliance and increases respiratory effort, often marked by gasping. This heighted effort results in more negative intrathoracic pressure, which increases both preload and afterload, adding strain to the already struggling LV.

Applying PEEP/CPAP helps to counter this negative inspiratory pressure. It effectively reduces both preload and afterload, moving the LV to a more efficient point of the Starling curve. This shift results in an increased SV and, therefore, increased CO.

Fact 1150:

What patterns can be observed on a **TEG** in cases of clotting factor deficiency, hypercoagulable states, thrombocytopenia and thrombolysis?

Clotting factor deficiency	↑ R time ↑ K time	↓ angle ↓ MA
Hypercoagulable states	↓ R time ↓ K time	↑ angle ↑ MA
Thrombocytopaenia	↑ K time ↓ MA	
Thrombolysis	↓ MA – continuously decreasing LY30 > 7.5% LY60 > 15%	

Fact 1151:

Why should gases be **humidified** in a ventilated patient?

- ↑ Mucociliary clearance
- Helps ↓ heat loss and maintains normothermia
- Provides a moist physiological surface for gas exchange at an alveolar level

Some methods of humidification include:

- Water baths – cold or heated
- Heat and moisture exchangers (HMEs)
- Heated nebulisers
- Ultrasonic nebulisers

Fact 1152:

Why is **magnesium sulphate** relatively contraindicated in myasthenia gravis (MG)?

- Magnesium inhibits the release of acetylcholine at the NMJ.
- In MG, this may worsen muscular weakness and, in some cases, can induce a myasthenic crisis.

Fact 1153:

What does this **arterial waveform** represent?

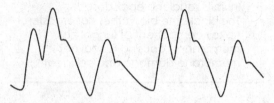

Intra-aortic balloon pump (IABP) counterpulsation with a 1:2 ratio (every other beat there is counterpulsation)

- The balloon inflates at the start of diastole (dicrotic notch) and remains inflated in diastole → ↑ diastolic pressure → ↑coronary perfusion pressure.
- It deflates during isovolumetric contraction before ejection of blood from LV → ↓ afterload → ↑ CO.

Fact 1154:

How may **phenytoin** influence the plasma levels of drugs that undergo hepatic metabolism?

Phenytoin may ↓ plasma levels of hepatically metabolised drugs by inducing cytochrome P450 enzymes.

Fact 1155:

What may happen to the LV if there is inadequate preload in someone with an **LVAD**?

- Inadequate preload reduces the amount of blood available for the LVAD to assist in pumping, leading to ↓ cardiac output and potential LV collapse as the LVAD tries to pull blood from the LV to the aorta.
- The LVAD may detect this and subsequently ↓ pump speed.

Fact 1156:

What is the optimal approach for treating a **post-operative oliguric patient** with a base excess of −12 mEq/L, hyperkalaemia of 6.5 mmol/L and a positive fluid balance of 5 L?

Renal replacement therapy

Fact 1157:

What is the rationale for an underwater seal chest drainage system in a **pneumothorax** and what are the characteristics of the drainage tube in a one-bottle system?

Rationale:

- Allows drainage of the pleural space using an airtight system to maintain subatmospheric intrapleural pressure.
- The underwater seal acts a one-way valve to allow unidirectional flow of air from the pleural cavity

Drainage tube:

- The first tube connecting the drain to drainage bottles must be wide to ↓ resistance.
- The volume capacity of this tube should be >50% of the patient's maximum inspiratory volume to stop water being aspirated into the chest during inspiration.
- The end of the tube submerged below the surface of water should not exceed 5 cm as inadequate submersion can impede drainage.
- The volume of water above the end of the tube should be >50% of the patient's maximum inspiratory volume to stop water being aspirated into chest during inspiration.
- The drain should always be ≥ 45 cm below the patient to prevent fluid that was removed or water from refluxing into the chest.

Fact 1158:

What are some strategies to optimise the **right ventricle**?

Optimise RV preload	• Closely monitored fluid challenges • Controlled diuresis/RRT if significant TR
Augment the RV	• Milirinone (inodilator): ↑ RV contraction, ↓ PVR • Others drug options: Dobutamine, adrenaline and levosimendan • With milirinone, there is a risk of systemic hypotension (↑ HR, ↑ myocardial work)→ NA/vasopressin may be added
↓ RV afterload	• Optimise all factors leading to hypoxic vasoconstriction, e.g. avoid hypoxia, avoid hypercapnia, avoid acidosis and avoid lung over/under distention (PVR is lowest when the lung is at FRC) • Pulmonary vasodilators: Inhaled nitric oxide (improves V/Q matching and oxygenation), inhaled Epoprostenol
Maintain systemic BP & coronary perfusion	• Noradrenaline • Vasopressin experimentally can lead to pulmonary vasodilatation (via NO dependent mechanisms) and can improve PVR/SVR ratio
Offload the RV	• Mechanical assist/ VA-ECMO can off-load the ventricle and improve pulmonary dynamics

---

Fact 1159:

Why should a tuberculosis test be performed prior to starting **infliximab** for Crohn's disease?

- Infliximab is a monoclonal antibody that neutralises TNF-α.
- Because it suppresses immune function, latent tuberculosis may become exacerbated.

Fact 1160:

Does a **bicuspid aortic valve** increase the risk of an aortic dissection?

Yes

Fact 1161:

Is CVVH beneficial in the treatment of a **tricyclic antidepressant (TCA)** overdose?

Nope

TCAs have a large volume of distribution and high protein binding. CVVH does not substantially eliminate it from the body.

Fact 1162:

What agent would you give for a clinically suspected **life-threatening PE**?

Alteplase 50 mg for immediate thrombolysis

Fact 1163:

What does this **flow volume loop** suggest in someone with vocal cord dysfunction?

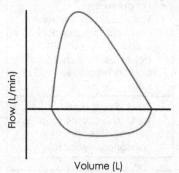

Volume (L)

Variable extra-thoracic obstruction:

* The inspiratory limb is flattened
* The expiratory limb is normal

There is abnormal adduction of vocal cords during inspiration but not expiration. This a functional disorder that is commonly mistaken for acute asthma. The diagnosis is confirmed by indirect laryngoscopy where there is complete adduction of the anterior ⅔ of the cords during inspiration with a 'glottic chink' posteriorly.

Fact 1164:

What is meant by drug **extravasation** and how do you manage it?

Accidental drug administration into tissues instead of into a blood vessel. This can cause tissue damage/ necrosis.

Important drugs implicated include:

* Vasoconstrictors
* Hyperosmolar drugs, e.g. high concentrations of glucose, calcium, potassium and TPN
* Cytotoxics
* Acidic and alkaline drugs

Management:

* Stop injection immediately
* Aspirate cannula
* Specialist advice, e.g. plastic surgery
* Remove cannula if not required by specialist
* Elevate limb to ↓ secondary injury from oedema
* Keep limb warm for vasodilation and drug absorption
* Consider the 'spread and dilute' method: This method is used when the risk of tissue necrosis is high. It involves creating stab wounds around the affected area, inserting a cannula into one of these wounds, and flushing it with saline to exit through the others, reducing drug concentration and minimising tissue damage. This approach is not used for cytotoxic drug extravasation.

Fact 1165:

What is the basic mechanism of action of the **antibiotic** classes?

Inhibit cell wall (peptidoglycan) formation	Penicillins (e.g. amoxicillin)	Bind to transpeptidase enzymes (penicillin-binding proteins) to block peptidoglycan cross-linking
	Cephalosporins (e.g. ceftriaxone)	Target penicillin-binding proteins, similar to penicillins
	Carbapenems (e.g. meropenem)	Inhibit cell wall synthesis by binding to penicillin-binding proteins
	Glycopeptides (e.g. vancomycin)	Bind to D-ala-D-ala terminus of peptidoglycan precursors
Inhibit protein synthesis	Aminoglycosides (e.g. gentamicin)	Bind to 30S subunit
	Tetracyclines (e.g. doxycycline)	
	Chloramphenicol	Bind to 50S subunit
	Clindamycin	
	Macrolides (e.g. erythromycin)	
	Linezolid	
Inhibit DNA synthesis	Quinolones (e.g. ciprofloxacin)	Inhibit DNA gyrase and topoisomerase IV
	Metronidazole	Causes DNA strand breakage
	Sulphonamides	Inhibit dihydropteroate synthase in the folic acid synthesis pathway
	Trimethoprim	Inhibits dihydrofolate reductase in the folic acid synthesis pathway
Inhibit RNA synthesis	<u>R</u>ifampicin	Binds to RNA polymerase beta subunit

Fact 1166:

Why is urgent operative management required in a **strangulated hernia**?

Strangulated hernias involve compromised blood supply to their contents, posing a high risk of bowel ischaemia and gangrene.

Fact 1167:

How do the **Valsalva manoeuvre** and **carotid sinus massage** affect the donor heart rate post-cardiac transplantation?

No effect – there is no vagal innervation to the heart and the efferent limb of the baroreceptor reflex is lost.

- The donor heart has its intrinsic SAN controlling its heart rate at 90–100 due to the loss of vagal tone.
- It relies on catecholamines and preload to compensate for the absence of autonomic innervation during changes in SVR, such as during induction or exercise.
- Drugs or manoeuvres that directly affect the heart are the only ones that have an impact, while parasympathomimetic drugs like <u>G</u>lycopyrrolate, <u>A</u>tropine and <u>D</u>igoxin have no effect.
- Sympathomimetic drugs like adrenaline and noradrenaline show an ↑ response due to denervation sensitivity. Direct-acting agents like dobutamine and isoprenaline maintain a normal response. Indirect-acting agents like ephedrine exhibit a ↓ response due to the absence of catecholamine stores in myocardial neurons.
- Although coronary arteries retain their vasodilatory responsiveness to metabolic demands and nitrates and can develop atherosclerosis, patients do not experience angina pain with ischaemia or infarction because of denervation.

Fact 1168:

Why is it crucial for the arterial transducer's **natural frequency** to substantially differ from the arterial pressure wave's frequency?

- Every system has a natural tendency to oscillate. When a system receives a slight push, it begins to vibrate at a specific frequency known as its natural or resonant frequency.
- The arterial transducer is designed to detect pressure changes from the arterial waveform, which can have frequencies as high as 40 Hz.
- If the resonant frequency of the blood pressure monitoring system is within the range of the arterial waveform frequency, it can lead to excessive oscillation or resonance. This phenomenon can result in the overestimation of systolic pressure and underestimation of diastolic pressure.
- To prevent resonance, the natural frequency of the transducer should be well above the highest frequency of the arterial waveform, ideally above 40 Hz.
- This can be achieved by using short, stiff and wide connecting tubing, to ensure that the natural frequency is higher than clinically encountered arterial waveform frequencies.

Fact 1169:

Which context best explains this arterial blood gas?

		Normal ranges
pH	7.60	7.36–7.44
PaO$_2$	3.78	10.5–13.1 kPa
PaCO$_2$	1.36	4.6–6 kPa
HCO$_3$	9.87	20–28 mmol/L
Lactate	1.8	1–2 mmol/L
SaO$_2$	78%	94-100 %
Hb	194	130–180 g/L

High altitude

- The primary abnormality is a chronic respiratory alkalosis secondary to hypoxia.
- Renal compensation has resulted in excretion of bicarbonate.
- Adaptation to chronic hypoxia has resulted in polycythaemia to improve oxygen carrying capacity.

Fact 1170:

What happens to the FiO$_2$ if you increase the oxygen flow rate beyond recommended value of a **Venturi mask**?

↑ Gas delivery but FiO$_2$ will not increase

Fact 1171:

What are some potential complications of an **endoscopic retrograde cholangiopancreatography (ERCP)**?

- Bleeding
- Infection, e.g. cholangitis
- Perforation
- Acute pancreatitis

Fact 1172:

How does **pralidoxime** function in the treatment of sarin (nerve gas) poisoning?

- Sarin is an organophosphate which irreversibly binds to acetylcholinesterase.
- Pralidoxime reactivates the acetylcholinesterase enzyme.

Fact 1173:

Why can acute **ethanol intoxication** cause a metabolic acidosis?

- *Lactate acidosis:*
  - ↑ Anaerobic metabolism: Ethanol metabolism impairs gluconeogenesis and fatty acid oxidation
  - ↓ Lactate clearance: Ethanol impairs conversion of lactate to pyruvate
- *Alcoholic ketoacidosis:* Occurs in poorly nourished chronic alcoholics a few days after a binge.

Fact 1174:

What typical alterations in **oesophageal Doppler monitoring** would be observed in cases of hypovolaemia, elevated afterload and left ventricular failure?

Hypovolaemia	↓ SV ↓ FTc
Elevated afterload	↓ SV ↓ FTc ↓ Peak velocity
Left ventricular failure	↓ SV ↓ Peak velocity ↓ Mean acceleration

Fact 1175:

How do various blood chemicals affect **pulse oximetry** readings?

- Significant methaemaglobinaemia can cause a falsely ↓ reading (80–85%).
- Carboxyhaemoglobin absorbs light at 660 nm, similar to oxyhaemoglobin, leading to a falsely ↑ reading.
- Dyes like methylene blue, fluoresceine and indocyanine green cause an erroneous ↓ reading.

Fact 1176:

What typically happens to the blood pressure and heart rate with **sodium nitroprusside (SNP)** use?

Venous and arterial vasodilatation → ↓ BP → reflex ↑ HR

SNP is an inorganic complex and prodrug. It initially appears as a reddish-brown powder but is dissolved in dextrose to create a straw-coloured solution. Exposure to sunlight can lead to brown/blue discoloration, releasing cyanide ions and potentially causing lactic acidosis and cyanide toxicity.

Fact 1177:

What is the difference between Phase 1 and Phase 2 reactions of **drug metabolism**?

Drug metabolism aids in drug clearance through two primary mechanisms (1) increasing solubility and (2) converting prodrugs into their active form. The liver is the principal, but not only site of most drug metabolism. The cP450 system is important because of the impact of inhibition or induction.

In phase I reactions, drug metabolism often creates sites for the attachment of larger polar side chains in subsequent phase II reactions. Both phase I and II reactions serve to enhance drug hydrophilicity, thus facilitating renal or hepatobiliary excretion.

Phase 1	Involves intramolecular modifications: Oxidation, reduction and hydrolysis, resulting in its conversion to a more polar molecule.
Phase 2	Conjugation of the drug with an endogenous substance by glucuronidation, sulphation, acetylation and methylation. This makes it water soluble and therefore able to be excreted by the kidneys.

The substances that result from metabolism may be inactive, or they may be similar to or different from the original drug in therapeutic activity or toxicity.

Fact 1178:

Why is it advisable to conduct an abdominal ultrasound when **acute pancreatitis** is confirmed?

To indicate the presence or absence of gallstones and/or dilation of the common bile duct (CBD).

Fact 1179:

What is **Bazett's formula** to correct the QT-interval and which common electrolyte abnormalities prolong this interval?

$$QTc = \text{measured } QT / \sqrt{RR}$$

- Measured QT interval is from the beginning of the QRS complex to the end of the T wave.
- Common electrolyte abnormalities include ↓ calcium ↓ magnesium ↓ potassium.

Fact 1180:

What is the effect of **positive pressure ventilation (PPV)** on intracranial pressure in someone with TBI?

PPV → ↑ intrathoracic pressure → ↓ cerebral venous drainage → ↑ ICP

Fact 1181:

What is the implication of each of the three **Lundberg waves** shown below:

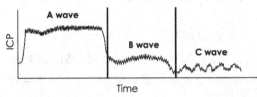

Lundberg waves refer to the ICP over time rather than the morphology of individual ICP waveforms.

	Amplitude	Duration	Description
A	50–100 mmHg above baseline ICP	5–20 minutes	These waves are always pathological and suggest ↓ brain compliance. Thought to be due to a reflex cerebral vasodilation in response to ↓ MAP. The pressure plateaus when maximum vasodilation is reached. May be terminated by increasing the MAP.
B	Up to 50 mmHg	<2 minutes	These waves signify normal autoregulation. Can be seen when there is unstable ICP (e.g. vasospasm), but are also observed in non-pathological states in normal individuals (e.g. REM sleep). Their absence following a head injury is a poor prognostic sign.
C	<20 mmHg	4–8 minute cycles	No clinical significance

Fact 1182:

What do the phases of a **capnography** trace represent?

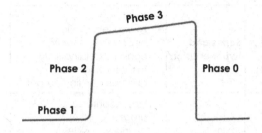

Phase I	Represents the start of expiration with the expiration of CO_2-free gas from anatomical dead space
Phase 2	Represents mixed gas from the airways and alveoli with a progressive ↑ in CO_2
Phase 3	Represents the expiration of pure alveolar gas. This usually has a minimal upward slope. This occurs due to variable mixing and time constants, e.g. alveoli with longer time constants empty later and have a higher concentration of CO_2
Phase 0	Represents the absence of CO_2 during inspiration

Fact 1183:

Why does atracurium help in the management of **ARDS**?

- ↑ Chest compliance
- ↓ Oxygen consumption
- Improved ventilation and ↓ dyssynchrony

Fact 1184:

How can healthcare providers implement the **STOP-AKI bundle** in patients identified as at risk of developing AKI?

S	Sepsis and hypoperfusion	• Treat sepsis • Avoid dehydration, treat hypovolaemia, consider holding anti-hypertensives/diuretics, optimise cardiac output
T	Toxins	• Stop nephrotoxic drugs, e.g. NSAIDs, aminoglycosides • Care with IV iodinated contrast
O	Obstruction	• Rule out obstruction with renal tract ultrasound +/– consider catheterisation
P	Prevent harm	• Identify the cause, e.g. screen for intrinsic renal disease, urine dip +/– immunological/viral infection screen • Identify drugs excreted through the kidneys and adjust drug doses promptly if AKI develops, e.g. LMWH, metformin, antibiotics • Prevent inadequate or excessive IV fluid administration

Fact 1185:

What action should be taken if the cricothyroid membrane cannot be felt in a **Can't Intubate Can't Oxygenate (CICO)** scenario?

Vertical skin incision + scalpel–bougie–tube technique

Fact 1186:

When would you start a statin after an **ischaemic stroke**?

• Patients already taking statins should continue
• Others should be considered after 48 hours

Fact 1187:

What is the **partial pressure of oxygen in the alveoli (P_AO_2)** if a person with healthy lungs and a normal diet is breathing 60% oxygen and has a $PaCO_2$ of 4.5 kPa?

$$P_AO_2 = FiO_2 \ (P_{atm} - P_{H2O}) - PaCO_2 / RQ$$

$$P_AO_2 = 0.6 \ (101 - 6.25) - 4.5 / 0.8 = \textbf{51.225 kPa}$$

A quicker and cruder way is $FiO_2 - 10 = 60 - 10 = 50$ kPa

Fact 1188:

What are some of the principles of peri-operative care in **sickle cell disease (SCD)**?

• Hydration, analgesia, normothermia, correcting acidosis and avoiding hypoxaemia
• Considering red blood cell transfusions
• Considering an exchange transfusion
• Thromboprophylaxis
• MDT involvement

Fact 1189:

Which condition does this **flow-volume loop** suggest in someone who had prolonged ventilation via an ETT?

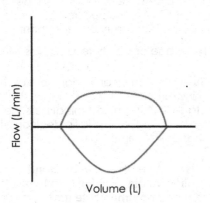

Tracheomalacia – trachea collapses during expiration but remains patent during inspiration

The flow volume loop shows variable intrathoracic obstruction (normal inspiratory limb and a flattened expiratory limb).

Tracheomalacia arises due to damage to tracheal tissue, initially caused by reduced blood supply, leading to chondritis and eventual breakdown/necrosis of the supporting tracheal cartilage. Clinical presentation often involves difficulties in weaning from mechanical ventilation. Diagnostic tools like bronchoscopy and dynamic CT scans can reveal tracheal narrowing during expiration.

Management options include tracheal excision, tracheoplasty or stenting.

Fact 1190:

What is the difference in pathophysiology between a **pseudobulbar** and **bulbar palsy**?

Pseudobulbar	Bulbar
Bilateral damage to the corticobulbar tracts to the nerve nuclei of CNs 5, 7, 9, 10, 11, 12	Bilateral damage to the CNs 9, 10, 11, 12 or to their nuclei in the medulla
This leads to UMN features of the respective muscles, e.g. spastic paralysis of the tongue and exaggerated gag and jaw jerk reflexes	This leads to LMN features of the respective muscles, e.g. flaccid paralysis, atrophy and fasciculations of the tongue and an absent gag reflex

- Note that the same nerves are involved in both of these conditions. In pseudobulbar there is also CN 5 and 7.
- Since the cranial nerve nuclei in the brain stem are paired, unilateral lesions are often asymptomatic.

Fact 1191:

Can **portal vein thrombosis** lead to acute liver failure?

No, acute liver failure is caused by hepatic vein thrombosis (Budd–Chiari syndrome) instead of portal vein thrombosis.

Fact 1192:

Which clinical situations can account for this ETCO$_2$ trace:

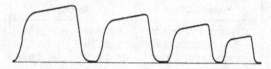

This is a rapid ↓ ETCO$_2$ over the course of a few breaths. This can occur because of:

- Oesophageal intubation: May initially register CO$_2$ especially if carbonated beverages were consumed
- ↑ V/Q → ↑ dead space:
  - o   Large air or pulmonary embolism
  - o   ↓ BP/↓ cardiac output of any cause (cardiogenic shock, massive haemorrhage, anaphylaxis) → ↓ alveolar perfusion

Fact 1193:

Why is **alfentanil** useful for pain relief in renal impairment?

- It is a potent short-acting opioid.
- It does not accumulate in renal failure.
- It is metabolised by CYP3A4 in the liver.

Fact 1194:

What are the basic principles of the **Mental Capacity Act**?

Capacity is presumed in all individuals unless proven otherwise. It is decision-dependent and can be temporary or permanent.

The two-stage capacity test involves:

- Stage 1: Identify an impairment of the mind/brain
- Stage 2: Determine if this affects the ability to make a specific decision at that point in time

Patients must be able to **understand** information, **retain** it, **weigh** it up to make a decision and **communicate** that decision. Efforts should be made to support them in achieving capacity, and if they lack it, decisions are made in their best interests. Emergency treatment can be provided without prior knowledge of preferences, prioritising the least restrictive and invasive option. Consultation with family, friends, carers or a valid advanced directive helps clarify wishes and informs best-interest decisions.

An appointed Lasting Power of Attorney (LPA) or Court of Protection-appointed deputy may consent on behalf of a patient who lacks capacity. An LPA can make decisions on life-sustaining treatment only if it's explicitly documented in the agreement. They cannot demand treatments if not in the patient's best interests. In cases without an advocate, an IMCA (Independent Mental Capacity Advocate) should be consulted, especially for significant medical decisions.

Fact 1195:

How many values fall between 4.3 and 4.9 mmol/L in a group of 1,000 patients taking an ACE inhibitor, where the mean potassium level is 4.6 mmol/L and the standard deviation (SD) is 0.3 mmol/L?

- Given that 1SD is equal to 0.3 mmol/L, both 4.3 and 4.9 are situated 1 SD away from the mean.
- In a normally distributed variable, approximately **68.3%** of values fall within 1 standard deviation of the mean.

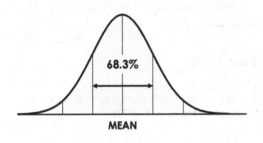

Fact 1196:

Which vascular structure is most likely to be damaged while cannulating the **subclavian vein**?

Subclavian artery – positioned posteriorly and partially superior to the vein. When trying to cannulate the vein, there's a risk of accidentally puncturing the subclavian artery, which is problematic to control due to its location.

Fact 1197:

What are some of the roles of **Vitamin C and thiamine**?

Vitamin C	Thiamine
Both are water-soluble and require external supplementation as they cannot be synthesised endogenously.	
Absorbed by sodium-dependent transporters in the gut	Absorbed in the jejunum, mostly by active transport
<ul><li>Free radical scavenger: ↓ ROS</li><li>↓ Cytokines from B-cells</li><li>↑ Lymphocytes and ↑ IFN → bacterial death</li><li>Co-factor for vasopressin and catecholamine synthesis → ↑ catecholamine sensitivity</li><li>↑ Wound healing, protects endothelial barrier and maintains microcirculatory patency</li></ul>	<ul><li>Essential co-factor in Krebs cycle and is important for carbohydrate metabolism</li><li>Involved in neuronal signalling</li><li>Necessary for the normal function of the nervous system and heart</li></ul>

Fact 1198:

Where is the lesion if someone has **hemiballismus**?

Subthalamic nucleus in the basal ganglia

Fact 1199:

What is the difference between Type A and Type B **lactic acidosis**?

- Type A: Tissue hypoperfusion, e.g. due to shock, anaemia and mesenteric ischaemia
- Type B: Normal tissue perfusion:

B1	B2	B3
Underlying disease	Drugs + Toxins	Inborn errors of metabolism
Renal failure Liver failure Malignancy, e.g. leukemia, lymphoma HIV/AIDS Ketoacidosis Phaeochromocytoma	**Drugs:** Adrenaline β_2-agonists HIV/HAART meds Isoniazid Linezolid Nitroprusside Niacin Metformin Propofol Paracetamol Salicylates **Toxins:** CO, cyanide, ethanol, methanol, ethylene glycol	G6PD Pyruvate DH deficiency

Fact 1200:

How do you classify **dead space**?

Dead space refers to the volume of inhaled air that does not participate in gas exchange:

- *Anatomical*: Mouth, nose, pharynx to large airways not lined with respiratory epithelium
- *Alveolar*: Refers to areas of the ventilated lung that are not adequately perfused, representing an extreme V/Q mismatch.
- *Physiological*: Anatomical + alveolar dead space

Fact 1201:

What are the potential consequences of improperly adjusting **sensitivity** during temporary pacing?

- Systems with low sensitivity may carry a risk of AF or VF if pacing is administered late in the depolarisation.
- In excessively sensitive systems, artefacts (e.g. respiration, shivering) or lower-amplitude activity (e.g. T-waves) may be interpreted as native electrical activity, potentially causing inappropriate inhibition of pacing.

Fact 1202:

What components make up the 4Ts scoring system for **type 2 heparin-induced thrombocytopaenia (HIT)**?

The 4Ts scoring system is based on four elements:

	0 points	1 point	2 points
Thrombocytopenia	<30% fall	30–50% fall	>50% fall
Time to thrombocytopenia	<4 days	>10 days	5–10 days
Thrombosis	None	Suspected, progressive or recurrent thrombosis; non-necrotising skin lesions	New thrombosis; skin necrosis
o**T**her causes of thrombocytopenia	Definite	Possible	None

- Low probability: 1–3
- Intermediate probability: 4–5
- High probability: 6–8 (~64% probability of HIT)

Fact 1203:

What clinical features are necessary for diagnosing **acute liver failure**?

- The absence of chronic liver disease
- Rapid decline in liver function ($\uparrow$ AST/ALT) with jaundice ($\uparrow$ bilirubin), coagulopathy ($\uparrow$ INR) and encephalopathy
- Presents within 12 weeks
- Classified by O'Grady as hyperacute, acute and subacute

In the developed world, paracetamol overdose is the most common cause. Worldwide, viral aetiologies and seronegative hepatitis are more prevalent.

Fact 1204:

If someone has a 4T score which demonstrates a high pre-test probability for **HIT**, what should you do?

- Stop heparin
- Start an alternative anticoagulant, e.g.
  - o   Direct thrombin inhibitors (lepirudin, argatroban, bivaluridin)
  - o   Anti-thrombin-dependent factor Xa inhibitors (danaparoid, fondaparinux)
- *HIT screen*: Can be functional (assessing heparin-dependent platelet activation by the heparin/PF4 antibody) or by using immunoassays (measuring antibody levels in the blood).

Fact 1205:

When applying **Fick's law** to a gas, how will molecular flux change if the diffusion coefficient is quadrupled?

Molecular flux will increase fourfold

$$V_{gas} = \frac{D \times (P_1 - P_2) \times A}{T}$$

V_{gas}: Molecular flux/flow

D: Diffusion coefficient

$(P_1 - P_2)$: Partial pressure gradient

A: Surface area

T: Thickness of barrier

Fact 1206:

What are the recommendations in the BTS guidelines for dealing with pleural effusions that are likely to be **transudates**?

Identify and treat the underlying cause.

If resolution doesn't occur or if an exudate is suspected, it is advised to consult a respiratory specialist and conduct a diagnostic pleural tap.

Fact 1207:

How do you classify **antifungals**?

Attack cell membrane	**Azoles** (inhibit ergos-terol synthesis)	**Triazole**	Fluconazole
			Itraconazole
			Voriconazole
			Posaconazole
		Imida-zole	Ketoconazole
			Miconazole
	Polyenes (bind to ergosterol)		Amphotericin B
			Nystatin
	Allylamines (inhibit squalene epoxidase)		Terbinafine
Attack cell wall glucan synthesis	**Echinocandins** (inhibit β-glucan synthesis)		Anidulafungin
			Caspofungin
			Micafungin
Act intra-cellularly	Griseofulvin (inhibits mitosis)		
	Flucytosine (inhibits DNA/RNA synthesis)		

Fact 1208:

What is the difference between **cleaning, disinfection** and **sterilisation**?

- *Cleaning*: The process of eliminating visible contaminants.
- *Disinfection*: The removal of microorganisms that can potentially cause infections, except for spores and certain viruses.
- *Sterilisation*: The complete elimination of all microorganisms, including spores.

Fact 1209:

How often do you deflate the oesophageal balloon on an **Sengstaken–Blakemore tube (SBT)**?

Every 4 hours for 15 minutes to prevent necrosis

The tube is usually removed within 36–48 hours.

Fact 1210:

How would you manage a haemodynamically stable patient with a **saddle pulmonary embolism,** right heart strain and a history of breast cancer with cerebral metastases?

Anticoagulation and consider referral to interventional radiology to consider, e.g. catheter embolectomy, rheolysis (clot dissolution) or localised thrombolysis.

It's important to note that while there is limited evidence supporting thrombolysis for an intermediate-risk PE (a sub-massive PE), the presence of intracerebral metastases contraindicates this approach.

Fact 1211:

What treatment would you give to the following patient:

- Rescued from a **housefire**
- Intubated and ventilated at the scene due to low SpO_2, a GCS of 3, and fixed unreactive pupils
- After intubation, maintains an SpO_2 of 99% on FiO_2 1.0 and received IV fluids for hypotension
- Post-intubation ABG shows: pH 7.1, PO_2 54.3 kPa, PCO_2 4.5 kPa, HCO_3 15 mmol/L, base excess −8 mmol/L, lactate 14 mmol/L and COHb 15%

Hydroxocobalamin (B12)

This is the first-line antidote for cyanide poisoning. Second-line antidotes include sodium thiosulphate, dicobalt edetate and sodium nitrite.

Cyanide inhalation during combustion of materials like wool, silk, polyurethane and rubber impairs aerobic respiration by binding to mitochondrial cytochrome α3 oxidase. Severe poisoning results in a HAGMA with ↑ lactate (>7 mmol/L), ↓ AV oxygen gradient and neurological/cardiovascular compromise. Cyanide levels aid in confirming the diagnosis retrospectively.

Fact 1212:

What are some examples of **IL-6 inhibitors** that can be used in the management of COVID-19 pneumonitis?

Tocilizumab and sarilumab

Fact 1213:

What are some features of an **aspirin** overdose?

Dose ingested	Levels	Clinical features
<150 mg/kg (mild)	<2.5 mmol/L	Nil
150–300 mg/kg (moderate)	2.5–5.1 mmol/L	Hyperventilation Respiratory alkalosis Pyrexia Sweating Tinnitus Vomiting Hypoglycemia
>300 mg/kg (severe)	>5.1 mmol/L	Metabolic acidosis Seizures Altered consciousness Coma

Fact 1214:

How do you diagnose **latent tuberculosis** in someone previously vaccinated with BCG to minimise the risk of a false-positive result?

IFN-γ release assay

Fact 1215:

What were the results of the **'TracMan' study (2013)** when comparing early (≤4 days) and late (≥10 days) tracheostomy insertion?

- No difference in 30-day mortality
- No difference in the duration of mechanical ventilation, length of stay and antibiotic therapy
- ↓ Sedation in those with early tracheostomy

Fact 1216:

What is the most likely diagnosis if a 35-year-old admitted for a tooth extraction develops **prolonged bleeding** which requires suturing?

Von Willebrand's disease – this is one of the most common bleeding disorders.

Von Willebrand's disease is caused by ↓ or structurally abnormal von Willebrand's factor, vital for platelet function and coagulation factor 8 stability. It is inherited in an autosomal dominant fashion.

Mild cases can improve with DDAVP (↑ release of vWF from Weibel–Palade bodies of the endothelium), while others may require clotting factor concentrates.

Fact 1217:

What action should be taken if a patient with **acute pancreatitis** exhibits a dilated common bile duct (CBD) and the presence of 'sludge' in the gallbladder on ultrasound?

Therapeutic endoscopic retrograde cholangiopancreatography (ERCP)

Fact 1218:

What may abdominal breathing suggest in someone with a **spinal cord injury**?

It could indicate a failure of the thoracic muscles to assist with breathing, which may signal the impending need for respiratory support.

Fact 1219:

Can an **intra-aortic balloon pump (IABP)** be used to manage haemodynamic instability in severe acute mitral regurgitation due to papillary muscle dysfunction?

Yes, as a bridge to definitive surgery

Fact 1220:

What **American Spinal Injury Association (ASIA) grade** corresponds to this patient's condition:

- Complete loss of motor function below the level of injury, identified as T10
- Below T10, sensation is diminished but present, including the sacral segments S4–S5

This corresponds to ASIA B classification, indicating an incomplete spinal cord injury.

ASIA grade	Features	Injury type
A	No motor or sensory function below lesion level	Complete
B	**Sensory but not motor function is preserved below lesion level in at least the sacral segments**	**Incomplete**
C	Muscle grade < 3 out of 5 below lesion level	Incomplete
D	Muscle grade ≥ 3 out of 5 below lesion level	Incomplete
E	Normal function	None

Fact 1221:

What consideration should you keep in mind when utilising **TEGs** in cases of hypothermia?

TEGs may not effectively detect coagulopathy in cases of hypothermia.

TEGs assess clot firmness over a 60-minute test by heating a whole blood sample to 37°C. However, hypothermia can interfere with this process, potentially masking in-vivo coagulopathy.

Fact 1222:

How many milligrams (mg) are present in 1 mL of a typical 1:1,000 **adrenaline** vial?

1:1,000 = 1 in 1,000 = 1 g in 1,000 mL

1 g in 1,000 mL = 1,000 mg in 1,000 mL

= **1 mg/mL**

Fact 1223:

How does **hypertonic 8.4% sodium bicarbonate** work in a TCA overdose?

1. Provides a large sodium load to overcome sodium channel blockade
2. Buffers acidosis
3. Facilitates excretion via urinary alkalisation–ionised TCA accumulates in the renal tubules and cannot be reabsorbed (a phenomenon known as 'ion trapping').

Fact 1224:

What is the albumin difference in an **exudative pleural effusion**?

[Serum albumin]–[effusion albumin] <1.2 g/dL indicates the likelihood of an exudative pleural effusion

Fact 1225:

What is the most common pathological basis of an **intracerebral haemorrhage**?

Spontaneous rupture of small intracerebral arteries or arterioles due to hypertension

Fact 1226:

What is the most probable reason for a decrease in GCS from 15 to 12, 8 hours after a deliberate ingestion of 30 g of **paracetamol**?

Hepatic encephalopathy due to paracetamol toxicity

Fact 1227:

What are some long-term pancreatic complications that can arise as a consequence of **acute pancreatitis**?

Exocrine deficiency necessitating pancreatic digestive enzyme supplementation and the development of diabetes mellitus.

Fact 1228:

Which reflexes may still be present in **brainstem death testing**?

Spinal reflexes may still be present.

Fact 1229:

Which NICE criteria must be met to consider performing a **decompressive hemicraniectomy** for acute ischaemic stroke?

- Age 18–60 years
- <48 hours of symptom onset
- NIHSS score >15
- ↓ GCS (≥1 in item 1a of the NIHSS)
- CT infarct ≥ 50% MCA territory

Fact 1230:

What are some complications that may arise following an **ST-elevation myocardial infarction (STEMI)**?

- **D**eath
- **A**rrhythmias
- **R**upture (ventricular free wall, ventricular septum, papillary muscles)
- **T**amponade
- **H**eart failure (acute or chronic)
- **V**alve disease
- **A**neurysm of ventricle
- **D**ressler's syndrome
- thrombo**E**mbolism (mural thrombus)
- **R**ecurrence/ mitral **R**egurgitation

Fact 1231:

Which anatomical positions do these pressure waveforms correspond to as a **pulmonary artery catheter** is advanced?

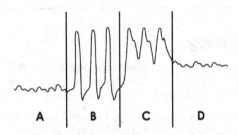

	Anatomical position	Expected depth	Normal values (mmHg)
A	Right atrium		2–6
B	Right ventricle	**25–30 cm**	Systolic 20–30
			Diastolic 0–5
C	Pulmonary artery (dicrotic notch, step-up in diastolic pressure)	**35–40 cm** (5–10 cm beyond RV)	Systolic 20–30
			Diastolic 8–12
			Mean 10–20
D	Pulmonary artery occlusion pressure	**45** cm (10 cm beyond PA)	4–12

Fact 1232:

How do you calculate **maintenance fluid** requirements for a child using the 4:2:1 method?

	4 mL/kg/hr for the first 10 kg
ADD:	2 mL/kg/hr for the second 10 kg
AND THEN ADD:	1 mL/kg/hr for each kg over 20 kg

e.g. for a 28 kg child:

4 mL/kg/hr for the first 10 kg	40 mL/hr
2 mL/kg/hr for the second 10 kg	20 mL/hr
1 mL/kg/hr for the remaining weight	8 mL/hr
Total	68 mL/hr

Fact 1233:

What are the four phases of **fluid resuscitation**?

Rescue, optimisation, stabilisation and de-escalation

Fact 1234:

What is meant by **pituitary apoplexy** and why may patients have meningism, cranial nerve palsies and visual field defects?

Pituitary apoplexy results from haemorrhage into or infarction of a pre-existing pituitary tumour. It is almost always associated with hypopituitarism.

- Meningism: If blood escapes into the subarachnoid space
- Cranial nerves: Compression of the cavernous sinus, which is adjacent to the pituitary gland, can lead to CN 3, 4 and 6 palsies, causing unilateral eye movement abnormalities
- Visual field/acuity deficits: Can occur from compression of the optic chasm, located just above the pituitary fossa

---

Fact 1235:

What are some quality indicators in the **Intensive Care National Audit and Research Centre (ICNARC)** Quarterly Quality Report (QQR)?

Admission risks	• High-risk admissions from the ward • High-risk sepsis admissions from the ward
Acquired infections	• Unit-acquired infections in blood
Discharges	• Out-of-hours discharges to the ward (not delayed) • Delayed discharges (>8 and >24 hours delay) • Discharges direct to home
Transfers and readmissions	• Non-clinical transfers to another unit • Unplanned readmissions within 48 hours
Mortality metrics	• Risk-adjusted acute hospital mortality • Risk-adjusted acute hospital mortality – predicted risk of death <20%

Fact 1236:

When do you given adrenaline and amiodarone in a **ventricular fibrillation arrest**?

After the third shock

Dose of amiodarone: 300 mg

Dose of adrenaline: 1 mg (and then every 3–5 minutes)

Fact 1237:

What are some consequences of **over-sedation**?

↑ Duration of mechanical ventilation
↑ Duration of recovery
↑ Risk of delirium
↑ Risk of myopathy and muscle wasting
↑ Risk of hypotension

Sedation holds are essential for regularly reassessing and adjusting sedation levels, ideally conducted daily unless contraindicated. The objective is to administer the lowest dose required to attain the appropriate sedation level, while recognising that deeper sedation may be needed at times.

Fact 1238:

What is the typical location for placing a **PICC line**?

Basilic vein – medial aspect of upper arm. It joins the brachial veins to form the axillary vein.

The cephalic can also be used but is more tortuous and enters axillary vein at acute angle.

Some complications of a PICC include thrombosis, phlebitis, CRBSI, malposition and tip migration. There is less risk of pneumothorax and arterial bleeding when compared to CVCs.

Fact 1239:

What is the **absolute risk reduction (ARR)**, **relative risk reduction (RRR)** and **number needed to treat (NNT)** for a mortality rate of 20% in the intervention group and 30% in the control group of a study?

- ARR is the difference between the groups:
  30–20% = 10%
- RRR is ARR/mortality rate in the control group:
  10/30 = 33%
- NNT is the number of people that would need to be subject to the intervention for one person to benefit. It is 100/ARR:
  100/10 = 10

Fact 1240:

Why might you consider giving **magnesium sulphate** to someone who normally takes bendroflumethiazide and is currently experiencing refractory ventricular fibrillation, despite receiving multiple shocks, adrenaline and amiodarone according to the ALS algorithm?

This is recommended in refractory VF if there is anything to suggest hypomagnesaemia, e.g. a thiazide diuretic.

Fact 1241:

What is meant by **functional (or true) warm ischaemic time** in organ donation?

- The functional warm ischaemic period starts when there is inadequate oxygenation/perfusion during withdrawal of life-sustaining treatment and extends until the initiation of cold perfusion.
- This time is important because organs suffer ischaemic damage that affects graft function.
- It is defined as a SBP < 50 mmHg for ≥2 minutes +/− SpO_2 < 70%.
- The accepted warm ischaemic times are:
  o *Liver and pancreas*: 30 minutes
  o *Lungs*: 60 minutes
  o *Kidneys*: 120 minutes

Fact 1242:

What are the six main types of **healthcare-associated infections** that account for the majority of these infections?

- Respiratory tract infections (22.8%)
- Urinary tract infections (17.2%)
- Surgical site infections (15.7%)
- Clinical sepsis (10.5%)
- Gastrointestinal infections (8.8%)
- Bloodstream infections (7.3%)

Fact 1243:

In addition to renal function, trace elements and electrolytes, what other biochemical tests should be monitored in patients receiving **parenteral nutrition**?

Liver function tests, glucose, lipids

Fact 1244:

What are some examples of congenital **acyanotic** and **cyanotic** heart disease?

Acyanotic heart disease	Cyanotic heart disease
Obstructive lesions or left to right shunting of blood	Right to left shunting of blood
Atrial and ventricular septal defects Patent ductus arteriosus Coarctation of the aorta Aortic or pulmonary stenosis	5Ts: • Tetralogy of Fallot • Transposition of the great vessels • Total anomalous pulmonary venous drainage • Truncus arteriosus • Tricuspid atresia Pulmonary atresia Hypoplastic left heart syndrome

Fact 1245:

If a low FTc of 290 ms increases to just 310 ms following a 250 mL fluid challenge, what does this suggest about **vascular resistance**?

The ↓ FTc reflects an ↑ SVR (↑ afterload)

- FTc acts as an indirect indicator of preload.
- ↑ FTc after a fluid bolus, accompanied by a notable ↑ in SV, may indicate the need for additional fluid.
- However, if there is minimal change in FTc after a fluid bolus, administering more fluid could be detrimental. This is particularly true in cases where there is an ↑ afterload (resulting in ↓ FTc) despite adequate preload, such as in hypothermia and cardiac failure.

Fact 1246:

What are the potential drawbacks of using a **heat and moisture exchanger (HME)** and in which clinical circumstances may its performance be suboptimal?

Potential drawbacks	Suboptimal performance
• ↑ Dead space • ↑ Expiratory resistance • Partial/complete airway obstruction, e.g. due to secretions, blood, vomit	• High minute ventilation • Hypothermia • Large bronchopleural fistulae

Fact 1247:

Can you prevent delirium with **haloperidol**?

No – it treats it, not prevents it

Fact 1248:

What is the clinical definition of **septic shock**?

Hypotension requiring vasopressors to maintain a mean arterial pressure ≥ 65 mmHg with a lactate ≥2 mmol/L in the absence of hypovolaemia.

Fact 1249:

Why is **delirium** important on intensive care?

- ↑ Incidence of adverse events (e.g. unplanned extubation, removal of NGTs/lines/catheters)
- ↑ Mechanical ventilation and therefore associated complications, e.g. VAP, CINM, ↑ sedation
- ↑ LOS
- ↑ Incidence of PTSD and post-ICU cognitive impairment
- ↑ Post-ICU rehabilitation
- ↑ Mortality

Fact 1250:

What is the most likely diagnosis if:

- A 57-year-old with a history of hypertension develops chest pain radiating through to his back and low GCS.
- On examination he is pale and sweaty.
- He has a BP of 215/120 mmHg in the left arm and a weak right radial pulse.

A dissecting aortic aneurysm

Fact 1251:

What volume of fluid is given as a bolus for resuscitation in a paediatric patient showing signs of **septic shock**?

- An immediate crystalloid fluid bolus 20 mL/kg IV/IO
- Reassess and repeat if necessary

Fact 1252:

What are some non-radiological early indicators of an unfavourable prognosis in **traumatic brain injury (TBI)** as outlined by the Brain Trauma Foundation?

- Age
- GCS post-resuscitation (especially motor component)
- Bilateral absent pupillary light reflex
- Hypotension (SBP < 90 mmHg)

Fact 1253:

What do these **lung function tests** show:

	% Predicted	Interpretation
FEV$_1$ (L)	80	Low
FVC (L)	64	Low
TLC (L)	70	Low
DLCO (mL/mmHg/min)	30	Low
FEV$_1$/FVC ratio	82	Normal to high

This is a restrictive defect

The DLCO (lung diffusion capacity for carbon monoxide) is a surrogate marker of the ability for oxygen to diffuse across the alveoli to erythrocytes. The severely ↓ DLCO suggests pulmonary parenchymal disease, e.g. pulmonary fibrosis.

Fact 1254:

What are the Resuscitation Council (UK) guidelines for **chest compression** depth and rate in adults?

- *Depth*: 5–6 cm or 1/3 of the depth of the chest
- *Rate*: 100–120 compressions/minute

Fact 1255:

What does an **oesophageal Doppler probe** measure?

Blood flow velocity in the descending aorta

Fact 1256:

In which type of poisoning can excessive **oxygen** administration exacerbate lung toxicity?

Paraquat (a highly toxic herbicide)

- Paraquat induces reactive oxygen species, leading to pneumonitis and secondary lung fibrosis.
- Administering additional oxygen may enhance the generation of oxygen free radicals, which can worsen lung injury.
- Fuller's earth is a recognised treatment but not a specific antidote.

Fact 1257:

What is the typical manufacturer's recommendation for the frequency of **tracheostomy tube replacement** in patients with an established stoma?

Most recommend that tracheostomy tubes be changed approximately 30 days after placement.

Fact 1258:

How can you differentiate **between left anterior hemiblock (LAHB)** and **left posterior hemiblock (LPHB)** on an ECG, and what are the diagnostic criteria for **bifascicular block** and **trifascicular block**?

- LAHB causes left axis deviation
- LPHB causes right axis deviation

The bundle of His consists of three fascicles:

- The right bundle branch
- Anterior fascicles of the left bundle branch
- Posterior fascicles of the left bundle branch

Bifascicular block = RBBB + LAHB/LPHB

Bifascicular block may progress to trifascicular block and may be an indication for the insertion of a permanent cardiac pacemaker:

- *Incomplete Trifascicular Block:* Bifascicular Block + first or second degree heart block
- *Complete Trifascicular Block:* Bifascicular Block + third degree heart block

Note that RBBB in isolation is a normal variant. LBBB is always pathological.

Fact 1259:

How is **pulmonary artery hypertension (PAH)** classified?

Group		Examples
1 **Pulmonary artery hypertension**		Idiopathic, heritable and drug-induced
	Associated with diseases	• Connective tissue diseases • HIV infection • Congenital heart diseases • Schistosomiasis
	Special cases	PPHN (persistent pulmonary hypertension of the newborn)
2 **Left heart disease**	Heart failure	Preserved/reduced ejection fraction
	Structural heart problems	• Valvular heart disease • Left heart inflow/outflow tract obstruction (congenital/acquired) • Congenital cardiomyopathies
3 **Lung diseases and/or hypoxia**	Chronic conditions	• COPD • Interstitial lung disease • Mixed restrictive and obstructive lung disease • Developmental lung diseases
	Specific contexts	• Sleep-disordered breathing • High altitude
4 **Chronic thromboembolic pulmonary hypertension**	Thrombo-embolic	Chronic thromboembolic obstruction (proximal/distal)
	Non-thrombo-embolic	Non-thrombotic embolism (tumours, parasites)
5 **Unclear and/or multifactorial mechanisms**	Haemato-logic	• Myeloproliferative disorders • Splenectomy
	Systemic disorders	• Sarcoidosis, • Langerhans cell histiocytosis • Lymphangioleiomy-omatosis
	Metabolic	• Glycogen storage diseases • Gaucher disease • Thyroid disorders
	Other con-ditions	• Fibrosing mediastinitis • Chronic renal failure on dialysis

Fact 1260:

Why might someone on co-trimoxazole for *Pneumocystis jirovecii* **pneumonia (PJP)** have an SpO_2 of 85% and a PaO_2 of 11 kPa on 45% oxygen?

Methaemoglobinaemia caused by co-trimoxazole

Fact 1261:

What are the major mechanisms of injury in **blunt abdominal trauma**?

- Compression, e.g. from seatbelt
  - o Subcapsular haematomas to solid organs
  - o ↑ Intraluminal pressure → rupture of hollow viscera
- *Deceleration*: Shearing between free and fixed structures
  - o A hepatic tear along the ligamentum teres
  - o Intimal injuries to the renal arteries
  - o Mesenteric tears

Fact 1262:

How do you treat **myxoedema coma**?

- Management of underlying precipitating disease and supportive care as indicated
- Corticosteroid replacement prior to thyroid hormones (most have adrenal impairment)
- Thyroid hormone replacement
  - o Enteral T4: Levothyroxine sodium
  - o IV T3: Liothyronine sodium (second line)

Fact 1263:

What advantages does a **subglottic suction port** offer in a cuffed tracheostomy?

- Removing oropharyngeal secretions from the proximal trachea → ↓ risk of VAP
- Using the subglottic suction port for air insufflation enables phonation

Fact 1264:

What are the Guidelines for the Provision of Intensive Care Services recommendations for **staffing** levels in ICU?

MEDICAL	NURSING
• 1 daytime consultant for 8–12 patients • 1 daytime resident for up to 8 patients • 1 night-time resident for up to 8 patients • All staff on resident rota should have basic airway skills with 24/7 access to a doctor/ACCP with advanced airway skills	• Level 3 patients: 1:1 nursing (minimum) • Level 2 patients: 1:2 nursing (minimum) • 1 supernumerary coordinating nurse (band 6/7) • 1 additional supernumerary nurse for every 10 patients

Fact 1265:

What are some causes of **thrombocytopenia** in the critically ill?

De-creased produc-tion	• Sepsis • Drugs, e.g. vancomycin, linezolid, chemotherapy • Alcohol excess • Critical illness marrow suppression
Con-sumption	• Vaccine-induced immune thrombotic thrombocytopaenia (VITT) • Thrombotic thrombocytopaenic purpura (TTP) • Pulmonary embolism • Major trauma • HELLP syndrome
Dilutional	Fluid resuscitation and unbalanced transfusions
Distribu-tive	• Hypersplenism • Hypothermia
Destruc-tion	**Immune** • Heparin-induced thrombocytopaenia (HIT) • Immune thrombocytopaenic purpura (ITP) • Systemic lupus erythematosus (SLE) • Antiphospholipid syndrome **Non-immune** • Disseminated intravascular coagulation • Intravascular devices (ECMO, IABP, LVAD, PAC)

Fact 1266:

What are some causes of **adrenal insufficiency**?

Primary (Addison's disease)	Secondary	Tertiary
Adrenal pathology	ACTH deficiency	Hypotha-lamic
• Autoimmune • TB • Metastasis • Adrenalectomy • Critical illness • Haemorrhage into gland (e.g. Water-house–Friedrich-sen syndrome) • Drugs (e.g. **m**etyrapone, **e**tomidate, **k**eto-conazole)	Hypopituita-rism Withdrawal of long-term corticoster-oids	Infarction Malig-nancy

Fact 1267:

Why is transthoracic echocardiography not the best modality for detecting **infective endocarditis**?

• TTE has a high level of false positives and false negatives.
• TOE is the imaging modality of choice.

Fact 1268:

What is the usual **blood gas profile** in a full-term pregnant woman who is not in labour?

Mild compensated respiratory alkalosis

Progesterone, oestradiol and prostaglandins influence the hypothalamus → ↑ TV with little change in RR → ↓ $PaCO_2$ → less bicarbonate reabsorption by kidneys.

Fact 1269:

Which autoantibodies are implicated in **Stiff person syndrome**?

Autoantibodies against glutamic acid decarboxylase, which is important in the synthesis of GABA.

This causes ↓ GABA levels (principal inhibitory neurotransmitter) → ↑ signalling to muscles → ↑ muscular contractions → stiffness and spasms.

Treatment is with benzodiazepines, which act as GABA agonists to compensate for ↓ GABA in the CNS and to counteract the excitatory signalling mediated by glutamate.

Fact 1270:

How can DDAVP administration during a **water deprivation test** differentiate between central and nephrogenic diabetes insipidus (DI)?

- *Central DI*: Urine osmolality will ↑ with DDAVP administration > 750 mOsm/kg.
- *Nephrogenic DI*: Urine osmolality remains low < 300 mOsm/kg in spite of DDAVP administration.

Fact 1271:

What are some metabolic consequences of **nephrotic syndrome**?

↑ **Susceptibility to infection**	Urinary loss of immunoglobulins and complement; protein deficiency; ↓ leucocyte bactericidal activity
Hypovolaemia	↓ Albumin → ↓ plasma oncotic pressure → ↓ circulating volume
Hyperlipidaemia and atherosclerosis	↓ Oncotic pressure → reactive hepatic protein and lipid synthesis
Hypercoagulability and risk of VTE	Urinary loss of antithrombin III and plasminogen (anticoagulant factors); ↑ procoagulant factors
Hypocalcaemia and bone abnormalities	Caused by ↓ serum albumin and urinary loss of vitamin D-binding proteins

Fact 1272:

Which **primary afferent neurons** take painful stimuli to the spinal cord?

Pain → Nociceptors → **Aδ & C fibres** → spinal cord

Fact 1273:

What grade of **intraabdominal hypertension (IAH)** has occurred if someone has high NG aspirates and an intra-abdominal pressure of 18 mmHg following an AAA repair?

Grade 2 IAH

IAH is an IAP > 12 mmHg. Grades of IAH (mmHg):

Grade 1	12–15
Grade 2	16–20
Grade 3	21–25
Grade 4	≥26

Abdominal compartment syndrome is sustained ↑ in IAP > 20 mmHg (Grade 3–4), with new organ dysfunction.

Fact 1274:

What can be achieved by a **case conference**?

Conflict resolution
Aims and goals of further management
Progress with treatment so far
Roles and responsibilities of the team/family
Interests of the patient (best interests)
Stumbling blocks and overcoming them

Fact 1275:

What are the goals of a **clinical trial**?

Phase 1	• Determines pharmacokinetics, pharmacodynamics and side effects prior to larger studies • Conducted on healthy volunteers
Phase 2	• Assesses efficacy and optimal dosage in a sample of patients with the disease
Phase 3	• Assesses effectiveness in hundreds to thousands of people with the disease often as part of a RCT, comparing the new treatment with established treatments
Phase 4	• Post-marketing surveillance to monitor long-term effectiveness and side effects

---

Fact 1276:

Which echocardiographic finding aids in distinguishing between acute and chronic **cor pulmonale**?

The presence of right ventricular hypertrophy – this is a feature of chronic cor pulmonale.

RVH can produce elevated systolic pressures (>35 mmHg) and tricuspid regurgitation jets (>60 mmHg), distinguishing it from acute cor pulmonale.

A dilated RV, on the other hand, can indicate either acute or late chronic cor pulmonale.

Fact 1277:

Which ECG changes may be seen in **hypothermia**?

- Prolonged PR, QRS and QT intervals
- Osborn (J) waves when temperature < 33°C
- Ventricular ectopics
- Artifact due to shivering
- Any type of bradyarrhythmia, e.g. sinus bradycardia, AV block, slow AF, slow junctional rhythms
- Cardiac arrest due to asystole, VF or VT

Fact 1278:

What did the **TRICC and TRISS studies** show about transfusion thresholds?

	TRICC (1999)	TRISS (2014)
Population	Patients admitted to ICU	Septic shock patients
Intervention (transfusion threshold)	Hb 70 g/L versus 100 g/L	Hb ≤ 70 g/L versus 90 g/L
Primary outcome	30-day mortality: No difference	90-day mortality: No difference
Secondary outcome	In-hospital mortality: Significantly lower (22% vs. 28%)	• Median number of transfusions: Significantly lower • Patients not undergoing transfusion: Significantly higher

---

Fact 1279:

How does a persistently raised **ICP** correlate with mortality?

↑ ICP → ↑ mortality

Fact 1280:

How do you assess **readiness to wean** from mechanical ventilation?

Clinical assessment
<ul><li>Improved underlying condition</li><li>General physiology optimised</li><li>Identifying airway and breathing concerns:<ul><li>Satisfactory airway reflexes, manageable secretions, cuff leak present</li><li>Spontaneously breathing, adequate strength, $FIO_2 \leq 0.4$, and minimal PEEP</li></ul></li><li>Haemodynamically stable with minimal vasoactive medication</li><li>Ideally obeying commands</li></ul>
Objective numerical indices to predict the likelihood of success with a spontaneous breathing trial
<ul><li>Respiratory rate (RR) < 30</li><li>Tidal volume (VT) > 5 mL/kg</li><li>Forced vital capacity (FVC) > 15 mL/kg</li><li>Minute ventilation (MV) < 15 L/min</li><li>Maximum inspiratory pressure (PI_{max}) < 30 cmH$_2$O (indicator of respiratory muscle strength)</li><li>Rapid shallow breathing index (RSBI) < 105 (RSBI = RR/VT)</li><li>P0.1/PI_{max} > 0.3 (reflects central respiratory drive; P0.1 is the initial negative airway pressure during the first 0.1 second of blocked inspiration)</li></ul>

Fact 1281:

How should you manage an **asystolic cardiac arrest** in a full-term pregnant woman on the delivery suite?

- Confirm the arrest, initiate CPR (30:2 ratio) with supplemental oxygen, manually displace the uterus or perform a left lateral tilt (15–30 degrees) and administer 1 mg of adrenaline IV/IO.
- Activate the maternal cardiac arrest team, considering a perimortem caesarean section if there is no ROSC after 4 minutes.
- Assess and address reversible causes (4Hs, 4Ts: **h**ypoxia, **h**ypokalaemia/ hyperkalaemia, **h**ypothermia/ hyperthermia, **h**ypovolaemia, **t**ension pneumothorax, **t**amponade, **t**hrombosis, **t**oxins).

Fact 1282:

Does increased PEEP compared to reduced PEEP affect mortality in **ARDS**?

No

Atelectrauma, characterised by the repetitive opening and closing of alveoli during the respiratory cycle, results in lung damage and the release of cytokines, which can contribute to lung injury. Generally, PEEP is used to ↓ the effects of atelectrauma.

Fact 1283:

What is the **pulmonary vascular resistance** in dynes/s/cm^5 if a pulmonary artery catheter generates these results:

- Mean pulmonary artery pressure (MPAP) = 10 mmHg
- Pulmonary artery occlusion pressure (PAOP) = 5 mmHg
- Cardiac output (CO) = 5 L/minute

PVR = [(MPAP − PAOP) / CO] × 80

PVR = [(10 − 5) / 5] × 80 = **80 dynes / s / cm^5**

A correction factor of 80 is used to convert to dynes/s/cm^5

Fact 1284:

What are the reasons for minimising the use of large volumes of **crystalloid** in trauma patients?

May result in dilutional coagulopathy by reducing platelet and clotting factor concentrations, which can potentially worsen bleeding. Management involves:

- Low-volume resuscitation.
- Permissive hypotension: Tailor circulatory support to central pulse, e.g. SBP = 80–100, unless TBI is suspected.
- Early blood product administration.
- Prompt bleeding control.

Fact 1285:

Are the findings seen in this **forest plot** significant?

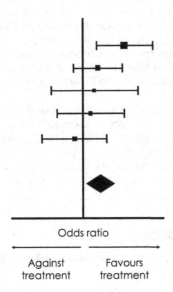

Odds ratio

Against treatment ← → Favours treatment

Yes – the diamond does not cross the y-axis

- Forest plots are employed in meta-analyses to evaluate overarching patterns using averages and confidence intervals derived from multiple studies.
- The y-axis is the line of no effect. If the diamond crosses this line, the overall outcome is not significant. The diamond's width represents the confidence interval (CI) for the combined odds ratio (OR).
- In this example with five studies, each square's position shows the OR, the square size reflects its weight (power) in the meta-analysis and the horizontal lines extending from each square indicates their respective CI.

Fact 1286:

How do you classify **cardiomyopathy**?

Dilated	LV dilatation and systolic dysfunction without abnormal loading conditions
Restrictive	Ventricular restriction with normal/↓ volumes and normal wall thickness
Hyper-trophic	Myocardial hypertrophy in the absence of haemodynamic stress
Arrhythmo-genic right ventricular	Replacement of RV myocardium with adipose and fibrous tissue in the triangle of dysplasia (apex, RV inflow/outflow tracts)
Unclassi-fied	Does not fall into any of the above

Fact 1287:

What are some ECG changes that are seen in severe **hypokalaemia**?

- ↑ Amplitude and width of the P wave
- ↑ PR interval
- ↓ T-wave (flattening and inversion)
- ↓ ST (ST depression)
- U waves
- Arrhythmias – many different types including supraventricular and ventricular

Fact 1288:

What is the microbial classification of **necrotising fasciitis (NF)**?

Type 1	Polymicrobial infections	A mixture of anaerobic and aerobic Gram-positive and Gram-negative organisms
Type 2	Monomicrobial	• Group A β-haemolytic Streptococcus (GAS) • *Staphylococcus aureus*
Type 3	Gram negative	Vibrio spp. (marine-related)
Type 4	Trauma-associated	• Candida spp. • Zygomycetes

The most common type is Type 1 (polymicrobial)

Fact 1289:

What are the **King's College criteria** used to select patients for liver transplant in cases of paracetamol-induced acute liver failure?

Any one of the following:

- pH < 7.3 (after resuscitation, >24 hours post-ingestion)
- Lactate > 3 mmol/L after fluid resuscitation
- All three of the following:
  - o   PT > 100 seconds (or INR > 6.5)
  - o   Serum creatinine > 300 µmol/L
  - o   Grade 3 or 4 encephalopathy

Fact 1290:

What is the expected **oxygen consumption** in a 25-year-old receiving a 24-hour ethyl alcohol infusion with a respiratory quotient (RQ) of 0.67, given her measured carbon dioxide production is 200 mL/min?

300 mL/min

$RQ = CO_2$ produced$/O_2$ consumed

$0.67 = 200/O_2$ consumed

$O2$ consumed $= 200/0.67 =$ **300 mL/min**

The RQ will vary with the energy substrates in the diet. A mixed diet usually produces a RQ of 0.8 because:

- CO_2 produced = 200 mL/min
- O_2 consumed = 250 mL/min

Lipids and alcohol require more oxygen than carbohydrates for complete oxidation.

Substrates	RQ
Glucose & other hexose sugars	1
Fats	0.7
Proteins	0.9

Fact 1291:

What is meant by the **Doppler effect**?

- The Doppler effect is the change in frequency or pitch of a sound wave when the source of the sound is in motion relative to an observer.
- When an object producing sound moves towards you, the frequency of the sound wave ↑, leading to a higher pitch.
- If an object producing sound moves away from you, the frequency of the sound wave ↓, leading to a lower pitch.
- This is similar to the observed pitch of sound of a car approaching and passing by a stationary observer.

Fact 1292:

How do you diagnose **primary biliary cirrhosis**?

- Antimitochondrial antibody positive (M2 subtype is highly specific)
- ↑ Immunoglobulins (particularly IgM)
- ↑ ALP & GGT
- ↑ AST/ALT (mildly)
- Liver biopsy shows granulomas around bile ducts (although a biopsy is not always required)

Fact 1293:

Why do the symptoms of **carcinoid syndrome** typically only manifest after metastasis of the primary neuroendocrine tumour to the liver?

- Carcinoid tumours, often located in the small bowel, release biologically active substances.
- Carcinoid syndrome symptoms, such as intermittent skin flushing, diarrhoea, wheezing and abdominal cramps, only manifest when these substances escape first-pass metabolism in the liver.
- If the primary tumour has metastasized to the liver, these products can be released directly into systemic circulation, or they can escape inactivation due to impaired liver function.

Fact 1294:

What is the equation for **therapeutic index (TI)**?

TI = LD50 (median lethal dose)/ED50 (median effective dose)

LD50 is the dose causing 50% mortality, while ED50 is the dose yielding a therapeutic effect in 50% of subjects. Drugs with a high TI are safer for clinical use due to a substantial gap between the effective and toxic doses.

Fact 1295:

What happens to **insulin** levels in starvation?

Levels are ↓

Fact 1296:

What is the next step in the emergency management of someone without a patent upper airway who is not breathing and in whom you have removed the **laryngectomy tube**?

- Call for expert help
- Oxygenate via laryngectomy stoma with a paediatric facemask or using a supraglottic airway device
- If this fails, attempt intubation of laryngectomy stoma which may require a fibreoptic bronchoscope or other airway equipment

Fact 1297:

What type of hypersensitivity reaction is responsible for **DRESS (drug rash with eosinophilia and systemic symptoms) syndrome?**

- A type 4 delayed hypersensitivity reaction where a drug or its metabolite triggers autoimmune reactions through the activation of T cells.
- This leads to generalised inflammation and the characteristic symptoms of DRESS, including a widespread rash, fever, eosinophilia and involvement of multiple organ systems.
- The most frequently implicated drugs include anticonvulsants, allopurinol, sulphonamides, antibiotics and antiretrovirals.
- Management involves discontinuing the causative drug and providing supportive treatment. Corticosteroids are often used, but the evidence regarding their effectiveness is limited.

Fact 1298:

What is first-line antifungal for treating **invasive aspergillosis**?

Voriconazole (an azole) ± amphotericin (a polyene)

- Commonly occurs in immunocompromised patients.
- Risk factors include pre-existing lung disease, co-morbid status and critical illness.
- The commonest feature is persistent fever.
- Respiratory features are seen in pulmonary involvement and neurological signs and seizures may occur with neurological involvement.
- The classical 'halo sign' (a nodule surrounded by ground-glass opacification) is seen on CT chest.

Fact 1299:

What is the best initial treatment to offer to an elderly man who **fell** and was on the floor for several hours, was hypothermic at 32°C and had blood tests which showed an acute kidney injury and a CK of 10,000 IU?

IV warmed crystalloid

Active rewarming without volume correction can lead to vasodilation and hypotension.

Fact 1300:

What is the most likely diagnosis if a pregnant lady during the **spontaneous onset of labour** complains of a headache and chest pain and then quickly becomes tachycardic, hypotensive, tachypnoeic, starts oozing from her peripheral cannula sites, desaturates to SpO$_2$ 83% on air and then has a brief tonic-clonic seizure?

Amniotic fluid embolism (AFE)

- AFE presents with a sudden, profound and unexpected maternal collapse associated with hypotension, hypoxaemia and DIC due to foetal antigens in the amniotic fluid entering the maternal circulation.
- The key factors in the management are early recognition, prompt resuscitation and delivery of the fetus.

Fact 1301:

Who can perform **brainstem testing (BST)** in a child older than two months of age?

- Two doctors competent in performing BST.
- One should be a consultant and the other should be registered with GMC (or an equivalent professional body) for >5 years.
- One of them should be a paediatrician and the other should not be directly involved in the child's care.

Fact 1302:

What is the commonest ECG abnormality seen in a **pulmonary embolism?**

Sinus tachycardia

Other changes that may be seen include:

- It may be normal
- RV strain TWI in V$_{1-4}$ ± the inferior leads
- S$_1$Q$_3$T$_3$
- RBBB (complete/incomplete)
- Right axis deviation

Fact 1303:

Is **stress ulcer prophylaxis** necessary for someone who is already established and maintained on full enteral feeding?

No

Continuous enteral feeding is superior to PPI/H2RBs in raising intragastric pH.

Liquid enteral feed buffers gastric acid, enhances mucosal blood flow and stimulates the secretion of cytoprotective prostaglandins and mucus.

Fact 1304:

How do you treat **necrotising fasciitis (NF)**?

- *Surgery*: Aggressive debridement is first priority and is time critical. Without it, NF is fatal as antibiotics alone cannot penetrate infected necrotic tissue.
- *Antibiotics*: Broad-spectrum to cover Gram-positive and Gram-negative aerobic and anaerobic organisms (e.g. Piperacillin-tazobactam or Meropenem) + antitoxin (e.g. clindamycin or linezolid).
- *Immunoglobulins (IVIGs) and hyperbaric oxygen (HBO)*: Limited evidence; may help in specific cases. IVIGs have been used to neutralise the exotoxins associated with Group A beta-haemolytic Streptococcus (streptococcal super-antigens), Clostridium and in Staphylococcal infections. HBO is controversial but may be beneficial in anaerobic Gram-negative necrotising fasciitis.

Fact 1305:

What is the benefit of using a **biphasic waveform** in a defibrillator over a monophasic waveform?

Biphasic waveforms defibrillate more effectively at lower energy than monophasic ones.

Fact 1306:

How do you manage **delirium** in critical care?

- Identify and treat contributing causes ('NEW CHIMP'):
  - o **N**utrition (hunger)
  - o **E**nvironment (noisy, dark, no clocks)
  - o **W**ithdrawal (alcohol, opioids)
  - o **C**onstipation
  - o **H**ypoxia, de**H**ydration, **H**ypotension
  - o **I**nfection
  - o **M**etabolic abnormalities
  - o **P**ain
- Avoid delirium-inducing drugs, e.g. benzodiazepines, anticholinergics, opioids, steroids
- Optimise sedation (RASS 0 to −1) and sedation holds
- *Non-pharmacological*: Use bedside sitters, create a comforting environment with familiar faces, ↓ noise, adjust lighting, use clocks, remove catheters/ lines, provide glasses/hearing-aids, maintain regular sleep ‑‑wake cycles, engage in cognitive activities and promote early mobilisation and physiotherapy.
- *Pharmacological treatment*:
  - o Atypical antipsychotics (e.g. haloperidol, quetiapine, olanzapine) for psychosis or to manage patients who pose danger to themselves or others.
  - o Dexmedetomidine may be considered especially if agitation affects weaning/extubation.

Fact 1307:

What is the most common cause of **acute kidney injury** in ICU?

Septic shock is the leading cause.

Other common causes, in descending order, include major surgery, cardiogenic shock, hypovolaemia and drug-related factors.

Fact 1308:

How can you shorten the half-life of **carbon monoxide (CO)**?

Administer 100% oxygen until COHb < 10%

- The half-life of CO breathing air is ~320 minutes.
- 100% oxygen ↓ half-life to ~80 minutes.
- Hyperbaric oxygen therapy (2.5 bar) will further ↓ half-life to ~23 minutes.

Fact 1309:

What is the rationale for giving **corticosteroids** to children with *Haemophilus influenzae* type B meningitis?

↓ Incidence of deafness

Fact 1310:

What is meant by **association** and what are the three different types?

Association occurs when one variable is more frequently observed in the presence of another.

There are three types of association:

- Spurious (chance)
- Indirect (confounding variable)
- Direct (true, not confounded)

The next step after establishing an association is to investigate whether it is causal.

Fact 1311:

How does mouth breathing with nasal cannulae capitalise on the **Venturi effect**?

Mouth breathing with nasal cannulae allows a Venturi effect to occur in the nasopharynx with oxygen-enriched air being entrained from the nose during inspiration.

Fact 1312:

What clinical findings may you see in a child with **anaphylaxis**?

A	Airway obstruction	e.g. tongue/lip swelling, stridor, hoarse voice
B	Bronchospasm	e.g. ↓ SpO$_2$, ↑ RR, ↑ work of breathing, wheeze
C	Shock	e.g. ↑ HR, ↓ BP, ↑ capillary refill time
D	↓ GCS	Altered consciousness
E	Skin changes	e.g. flushing, urticaria, angioedema

Fact 1313:

What are the components of **Virchow's triad**, and what are some factors that can predispose to venous thromboembolism?

Local injury to the vascular wall	• Vasculitis • Previous thrombosis • Catheter placement
↑ **Coagulability**	• Genetic, e.g. factor V Leiden • Acquired, e.g. cancer, pregnancy • Medications, e.g. contraceptive pill • Systemic diseases, e.g. antiphospholipid syndrome
Circulatory stasis	• Immobilisation • Heart failure • Venous insufficiency

Fact 1314:

How can bedside bronchoscopy help to stop **massive pulmonary haemorrhage (MPH)**?

- Lung lavage with cold saline
- Applying topical medications like adrenaline, ADH derivatives and fibrinogen–thrombin.
- Using balloon tamponade techniques with an endobronchial blocker or a Fogarty balloon catheter

Fact 1315:

What are some complications of **prone positioning**?

Instability	Patient injury
• Airway displacement, e.g. ETT obstruction, extubation, endobronchial intubation • Haemodynamic instability • ↑ Intra-abdominal pressure • ↓ Flow in CRRT and ECMO • Line/device displacement • Gastroesophageal reflux and aspiration	• Pressure sores/ulcers • Oropharyngeal swelling and macroglossia • Periorbital oedema, chemosis • Ocular injury, including corneal abrasion and blindness • Nerve compression and brachial plexus injury • Stroke when head rotation: Vertebral or carotid artery occlusion

Fact 1316:

Why can a patient with chronic respiratory disease develop **atrial flutter**?

- ↑ Pulmonary vascular resistance and right ventricular strain → right atrial dilation → atrial dysrhythmias.
- Hypoxia and respiratory acidosis → ↑ the incidence of dysrhythmias.
- At high doses, salbutamol has β$_1$ effects → tachycardia and ↓ threshold for atrial dysrhythmias.
- β-agonists and steroids used in management of respiratory disease may cause hypokalaemia which can produce arrhythmias.

Fact 1317:

What are some indications for emergency **renal replacement therapy**?

A	Refractory metabolic **A**cidosis
E	Refractory **E**lectrolyte disturbance, e.g. hyperkalaemia
I	**I**ngested poisons amenable to dialysis, e.g. lithium, salicylates, ethylene glycol, methanol
O	Refractory fluid **O**verload
U	**U**raemic pericarditis or encephalopathy

Fact 1318:

What causes **serotonin syndrome**?

Anything that causes ↑ serotonin

- Drug reactions, e.g. macrolides inhibiting the P450 enzymes (CYP3A4) → ↓ the metabolism of an SSRI
- Deliberate overdose of an SSRI
- Dose ↑ of an SSRI
- Introduction of an SSRI and concomitant administration of a second serotonergic drug, e.g. SSRIs, MAOi, pethidine, fentanyl, tramadol

Fact 1319:

How should you approach the management of a patient who develops hypotension and abdominal pain after initiating thyroxine therapy for **hypothyroidism**?

IV hydrocortisone and IV fluids

This suggests an Addisonian crisis.

Treatment with thyroxine may precipitate acute hypoadrenalism.

Fact 1320:

What is most likely diagnosis if an asymptomatic patient has:
- Anti-hepatitis B core IgG antibody: Positive
- Anti-hepatitis B core IgM antibody: Negative
- Anti-hepatitis B surface antibody: Positive
- Hepatitis B surface antigen: Negative

Previous infection with hepatitis B

Some other common examples to keep in mind:

Previous vaccination	Acute hepatitis B	Previous hepatitis B (not a carrier)
Surface antibody positive	Surface antigen positive	Surface antigen negative
Everything else negative	Core IgM positive	Core IgG positive

Fact 1321:

What do these pulmonary function tests show:

	% Predicted	Interpretation
FEV$_1$ (L)	38%	Low
FVC (L)	71%	Normal
TLC (L)	121%	High
FEV$_1$/FVC ratio	44%	Low

An obstructive defect

Examples include **A**sthma, **B**ronchiectasis, **C**OPD

↑ TLC suggests hyper-expansion.

Fact 1322:

Which microorganisms are associated with an unfavourable prognosis in **infective endocarditis**?

- *Staphylococcus aureus*
- Non-HACEK Gram-negative bacilli
- Fungi

Fact 1323:

What are some extrapulmonary complications associated with **Legionella spp infection**?

Thrombocytopenia
Renal failure and hyponatraemia
Abnormal LFTs and poly**A**thropathy
Pericarditis
Pancreatitis
Encephalitis
Diarrhoea

Fact 1324:

What are some common causes of **hypercalcaemia**?

Drugs	Calcium, thiazides, lithium, theophylline, vitamin D	
Hyper-parathyroidism	↑ PTH	
Malignancy	Solid tumours	• ↑ PTHrP (adenoma, squamous) • Bone lysis (breast cancer)
	Haema-tological	• ↑ Calcitriol (lymphoma) • Bone lysis (multiple myeloma)
Sarcoidosis	↑ 1,25-dihydroxyvitamin-D3	
Immobilisation	↑ Bone resorption	

Fact 1325:

What would your first intervention be if someone on **DDD temporary pacing** at a HR 90 bpm develops a HR of 35 bpm, BP of 72/40 mmHg and has an ECG which shows wide QRS complexes at a rate of 35 bpm and pacing spikes at a rate of 90 bpm?

↑ Voltage output from the pacemaker (↑ capture threshold)

This is failure to capture, the most common issue with temporary pacing, where electrical output occurs at the pacemaker wire tips (seen as pacing spikes on ECG) but does not lead to a cardiac contraction (no mechanical cardiac impulse on the arterial pressure waveform).

This often happens due to ↑ resistance at the wire/myocardium interface, typically caused by fibrosis around the pacemaker lead.

If the capture threshold is ↑, then there should be ↑ output from the pacemaker to cause mechanical capture and rectify the problem.

If the threshold continues to ↑, and the patient is dependent on the pacemaker, an alternative method of stimulation should be established before complete capture failure occurs.

Fact 1326:

What is the management of **calcium channel blocker (CCB) overdose**?

- Single dose of activated charcoal within 1 hour (or later if modified-release preparation).
- Atropine for symptomatic bradycardia.
- Cardiovascular support: Fluid resuscitation, calcium replacement, vasopressors ± inotropes.
- Consider ventricular pacing to bypass atrioventricular blockade.
- IV glucagon can serve as a positive inotrope and chronotrope by increasing cAMP and aiding calcium entry into myocytes via cardiac glucagon receptors.
- High-dose insulin euglycaemic therapy (HIET): ↑ myocardial contractility is achieved without elevating oxygen demand by improving glucose uptake and myocardial lactate oxidation.
- Intralipid can be considered in refractory cases.

Note that RRT may not work in this setting as CCBs are highly protein bound and have a ↑ Vd.

Fact 1327:

How does **thoracic impedance** relate to the delivered current from a defibrillator?

Delivered current is inversely proportional to thoracic impedance (current = 1/thoracic impedance).

Fact 1328:

What are some endogenous nephrotoxins that can cause **acute tubular necrosis**?

Uric acid	Acute uric acid nephropathy
Myoglobin	Rhabdomyolysis
Haemoglobin	Haemolysis
Light chains	Myeloma

Fact 1329:

Which patient groups are at risk of developing **hypercapnic respiratory failure**?

- Respiratory disorders, e.g. COPD, bronchiectasis, cystic fibrosis
- Chest wall deformities, e.g. kyphoscoliosis
- Respiratory muscle weakness, e.g. Guillain–Barré syndrome, myasthenia gravis
- Morbid obesity
- Respiratory depression, e.g. TBI, opioid overdose
- A late manifestation in conditions typically associated with type 1 respiratory failure, e.g. systemic sclerosis, pulmonary fibrosis and asthma with fatigue

Fact 1330:

What is the most likely diagnosis if a patient is hypotensive and oliguric after a CABG, with the following pulmonary artery catheter measurements:

- PAOP 5 mmHg (low-normal)
- Cardiac index 1.6 L/min/m^2 (low)
- SVR 2750 dynes/sec/cm^5 (high)

Hypovolemia

There is ↑ SVR, ↓ cardiac index and low-normal PAOP (filling pressure)

Fact 1331:

What are some possible causes of **post-laparotomy hypertension** within 1 hour of closure?

- Inadequately controlled pain/sedation
- Hypercapnia due to alveolar hypoventilation
- A full bladder due to urinary retention or a blocked catheter
- Diffusion hypoxia
- Malignant hyperpyrexia

Fact 1332:

What is the BTS guidance on **secondary spontaneous pneumothorax (SSP)** management?

Treat as SSP if there is underlying lung disease or if age > 50 years with a significant smoking history.

- All SSPs require a minimum 24-hour hospital admission and should receive supplemental oxygen if necessary.
- Patients experiencing breathlessness and/or a SSP > 2 cm should undergo chest drain placement.
- A smaller pneumothorax (1–2 cm) can be aspirated using a 16G or 18G cannula. If successful, a 24-hour observation is recommended. If unsuccessful, proceed with chest drain insertion.
- Patients with a pneumothorax < 1 cm on admission should be observed while receiving high-flow oxygen unless oxygen-sensitive.

Fact 1333:

What is the common mechanism of action for the **azole antifungal group**?

Inhibition of lanosterol 14-alpha-demethylase, which in turn prevents the conversion of lanosterol into ergosterol within the fungal cell membrane.

Fact 1334:

What are the mechanisms of laxatives?

- **B**ulk-forming agents (e.g. fibre, husk)
- **L**ubricants (e.g. mineral oil)
- **E**mollients (softeners) (e.g. sodium docusate)
- **S**timulants (e.g. senna, bisacodyl)
- **S**alts (e.g. magnesium salts)
- Hyperosmotics (e.g. lactulose, glycerin)

Fact 1335:

Which abnormality in parathyroid activity do you see in **chronic kidney disease (CKD)**?

Secondary hyperparathyroidism

This can later develop into tertiary hyperparathyroidism.

This occurs as a result of:

1. ↓ Vitamin D (the kidney converts 25-hydroxycholecalciferol to active 1,25-dihydroxycholecalciferol) → ↓ serum calcium
2. ↑ Serum phosphate due to ↓ renal clearance

↓ Calcium and ↑ phosphate → ↑ PTH → secondary hyperparathyroidism → tertiary hyperparathyroidism

Fact 1336:

Can increasing the FiO_2 improve peripheral oxygen saturations beyond 85–90% in an individual with **drug-induced methaemoglobinaemia**?

Not really

All available Hb may already be fully oxygenated.

Methaemoglobinaemia is a condition in which ferrous ions (Fe^{2+}) within haemoglobin are oxidised to the ferric state (Fe^{3+}), preventing them from binding to oxygen.

Fact 1337:

What is the intravenous **adrenaline** dose in a cardiac arrest?

The usual concentration provided is 10 mL of 1:10,000

Adults	Children
1 mg	10 mcg/kg
Give the full 10 mL of 1:10,000 solution	e.g. 20 kg child = 20 mcg = 0.2 mg (give 2 mL of 1:10,000 solution)

Fact 1338:

Which treatable haemodynamic states are poorly tolerated by patients with **severe aortic stenosis (AS)**?

- ↓ Preload
- ↓ Afterload
- ↑ HR
- Atrial fibrillation

In severe AS, the LV becomes hypertrophic and less compliant. This leads to diastolic dysfunction, ↑ filling pressures and a higher myocardial oxygen demand. Adequate cardiac output relies on an ↑ preload, and the 'atrial kick' contributes up to 40% of diastolic filling, helping to fill the stiff LV. Diastolic time and flow are essential for coronary perfusion.

Key points:

- Maintaining preload and preserving the 'atrial kick' is crucial, such as through rhythm control for AF. While diuretics can be used for fluid overload, caution is needed as they can ↓ preload and cardiac output.
- Tachycardia → ↓ ventricular diastolic time → ↑ dependence of ventricular filling on the atrial kick
- Tachycardia → ↓ coronary perfusion time → ↑ risk of ischaemia
- ↓ Afterload → ↓ coronary perfusion as the LV is hypertrophied → ↑ risk of ischaemia if DBP falls

Fact 1339:

What is the Stanford classification of **aortic dissections**?

Type A	Type B
Involves the ascending aorta	Involves the descending aorta only, distal to the origin of left subclavian artery
If hypotensive, give judicious fluid or blood, aiming for a target SBP of 110–120 mmHg to ensure organ perfusion without excessive resuscitation	
If hypertensive, aim to ↓ BP to a level that maintains organ perfusion while preventing dissection progression, typically targeting SBP 110–120 mmHg. Beta-blockers are first line as they control tachycardia and ↓ shear force around the dissection flap.	
Type A dissections require emergency surgical intervention, typically involving a median sternotomy and the use of cardiopulmonary bypass	Uncomplicated type B dissections are conservatively managed, while complicated cases may necessitate surgical approaches like a left lateral thoracotomy or endovascular intervention.

Fact 1340:

If you were alone and found a **collapsed five-year-old child** in the community, after calling for help, what is the next thing to do if they are not breathing?

- Open the airway
- Deliver five rescue breaths
- Assess for signs of life for no more than 10 seconds
  - o If signs of life are present, continue rescue breathing until normal breathing resumes.
  - o If no signs of life or uncertainty, initiate chest compressions at a ratio of 15:2.
- Perform 1 minute of CPR before going to call for further help if no one is nearby. To minimise interruptions in CPR, it may be possible to carry the child whilst summoning help.

Children are more prone to collapse due to respiratory distress rather than cardiac abnormalities. Resuscitation primarily prioritises efficient ventilation and oxygenation since a shockable rhythm is less probable.

Fact 1341:

How do you manage **fluid responders** in trauma?

Damage control surgery aimed at haemostasis

Fact 1342:

Why is monotherapy with **dobutamine** helpful in managing a BP = 72/35 with HR = 82 following an anterior STEMI if the SVR is 2,200 dynes/s/cm^5 and stroke volume is 30 mL, but monotherapy with enoximone, adrenaline or noradrenaline may not work?

This is cardiogenic shock with a ↓ cardiac index and ↑ SVR.

- Dobutamine is a $\beta_{1/2}$ agonist with minimal α effects. It will ↑ SV and ↓ afterload.
- PDE3i, e.g. enoximone (inodilator) causes an ↑ SV but ↓ SVR, potentially ↓ coronary perfusion pressure and worsening of myocardial ischaemia.
- Adrenaline and noradrenaline have α_1 and $\beta_{1/2}$ activity. Both will ↑ SVR further. The β-effects may ↑ myocardial work and can compromise myocardial oxygen supply (↑ HR → ↓ diastolic filling time).

Fact 1343:

How do drug dosages differ between **intraosseous** and **intravenous** routes?

The same doses are used.

Fact 1344:

What are the minimum mandatory requirements of a **portable ventilator** according to FICM guidelines?

- The ability to vary FiO_2
- The ability to supply PEEP
- The ability to alter RR
- The ability to change TV
- The ability to change the I:E ratio
- Disconnection and high-pressure alarms

The ability to provide pressure-controlled ventilation, pressure support and CPAP are desirable.

Fact 1345:

What factors influence the FiO_2 delivered by a **Hudson mask**, and what is the purpose of its side holes?

Factors influencing FiO_2	Purpose of its side-holes
Patient: • Peak inspiratory flow rate • Minute ventilation Equipment: • Oxygen flow rate • Mask fit	• To entrain ambient air when the patient's inspiratory flow exceeds the oxygen flow rate • To flush out exhaled gases with fresh gas flow

---

Fact 1346:

What is the main causative agent of **bronchiolitis**, and which children are more prone to severe disease?

Respiratory syncytial virus (RSV) – confirmed by immunofluorescence of nasopharyngeal aspirates

Children at higher risk of severe disease include:

- **S**moke exposure (passive)
- **P**rematurity, especially < 32 weeks
- **I**mmunodeficiency
- **N**euromuscular disorders
- **A**ge < 3 months
- **C**hronic lung disease
- **H**eart disease (congenital)

Fact 1347:

What happens to **peripheral deiodination of thyroid hormones** in critical illness?

↓ Most T3 is produced by peripheral deiodination of T4.

This process is also ↓ by fasting, malnutrition and drugs (propylthiouracil, steroids, propranolol and amiodarone).

Fact 1348:

What is the significance of a **pulmonary artery catheter (PAC)** tip being positioned below the level of the left atrium on a chest X-ray?

It is in the optimal position – this indicates that the PAC is situated in West zone 3, a dynamic zone influenced by pulmonary and alveolar pressure.

Note that if the tip is apically positioned on a chest X-ray, the PAOP may be falsely high due to alveolar pressure exceeding capillary pressure in that region.

Fact 1349:

What ECG changes would you expect to see in **hypermagnesaemia**?

There is some overlap with hyperkalaemia:

- ↑ PR, ↑ QT, ↑ QRS
- Peaked T waves and flat P-waves
- Complete AV block and asystole

Some features of hypermagnesaemia include GI symptoms (nausea, vomiting), neurological signs (↓ tendon reflexes, weakness, respiratory paralysis, coma) and cardiovascular complications (conduction abnormalities and cardiac arrest).

Fact 1350:

What is **ventilator-associated pneumonia (VAP)** and why is it significant?

Pneumonia in someone who has been intubated for at least 48 hours.

There is a lack of consensus definition to diagnose VAP. Scoring systems include Clinical Pulmonary Infection Score (CPIS), Johannson criteria and HELICS criteria.

VAP may have significant consequences:

- ↑ ICU LOS
- ↑ Patient ventilator days
- ↑ Mortality

Early VAP	Within 4 days of ventilation	Oropharyngeal flora, e.g. *Strep pneumoniae, H. influenzae*, MSSA
Late VAP	>4 days of ventilation	Gram-negative and/or drug-resistant organisms aspirated from gastrointestinal tract, e.g. MDR organisms such as pseudomonas, acinetobacter, MRSA

Fact 1351:

What is the likely diagnosis for a person displaying right-sided cerebellar ataxia, right-sided Horner's syndrome and left-sided spinothalamic sensory loss in the left arm and leg?

Lateral medullary syndrome (Wallenberg's syndrome)

Caused by a stroke involving the vertebral artery or the posterior inferior cerebellar artery.

Ipsilateral	Contralateral
Horner's syndrome **A**taxia (cerebellar) **S**ensory loss of face (pain and temperature	Spinothalamic sensory loss below the neck (pain and temperature)

Fact 1352:

What is the effect of **hypothyroidism** on prolactin levels?

↑ Prolactin levels

In patients with primary hypothyroidism, ↑ levels of thyrotropin-releasing hormone can cause ↑ prolactin release from the anterior pituitary, and some patients may experience galactorrhea.

Fact 1353:

How do you classify **burns**?

Superfi-cial	Epidermis		Red without blisters, accompanied by pain and tenderness
Partial thickness	Superficial	Epidermis and superficial dermis	Red or white with blisters, accompanied by severe pain
	Deep	Epidermis and deep dermis	
Full thick-ness	Epidermis, dermis and may involve subcutaneous tissue (including hair follicles, sebaceous glands)		White (no capillary return) and painless (nociceptors destroyed) but surrounding partial thickness will be painful

Fact 1354:

What are some important side effects associated with **anti-tuberculosis** treatment?

- *Hepatitis*: Caused by rifampicin, isoniazid and pyrazinamide
- *Optic neuritis*: Caused by ethambutol
- *Peripheral neuropathy*: Caused by isoniazid (pyridoxine is given to ↓ the risk)

Fact 1355:

What clinical feature should you monitor for magnesium toxicity in **pre-eclampsia**?

Tendon reflexes – ↓ tendon reflexes are an early sign of magnesium toxicity. It tends to occur at levels of 4–6 mmol/L.

Note that calcium antagonises the effects of magnesium and can be used as part of managing toxicity along with diuretics and RRT.

Fact 1356:

What are the mechanisms by which **tricyclic antidepressants (TCAs)** exert their toxic effects?

They block:

- Central and peripheral muscarinic Ach receptors
- NA and serotonergic reuptake at nerve terminals
- Histamine-1 receptors
- α-receptors
- Cardiac and nerve fast sodium channels

Fact 1357:

When assessing the post-repair outcome of a ruptured aortic aneurysm, which variables are included in the calculation of the **Glasgow Aneurysm Score**?

- **C**erebrovascular disease
- **R**enal disease
- **A**ge
- **M**yocardial disease
- **S**hock

Fact 1358:

What does an **IVC collapsibility index** greater than 36% indicate during spontaneous breathing?

An IVC collapsibility index exceeding 36% during spontaneous breathing can suggest fluid responsiveness. This measure is more variable and less reliable in mechanically ventilated patients.

Fact 1359:

How does the site of injection influence the risk of developing **local anaesthetic systemic toxicity**?

Toxicity occurs when an overdose of a LA enters the systemic circulation, e.g. inadvertent IV injection.

Vascular areas are more prone to systemic absorption. In order of most vascular to least vascular are:

- Intercostal and paracervical block
- Caudal epidural block
- Lumbar and thoracic epidural block
- Brachial plexus block
- Sciatic/femoral nerve block
- Subcutaneous infiltration

The likelihood of LA toxicity is also dependent on:

- Drug type, dose and concentration
- Use of vasoconstrictors
- Procedural factors, e.g. operator
- Changes in protein binding in relation to intracellular pH

Fact 1360:

Why may **cytokine release syndrome (CRS)** occur in Chimeric Antigen Receptor T-Cell (CAR-T) therapy?

CAR-T therapy is a form of immunotherapy where a patient's T cells are genetically engineered to express a chimeric antigen receptor that targets specific proteins on cancer cells. When these modified CAR-T cells are reinfused into the patient and engage with their target cancer cells, they become activated. This activation leads to the rapid and massive release of cytokines. This storm can lead to CRS, which, in severe cases can lead to multi-organ dysfunction. Treatment for CRS typically includes supportive care and may involve immunosuppressive agents like corticosteroids or cytokine blockers (e.g. tocilizumab, an IL-6 receptor antagonist).

Fact 1361:

What are some ECG changes in **hyperkalaemia**?

- ↑ T waves (peaked)
- ↑ PR interval
- ↑ QRS widening
- ↓ P waves (widening/flattening)
- Heart block and bradyarrhythmias

Fact 1362:

What are some signs of poor prognosis in **infective endocarditis**?

Background	Old age, severe comorbidities, insulin-dependent diabetes mellitus
Type of endocarditis	Prosthetic valve endocarditis
Organisms	*Staphylococcus aureus*, fungal, non-HACEK Gram-negative bacilli
Complications	Heart failure, renal failure, stroke, septic shock and peri-annular issues
Echocardiographic findings	Severe left sided valve regurgitation, ↓ LVEF, pulmonary HTN, large vegetations, severe prosthetic valve dysfunction

Fact 1363:

What is the definition of **cardiogenic shock (CS)** according to haemodynamic criteria?

- SBP < 90 mmHg
- Cardiac index < 2.2 L/min/m^2
- PCWP ≥ 15 mmHg

Cardiac dysfunction → inadequate tissue perfusion

Fact 1364:

What are the features of **pericardial tamponade** using point of care echocardiography?

Early signs	Late sign	Very late sign
• Dilated non-collapsing IVC • RA collapse	RV early diastolic collapse	LV/LA collapse

Fact 1365:

What are the most likely significant complications of inserting a **radial arterial line**?

• Arterial occlusion
• Bleeding/haematoma formation

Fact 1366:

What is the most appropriate course of action for a haemodynamically unstable trauma patient with **intraperitoneal-free fluid** on a FAST scan who has shown no response to fluids or blood products?

Immediate transfer to theatre for 'damage control laparotomy'

This is to identify and treat sources of internal bleeding points through packing/ resection/ vascular intervention. Operative time should be kept to <90 minutes, with definitive surgery planned for a later time after a period of stability on the critical care unit.

Fact 1367:

Which gas is released if an **MRI scanner** is stopped rapidly?

Helium gas

MRI scanners use liquid helium for superconducting magnets, and a sudden stop can release helium for system protection. Helium, while non-toxic, displaces oxygen and requires proper ventilation and safety measures to prevent asphyxiation in case of release.

Fact 1368:

What is the single best method of preventing **acidaemia** during a cardiac arrest?

Chest compressions

Bicarbonate is only recommended in a cardiac arrest when associated with certain drug overdoses or in hyperkalaemia.

Bicarbonate can cause:

• A paradoxical intracellular and CSF acidosis through CO_2 production
• Negative inotropy to an ischaemic myocardium
• Shifts the oxygen dissociation curve to the left, which could impair tissue oxygenation
• ↑ Osmotic and sodium load → ↑ risk of volume overload

Fact 1369:

What shifts the **oxygen dissociation curve** to the left and to the right?

Shifts to left = ↓ oxygen delivery	Shifts to right = ↑ oxygen delivery
• ↓ [H+] (alkali) • ↓ pCO_2 • ↓ 2,3-DPG • ↓ Temperature • HbF, MethCO, COHb	• ↑ [H+] (acidic) • ↑ pCO_2 • ↑ 2,3-DPG • ↑ Temperature

Fact 1370:

Which factors increase the risk of **vasospasm** after a subarachnoid haemorrhage, and what are the strategies for prevention and management?

Risk factors	Prevention	Management
Poor grade Age < 50 years Hypertension Smoking Alcohol excess Cocaine use	Avoid: • Hypovolaemia • Hypotension • Hypoxia • Hyperthermia Pharmacological: L-type calcium channel antagonists, e.g. nimodipine	• Nimodipine • Haemodynamic optimisation: Euvolaemia, individualised BP targets, avoidance of anaemia • Endovascular intervention: Early coiling, balloon angioplasty, intra-arterial vasodilator infusions

Note that triple H therapy (hypervolemia, hypertension and haemodilution) is no longer recommended, and the MASH-2 trial (2012) found no evidence to support magnesium prophylaxis.

Fact 1371:

What types of infections might **post-splenectomy** patients be susceptible to, and which vaccinations are recommended for them?

Organisms	Vaccines
• Pneumococcus • Haemophilus • Meningococcal • Capnocytophaga canimorsus	• Influenza vaccine every 1 year • Pneumococcal vaccine every 5 years • Hib and meningococcal C vaccines if not received in childhood • Meningococcal ACWY vaccine if travelling to high-risk areas

After splenectomy, individuals are at a higher risk of infections, especially those caused by encapsulated bacteria like *Streptococcus pneumoniae*. Therefore, patients typically take lifelong Penicillin V.

Fact 1372:

Which autoimmune conditions can lead to **dilated cardiomyopathy**?

- **G**ranulomatosis with polyangiitis
- **A**myloidosis (also causes restrictive cardiomyopathy)
- **S**arcoidosis
- **P**olyarteritis nodosa
- **S**ystemic lupus erythematosus

Fact 1373:

What is the effect of **hepatic drug metabolism** in sepsis?

Sepsis leads to splanchnic vasoconstriction and ↓ liver blood flow:

- Drugs that are 'flow-limited' with high extraction ratios, like midazolam, will accumulate significantly.
- Drugs that are 'metabolism-limited' with low extraction ratios, such as phenytoin, will not be impacted by ↓ liver blood flow because enzymes are already functioning at their maximum capacity. This process is only affected when liver blood flow ↓ to the point of causing hepatocellular injury and reducing enzyme function.

Fact 1374:

What are the most likely causes for **intrinsic renal failure** in someone being managed for infective endocarditis (IE)?

Renal tubules	Acute tubular necrosis secondary to antibiotics, e.g. vancomycin, gentamicin
Glomerulus	Glomerulonephritis secondary to IE
Blood vessels	Vasculitis secondary to IE
Interstitium	Interstitial nephritis secondary to antibiotics, e.g. penicillins, cephalosporins

Fact 1375:

What are some variables that influence the spread of neural blockade in a **thoracic epidural**?

Patient factors	Non-patient factors
• Age • Patient position • Intra-abdominal pressure • Epidural adhesions	• Anatomical level of epidural catheter • Catheter tip position • Mass/volume/dose of drug/s injected

Fact 1376:

How are **pericardial effusions** categorised by size on echocardiography?

Mild	Moderate	Severe
<10 mm	10–20 mm	>20 mm

Fact 1377:

What is the most serious complication of bronchial artery embolisation in the management of **pulmonary haemorrhage**?

Spinal cord infarction

Fact 1378:

How are **ventricular assist device (VAD)** classified?

Ventricle supported	• RVAD • LVAD • BiVAD
Mechanism	• Pulsatile (first generation) • Non-pulsatile (second and third generation)
Location	• Short-term: Extracorporeal, paracorporeal • Long-term: Intracorporeal
Drive train	• Pneumatic • Electrical • Magnetic

Fact 1379:

What are some complications linked to the use and care of a **pulmonary artery catheter**?

- **P**ulmonary artery pseudoaneurysm or perforation
- **L**ung infarction
- **A**ir embolism
- **I**nfections, e.g. CRBSI, endocarditis
- **T**hrombosis

Fact 1380:

Which factors indicate an unfavourable neurological outcome after a **cardiac arrest**?

- Absent bilateral pupillary reflexes ≥ 72 hours
- Absent bilateral corneal reflexes ≥ 72 hours
- GCS motor score ≤ 3 at ≥72 hours
- Bilaterally absent N20 SSEP wave after 24 hours
- Highly malignant EEG > 24 hours in the absence of sedation (generalised suppression, burst suppression or generalised periodic complexes)
- Myoclonic status epilepticus (MSE) ≤ 72 hours
- Serum neuron-specific enolase > 60 µg/L at ≥48 hours
- Imaging evidence of diffuse and extensive anoxic brain injury.

Fact 1381:

How would you identify the site of a **cerebellar lesion** from clinical findings?

The cerebellum is divided into a midline vermis and two cerebellar hemispheres:

- Disease of a hemisphere causes ipsilateral dysmetria, dysdiadochokinesis, intention tremor and fast-beat nystagmus towards the lesion.
- Disease of the vermis leads to truncal ataxia and ataxic gait.

Fact 1382:

How would you manage a case of **COPD** after 1 hour of medical treatment involving controlled oxygen, nebulizers, steroids and antibiotics, given the following ABG results: pH = 7.23, pCO_2 = 9.4 kPa and pO_2 = 7.6 kPa?

NIV in an HDU/ITU setting

A pH < 7.25 indicates an ↑ risk of treatment failure and the potential need for mechanical ventilation (hence the need to provide NIV in an HDU/ITU setting).

Fact 1383:

Which **central active warming techniques** can be employed for rewarming hypothermic patients?

- Warmed humidified inspired gases
- Infusion of warm intravenous fluids
- Body cavity lavage using warmed fluids, e.g. bladder, stomach, colon, peritoneal, pleural
- Extracorporeal warming, e.g. renal replacement therapy, ECMO, cardiopulmonary bypass.

Some reliable sites for recording temperature include pulmonary artery, oesophageal, rectal and bladder.

Fact 1384:

What are the risk factors for developing **refeeding syndrome** in critical care?

	At risk if ≥1 of:	At risk if ≥2 of:
BMI (kg/m²)	<16	<18
Unintentional weight loss in last 3–6 months	>15%	>10%
Days without food	>10 days	>5 days
Other	↓ K⁺, PO₄³⁻, Mg²⁺ prior to feeding	Alcohol abuse, insulin, chemotherapy, antacids, diuretics

In starvation, ↓ insulin secretion, ↓ gluconeogenesis and intracellular electrolyte depletion occur, even if serum levels appear normal. Refeeding leads to ↑ insulin, which causes in ↓ magnesium, ↓ potassium and ↓ phosphate.

Fact 1385:

To which patient groups would you consider giving **parenteral nutrition (PN)**?

- Malnourished or at risk of malnutrition + inadequate or unsafe enteral intake
- A gastrointestinal tract that is non-functioning, inaccessible or perforated.

Fact 1386:

Is there a likelihood that **haemodialysis (HD)** can effectively remove drug X with these characteristics:

- Weak base (pKa 9)
- Highly lipid-soluble
- 85% protein-bound
- Metabolised by the liver into inactive metabolites, with only 10% of the active drug excreted in urine

Nope – HD is unlikely to be effective for a drug with a high volume of distribution, significant protein binding and minimal renal excretion

Fact 1387:

With sufficient access pressures and no problems detected in the oxygenator and blender, how can you enhance oxygenation on **VV-ECMO** it the SaO_2 remains low at 79%?

↑ Pump speed (blood flow rate)

If oxygenation still does not improve, this may indicate potential recirculation of oxygenated blood within the circuit. Addressing this might require repositioning the cannulae, changing to a single dual-lumen cannula or transitioning to VA-ECMO.

Fact 1388:

What would you do to manage an intraarterial (IA) injection of **thiopentone**?

Unlike venous injection, IA injection of thiopentone results in crystal precipitation when it encounters the alkaline pH of arterial blood, potentially causing limb ischaemia.

Management includes:

- Stop injecting thiopentone
- Flush cannula with saline to dilute the drug and promote distal distribution
- Give analgesia to ↓ the sympathetic vasoconstrictive response
- Warm the limb to stimulate vessel dilation
- Elevate limb to improve venous drainage
- Additional options:
  o Consider heparin for anticoagulation to minimise ischaemic damage
  o Consider sympathetic blocks (e.g. stellate ganglion) to induce vascular dilation.

Fact 1389:

Despite thorough cleaning practices, which bacterium is most frequently reported in cases of **bronchoscopic contamination**?

Mycobacterium tuberculosis

Fact 1390:

What are some acute potential complications of **VAD** insertion?

- **C**annula obstruction
- **H**aemorrhage: VADs require systemic anticoagulation
- **A**ir embolus
- **R**V failure (common after LVAD insertion and many will subsequently need RVAD support)
- **M**ulti-organ failure
- **H**aemolysis
- **A**rrhythmias
- **R**ight-to-left shunting through a patent foramen ovale (LVAD)
- **M**alposition

Fact 1391:

What is the next step in treating hypoxia in someone with **pulmonary oedema** secondary to an NSTEMI who is already on 15 L/min oxygen via a non-rebreathe mask?

CPAP to ↑ oxygenation, ↓ work of breathing and ↑ cardiac output

This can potentially prevent the need for intubation.

Fact 1392:

Why must **aortic insufficiency** be excluded before inserting an LVAD and what is the effect of an LVAD on **mitral insufficiency**?

Aortic insufficiency:

- LVAD insertion increases the gradient between MAP and LVEDP.
- This worsens aortic regurgitation, recirculates blood through the LVAD and causes a ↓ CO.

Mitral insufficiency:

- MR often improves after LVAD insertion.
- This is due to decompression of the LV.

Fact 1393:

What is the rationale for urinary alkalinisation in **salicylate poisoning**?

Urinary alkalinisation in salicylate poisoning involves raising urine pH with intravenous sodium bicarbonate (a base) to convert salicylates (weak acids) into their ionised, water-soluble form, preventing reabsorption and enhancing excretion through the kidneys.

Haemodialysis is indicated if urinary alkalinisation fails or is not feasible due to conditions like renal failure or pulmonary oedema.

Fact 1394:

What are the physiological effects of **positive pressure ventilation** on cardiorespiratory system?

System	Effect	
Resp	↓ Atelectasis → recruitment of collapsed alveoli → ↑ FRC → ↑ surface area for oxygen transfer and ↑ V/Q matching	
	↑ Alveolar hydrostatic pressure → redistribution of extravascular lung water out of the lung interstitium	
CVS	**Right ventricle**	• ↑ Intrathoracic pressure → ↓ **RV preload** • ↑ Intrathoracic pressure → ↑ PVR → ↑ **RV afterload**
		Overall, there is a ↓ RV stroke volume
	Left ventricle	• ↑ Intrathoracic pressure → ↓ pulmonary venous pressure → ↓ **LV preload** • ↑ Intrathoracic pressure → ↓ LV end-systolic transmural pressure + ↑ pressure gradient between intrathoracic aorta and extrathoracic systemic circuit → ↓ **LV afterload**
		Overall, the net effect on SV can vary: • Failing LV: ↑ SV • Healthy LV: ↓ SV

Fact 1395:

What are some vascular, glomerular and interstitial causes of **intrinsic renal failure**?

Vascular	**Large vessel**	Renal artery/vein stenosis/thrombosis
	Small vessel	• Vasculitis • Thrombotic microangiopathies, e.g. HUS/TTP • Malignant hypertension • Emboli
Glomerular	Goodpasture	Anti-GBM antibodies
	IgA glomerulonephritis	Days after URTI/UTI/gastroenteritis
	Post-infectious glomerulonephritis	Weeks after streptococcal throat infection (ASOT positive)
	Lupus nephritis	ANA positive, dsDNA positive, ↓ complement
	Granulomatosis with polyangiitis	c-ANCA positive
Acute interstitial nephritis	**Drugs**	• Antibiotics, e.g. penicillin, cephalosporins • NSAIDs • PPIs • Phenytoin • Furosemide
	Infections	Streptococcus, Staphyloccus, TB, EBV, Legionella

Fact 1396:

How do you treat an acute attack of **hereditary angioedema** (HAE)?

• IV C1-inhibitor concentrate <u>or</u>
• Icatibant (a bradykinin B2 receptor antagonist)

If these are not available, then FFP can be given as an alternative.

HAE is an autosomal dominant condition associated with low plasma levels of C1 inhibitor protein.

Fact 1397:

What is the most likely diagnosis if someone has a **pansystolic murmur** best heard at the left sternal edge, giant V-waves in the JVP and pulsatile hepatomegaly?

Tricuspid regurgitation

In tricuspid regurgitation there is a pansystolic murmur, which is heard best at the left sternal edge in inspiration

In severe tricuspid regurgitation, the V wave of tricuspid regurgitation merges with the C wave forming a single prominent CV-wave.

Fact 1398:

Which autoantibodies are involved in **vaccine-induced immune thrombotic thrombocytopenia (VITT)** following one dose of an adenoviral-vectored COVID-19 vaccine?

Autoantibodies targeting platelet factor 4 (PF4) activate platelets through FcγIIa receptors, leading to thrombosis, similar to the mechanism seen in heparin-induced thrombocytopenia (HIT).

Fact 1399:

What blood results are classically seen in **dengue fever**?

- Leucopaenia
- Thrombocytopaenia
- Transaminitis

Dengue fever is an infection that is primarily transmitted by the female *Aedes aegypti* mosquito.

Fact 1400:

What anatomical landmark describes the insertion point of an **anterior apical chest drain**?

Second intercostal space, mid-clavicular line

Index

Printed in the United States
by Baker & Taylor Publisher Services